BASIC Essentials

BASIC Essentials

A Comprehensive Review for the
Anesthesiology BASIC Exam

Edited by

Alopi M. Patel, M.D.
Mount Sinai St. Lukes's and Mount Sinai West

Himani V. Bhatt, D.O., MPA.
Icahn School of Medicine at Mount Sinai

Sang J. Kim, M.D.
Hospital for Special Surgery

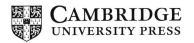

CAMBRIDGE
UNIVERSITY PRESS

CAMBRIDGE
UNIVERSITY PRESS

University Printing House, Cambridge CB2 8BS, United Kingdom

One Liberty Plaza, 20th Floor, New York, NY 10006, USA
477 Williamstown Road, Port Melbourne, VIC 3207, Australia
314–321, 3rd Floor, Plot 3, Splendor Forum, Jasola District Centre, New Delhi – 110025, India
103 Penang Road, #05-06/07, Visioncrest Commercial, Singapore 079906

Cambridge University Press is part of the University of Cambridge.

It furthers the University's mission by disseminating knowledge in the pursuit of education, learning, and research at the highest international levels of excellence.

www.cambridge.org
Information on this title: www.cambridge.org/9781108402613
DOI: 10.1017/9781108235778

First published 2019
3rd printing 2022

Printed in the United Kingdom by TJ Books Limited, Padstow Cornwall

A catalogue record for this publication is available from the British Library.

Library of Congress Cataloging-in-Publication Data

Names: Bhatt, Himani, editor.
Title: Basic essentials : a comprehensive review for the anesthesiology basic
    exam / edited by Himani Bhatt, Icahn School of Medicine, Alopi
    Patel, Mount Sinai St. Luke's Sang Kim, Mount Sinai Health System.
Description: Cambridge, United Kingdom ; New York, NY : Cambridge University
    Press, 2018. | Includes bibliographical references and index.
Identifiers: LCCN 2018011566 | ISBN 9781108402613 (pbk. : alk. paper)
Subjects: LCSH: Anesthesia—Examinations, questions, etc.
Classification: LCC RD82.3 .B38 2018 | DDC 617.9/6076—dc23
    LC record available at https://lccn.loc.gov/2018011566

ISBN 978-1-108-40261-3 Paperback

To my supportive family, loving husband and the
inspirational mentors who have paved the way …

Alopi

To my parents, without whom none of my success would
be possible.
To my husband, for his support and dedicated partnership
in life.
To my children, for their unconditional love that keeps me
grounded.
Love, Daughter, Wife and Mom

Himani

To my wife, Yina, for her patience and support.
To my parents, who provided me the opportunity that they
never had.

Sang Kim

Contents

Contents

Contributors

Jonah Abraham, M.D.
University of Pittsburgh Medical Center
Pittsburgh, PA

Douglas Adams, M.D.
University of Pittsburgh Medical Center
Pittsburgh, PA

Diana Anca, M.D.
Mount Sinai St. Luke's and Mount Sinai West
New York, NY

Christy Anthony, M.D.
Rutgers, New Jersey Medical School
Newark, NJ

Marshall Bahr, M.D.
University of Pittsburgh Medical Center
Pittsburgh, PA

Gabriel C. Baltazar, M.D.
The Mount Sinai Hospital
New York, NY

Ryan Barnette, M.D.
Mount Sinai St. Luke's and Mount Sinai West
New York, NY

Himani V. Bhatt, D.O.
Icahn School of Medicine
at Mount Sinai

Ethan Bryson, M.D.
The Mount Sinai Hospital
New York, NY

Maria Castillo, M.D.
The Mount Sinai Hospital
New York, NY

Brian Chang
Presbyterian-Columbia University Medical Center
New York, NY

Tyler Chernin, M.D.
Mount Sinai St. Luke's and Mount Sinai
West New York, NY

Jeffrey Ciccone, M.D.
The Mount Sinai Hospital
New York, NY

Dallis Clendeninn, M.D.
University of Texas Health Science Center at Houston
Houston, TX

Christopher R. Cowart, M.D.
Mount Sinai St. Luke's and Mount Sinai West
New York, NY

Jeffrey Derham, M.D.
Doylestown Anesthesia Associates
Doylestown, PA

Shane Dickerson, M.D.
Keck School of Medicine of University
of Southern California

Christian Estrada
Rutgers, New Jersey Medical School
Newark, NJ

Shaji Faisal, M.D.
The Mount Sinai Hospital
New York, NY

Devon Flaherty, M.D.
The Mount Sinai Hospital
New York, NY

Ellen Flanagan, M.D.
Duke University Hospital
Durham, NC

Michal Gajewski, D.O.
Rutgers, New Jersey Medical School
Newark, NJ

Jonathan Gal, M.D.
The Mount Sinai Hospital
New York, NY

Jacqueline Geier, M.D.
Mount Sinai St. Luke's and Mount Sinai West
New York, NY

Theresa A. Gelzinis, M.D.
University of Pittsburgh Medical Center
Pittsburgh, PA

Morgane Giordano, M.D.
The Mount Sinai Hospital
New York, NY

Andrew Glasgow, M.D.
The Mount Sinai Hospital
New York, NY

Andrew Goldberg, M.D.
The Mount Sinai Hospital
New York, NY

Nadia Hernandez, M.D.
University of Texas Health Science Center at Houston
Houston, TX

Bryan Hill, M.D.
The Mount Sinai Hospital
New York, NY

Samuel Hunter, M.D.
The Mount Sinai Hospital
New York, NY

Stefan A. Ianchulev, M.D.
Tufts Medical Center
Boston, MA

Christina L. Jeng, M.D.
The Mount Sinai Hospital
New York, NY

Claire Joseph, D.O.
Mount Sinai St. Luke's and Mount Sinai West
New York, NY

Daniel Katz, M.D.
The Mount Sinai Hospital
New York, NY

Yury Khelemsky, M.D.
The Mount Sinai Hospital
New York, NY

Hae-Young Kim, Dr PH
New York Medical College
Valhalla, NY

Jung Kim, M.D.
Mount Sinai St. Luke's and Mount Sinai West
New York, NY

Sang Kim, M.D.
Hospital for Special Surgery
New York, NY

Nakiyah Knibbs, M.D.
The Mount Sinai Hospital
New York, NY

Michael D. Lazar, M.D.
Mount Sinai St. Luke's and Mount Sinai West
New York, NY

Vanny Le, M.D.
Rutgers, New Jersey Medical School
Newark, NJ

Rebecca E. Lee, M.D.
The Mount Sinai Hospital
New York, NY

Matthew A. Levin, M.D.
The Mount Sinai Hospital
New York, NY

Hung-Mo Lin, Sc.D.
The Mount Sinai Hospital
New York, NY

Sanford Littwin, M.D.
University of Pittsburgh Medical Center
Pittsburgh, PA

Katherine Loftus, M.D.
The Mount Sinai Hospital
New York, NY

Anuj Malhotra, M.D.
The Mount Sinai Hospital
New York, NY

Daniel R. Mandell, M.D.
University of Pittsburgh Medical Center
Pittsburgh, PA

Aleksey Maryansky, D.O.
Mount Sinai St. Luke's and Mount Sinai
West New York, NY

Edward Mathney, M.D.
The Mount Sinai Hospital
New York, NY

Dion McCall
Rutgers, New Jersey Medical School
Newark, NJ

Jamie Metesky, M.D.
Mount Sinai St. Luke's and Mount Sinai
West New York, NY

Katelyn O'Connor, M.D.
Mount Sinai St. Luke's and Mount Sinai West
New York, NY

Poonam Pai, M.D.
Mount Sinai St. Luke's and Mount Sinai West
New York, NY

Denes Papp, M.D.
Rutgers – Robert Wood Johnson Medical School
New Brunswick, NJ

Thomas Palaia, M.D.
The Mount Sinai Hospital
New York, NY

Raj Parekh, M.D.
Mount Sinai St. Luke's and Mount Sinai West
New York, NY

Anant Parikh
Rutgers, New Jersey Medical School
Newark, NJ

Chang H. Park, M.D.
The Mount Sinai Hospital
New York, NY

Joseph Park, M.D.
The Mount Sinai Hospital
New York, NY

Bhoumesh Patel, M.D.
Rutgers – Robert Wood Johnson Medical School
New Brunswick, NJ

Jonathan A. Paul, D.O.
Mount Sinai St. Luke's and Mount Sinai West
New York, NY

Charles P. Plant, M.D., Ph.D.
Tufts Medical Center
Boston, MA

Kyle James Riley, M.D.
The Mount Sinai Hospital
New York, NY

Martha Schuessler, M.D.
Mount Sinai St. Luke's and Mount Sinai West
New York, NY

Andrew Schwartz, M.D.
The Mount Sinai Hospital
New York, NY

Ali Shariat, M.D.
Mount Sinai St. Luke's and Mount Sinai West
New York, NY

Marc Sherwin, M.D.
The Mount Sinai Hospital
New York, NY

Christopher Sikorski, M.D.
Mount Sinai St. Luke's and Mount Sinai West
New York, NY

Natalie Smith, M.D.
The Mount Sinai Hospital
New York, NY

Daniel G. Springer, M.D.
University of Pittsburgh Medical Center
Pittsburgh, PA

Petrus Paulus Steyn
Temple University Hospital
Philadelphia, PA

Agathe Streiff, M.D.
Mount Sinai St. Luke's and Mount Sinai West
New York, NY

Kathirvel Subramaniam, M.D., M.P.H.
University of Pittsburgh Medical Center
Pittsburgh, PA

Sriniketh Sundar, D.O.
Mount Sinai St. Luke's and Mount Sinai West
New York, NY

Ben Toure
The Mount Sinai Hospital
New York, NY

Sanjana Vig, M.D., M.B.A.
University of California
San Diego, CA

John Michael Williamson, Sc.D.
Centers for Disease Control and Prevention
Atlanta, GA

James Yeh, M.D.
The Mount Sinai Hospital
New York, NY

Connie Yue, M.D.
Mount Sinai St. Luke's and Mount Sinai West
New York, NY

Jeron Zerillo, M.D.
The Mount Sinai Hospital
New York, NY

Preface

The ABA Staged examinations consist of the BASIC, Advanced and Applied Exams. The BASIC Exam was first introduced in 2014 in a series of exams that eventually allows resident anesthesiologists to become American Board of Anesthesiology (ABA) certified. Candidates can take the BASIC exam after completing their Clinical Anesthesia (CA) for one year. This exam focuses on the scientific basics of clinical anesthetic practice with a focus on pharmacology, physiology, anatomy, anesthesia equipment and monitoring.

As with most examinations, the BASIC examination may induce a great deal of stress for resident anesthesiologists; however, with the appropriate resources, the candidates can pass the exam on their first attempt. Per the ABA, a diplomate of the Board must possess "knowledge, judgment, adaptability, clinical skills, technical facility, and personal characteristics sufficient to carry out an entire scope of anesthesiology practice without accommodation or with reasonable accommodation." The examination provides a means for the ABA to evaluate if a candidate has attained a certain level of proficiency to proceed with advanced training. The BASIC Essentials book is meant to provide a comprehensive review of the content for the ABA BASIC exam. Detailed information is also available on the ABA website (www.theaba.org) and the booklet of information published on the website.

Exam Structure

The BASIC examination is a computer-based test that is administered in numerous test centers across the country. The exam consists of 200 questions and examinees are given four hours to complete the examination. The questions consist of only A type. A-type questions are multiple choice questions with a single best answer out of four choices that require the application of knowledge as well as recall of factual information. The questions can be simply stated or include a brief clinical scenario. Some questions will require interpretation of an image.

Exam Content

The BASIC exam covers four content categories: basic sciences, clinical sciences, organ-based basic and clinical sciences, and special problems or issues in anesthesiology. The examination outline can be found on the ABA website. Per the ABA, the breakdown of the questions is as follows:

- Basic Sciences (24%): 44–52 questions
- Clinical Sciences (36%): 65–79 questions
- Organ-based Basic and Clinical Sciences (37%): 66–82 questions
- Special Problems or Issues in Anesthesiology (3%): 4–8 questions

Test Preparation

This comprehensive review for the BASIC examination is based on the ABA content outline. Each chapter contains a thorough summary of each of the required content categories and sub-categories. We recommend you to use this book to annotate into as you learn more high-yield information from various resources. This book is meant to be an ultimate source of high-yield information as you take notes into it over three years of anesthesiology residency. The BASIC exam will focus on many facets of anesthetic management from basic pharmacology and physiology to the application of these details to clinical management. This book is a good foundation to obtain high-yield information; however, use of multiple resources including textbooks, articles, and question banks is recommended.

The key to being prepared for the BASIC exam is to start studying early. Start reading textbooks, doing questions, and annotating into this review book early on in residency, so when time comes to really start studying you will be well equipped with a great source of information – all in one place!

Test Day Tips

Just like most exams you've taken thus far, this exam can be anxiety provoking. The key is to stay calm and have faith in your preparation. As with any exam, start your day by eating a well-balanced and nutritious breakfast. Wear something comfortable. Go through the tutorial the day of the exam. It may seem like a waste of time but can help ease you into the exam by preparing you for how to use the tools on the screen rather than trying to find them later. Pace yourself during the exam even if it means leaving a question "marked" so you can return to it later. There will be questions where you don't know the answers, and it is perfectly reasonable to return to those questions so you can move on to questions that you may know the answers. There is no penalty for guessing, so do **NOT** leave an answer blank. There is a 25 percent chance that you pick the correct answer even if you cannot eliminate any answer choices. Read each question carefully and look for key words. When time comes for the break, use it. There is no reason to power through the entire exam without taking a break. Use this time to hydrate, eat a snack, or use the restroom even if you don't feel like you need to because that mental break will help you stay focused for the second half. If you have time left at the end of the exam, use it to review your marked questions or even the entire exam if you have time. Be hesitant to change your answers and second guess yourself.

Anatomy

1

Dallis Clendeninn and Nadia Hernandez

Head and Neck

Vasculature

Internal jugular vein (IJ)
- Drains the blood that comes from the head, face, and brain
- Lies deep to the sternocleidomastoid (SCM) muscle and lateral to the carotid artery within the carotid sheath, coursing inferiorly to join with the subclavian vein (SCV) to become the brachiocephalic (or innominate) vein
- Easily accessed for central venous cannulation

External jugular vein (EJ)
- Carries deoxygenated blood from the face, and is most noticeable on the neck
- Superficial to the SCM muscle as it crosses obliquely from the angle of the mandible and dives posterior to the SCM and clavicle to join the SCV

Subclavian vein
- Posterior to the clavicle but anterior to the insertion of the anterior scalene muscle on the first rib, coursing laterally to become the axillary vein
- Accessed by placing a needle inferior to clavicle, 1–2 cm lateral to the midclavicular line, with the tip directed medially and superiorly toward the sternal notch (Figure 1.1)

Vertebral artery
- Branches from the subclavian artery, traveling cephalad to enter the spinal column deep to Chassaignac's tubercle
- Travels through the transverse foramen of C1–C6 before fusing to form the basilar artery, supplying the posterior Circle of Willis and the spinal cord
- Can be injected directly during an interscalene brachial plexus block

Carotid artery
- Arises from brachiocephalic artery on the right and the aortic arch on the left
- Travels in carotid sheath medial to IJ and anterior to cranial nerve (CN) X
- Bifurcates into internal and external carotid arteries at the level of the C4
  - Carotid sinus:
    - Located at bifurcation of carotid artery

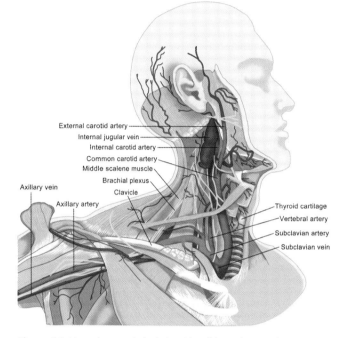

Figure 1.1 Normal anatomical relationships of the major vessels, nerves, bones, and muscles of the neck and axilla

- Compression during carotid endarterectomy can cause a baroreceptor reflex resulting in bradycardia.

Thoracic duct
- Primary endpoint for the lymphatic drainage of the body before joining the venous system
- Arises at the L2 level, courses through the diaphragm posterior to the esophagus, and ascends the thorax just right of the midline between the aorta and azygos vein
- Crosses to the left at T4–T5 and empties into the SCV just lateral to the IJ
- Can be damaged during attempts for central access to the left SCV or IJ, leading to chylothorax

Surface Landmarks

Thyroid cartilage
- In adults, located approximately at the level of C5. Marks the glottic opening, or the start of the larynx

1

- Motor and sensory innervation to the larynx is derived from CN X (vagus nerve) via the superior, inferior, and the recurrent laryngeal nerves bilaterally
- Musculature of the larynx is innervated entirely by the recurrent laryngeal nerve except for the cricothyroid muscle which is innervated by external branch of superior laryngeal nerve.

Cricothyroid membrane
- Palpable in the anterior neck just inferior to the thyroid cartilage and superior to the cricoid cartilage
- Located approximately at the C6 vertebral level
- Marks the access point for the cricothyroidotomy procedure

Chassaignac's tubercle
- Another name for the anterior tubercle of the transverse process of C6
- Lies just posterior to the carotid artery, which can be compressed upon this structure to increase vagal tone via carotid massage
- Marks the approximate location of the vertebral artery, which enters deep to this structure into the spinal column after rising from the subclavian artery
- Clinically used to identify the appropriate location to perform nerve blocks of the brachial plexus, cervical plexus, and stellate ganglion

Vertebrae prominens
- Another name for the spinous process of the C7 vertebral body
- This spinous process is the most prominent in the majority of patients (can be C6 or T1 in small subset of patients).

Stellate ganglion
- Named for its "star-like" appearance
- Is the fusion of the inferior cervical and first thoracic sympathetic ganglia
- Located lateral to the vertebral body of C7
- Blockade of this structure is clinically useful for the treatment of sympathetically mediated pain syndromes, such as complex regional pain syndrome (CRPS) or Raynaud's phenomenon.
  - Side effect associated with stellate ganglion blockade is Horner's syndrome (e.g., ptosis, anhidrosis, miosis), and may frequently occur following many of the cervical and brachial plexus nerve blocks.

Brachial plexus
- Provides cutaneous and motor innervation to the upper extremity
- Lies between the anterior and middle scalene muscles in the neck before running alongside the subclavian and axillary arteries

Radiological Anatomy
See Figure 1.2.

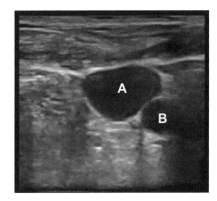

Figure 1.2 Ultrasound image of the lateral neck, displaying (A) the internal jugular vein and (B) the carotid artery

Chest
Surface Landmarks
Trachea
- Begins at C6 and continues inferiorly until it bifurcates at the primary *carina*
- This bifurcation occurs at the level of the *sternal angle*, or *Angle of Louis*, which is the joint between the sternum and manubrium and the connection of the T2 costal cartilages. This structure also marks the approximate level of the T4–T5 intervertebral disk.

Lungs
- Are divided into their lobes by the structures called fissures
- Three lobes on the right and two lobes on the left plus the lingual
- Fissures
  - Bilaterally, the oblique fissure divides the superior and inferior lobes on the left and superior and middle lobes on the right.
  - The fissures begin posteriorly at the level of T4, traveling caudally and laterally, and then around the torso to terminate anteriorly approximately at the level of the seventh rib on the midclavicular line.
  - The right lung is divided a second time by the *horizontal fissure*, which begins anteriorly approximately at the fourth costal cartilage and traverses laterally to the anterior axillary line, where it intersects with the oblique fissure at the level of the fifth rib. This fissure demarcates the border between the inferior and middle lobes.

Heart
- **Point of maximal impulse (PMI)**
  - Landmark for the apex of the heart located at level of the fifth intercostal space (ICS) 6–10 cm lateral to midline
- **Auscultation zones**
  - **Aortic:** Second ICS right upper sternal border
  - **Pulmonary valve:** Second ICS left upper sternal border
  - **Tricuspid valve:** Fourth left ICS on the sternal border
  - **Mitral valve:** Fifth left ICS midclavicular line

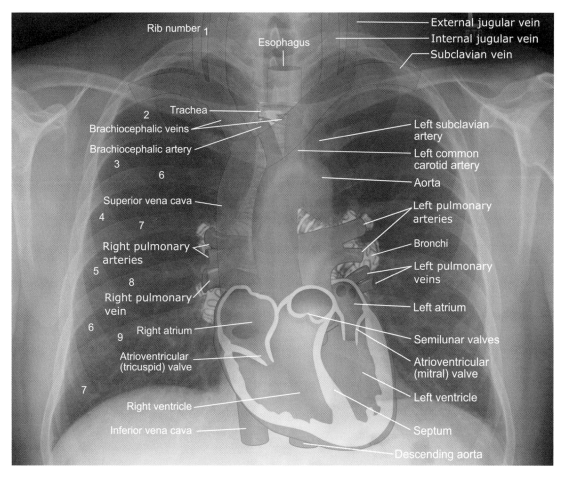

Figure 1.3 Normal radiograph of the chest. Superimposed on this image are outlines of some of the major topographical landmarks of the chest.

- **Coronary arteries**
  - ○ Left and right main arteries arise from the aorta behind the left and right aortic valve leaflets.
  - ○ Left main artery divides into the left anterior descending (LAD) and the circumflex (LCX).
  - ○ LAD supplies the anterior wall of the left ventricle (LV) and the anterior two-third of the interventricular septum (IVS).
  - ○ LCX supplies the lateral wall of the LV and part of the posterior wall.
  - ○ Right coronary artery (RCA)
    - ▪ Supplies most of the right side and usually both sinoatrial (SA) and atrioventricular (AV) nodes
      - • Posterior and anterior walls of the right ventricle (RV) except for the apex (LAD)
      - • Right atrium including SA node
      - • Upper half of the atrial septum
      - • Posterior one-third of IVS
      - • Inferior wall of LV
      - • AV node
  - ○ Posterior descending artery (PDA) arises from RCA in approximately 80 percent of patients. This is called "right-dominant" circulation.

Radiological Anatomy

See Figures 1.3–1.4.

Upper and Lower Extremities

Upper Extremity Vasculature

Basilic vein

- Travels from the medial posterior forearm at the ulnar head proximally to the anterior elbow, where it lies *medial to the tendon of the biceps brachii muscle*
- Becomes the axillary vein at the border of the *teres major muscle*
- Becomes the SCV at the outer border of the first rib

Cephalic vein

- Begins laterally at the wrist within the *anatomic snuffbox* – a triangle formed by the *radial head, the extensor pollicis longus tendon*, and the *extensor pollicis brevis tendon*.
- At the elbow, it is most commonly found lateral to the biceps tendon. It then continues proximally in the arm lateral to the biceps brachii muscle before crossing anterior to the deltoid and diving deep to join with the axillary vein under the clavicle.

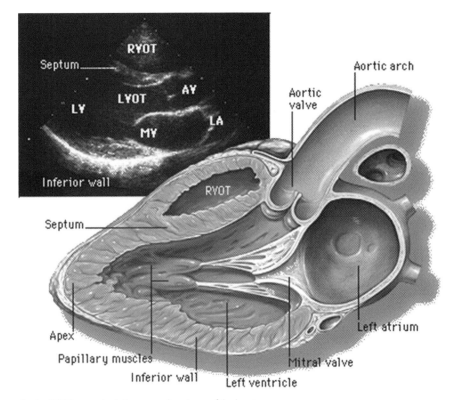

Figure 1.4 Transesophageal echo (TEE) image depicting normal anatomy of the heart

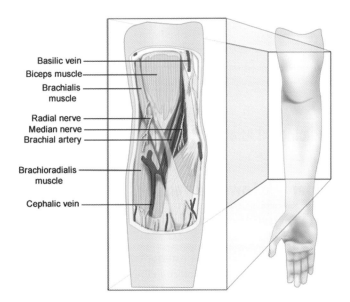

Figure 1.5 Normal anatomical relationships of the major vessels and nerves, bones, and muscles of the antecubital fossa

Box 1.1 Upper extremity nerve block landmarks

Interscalene (i.e., brachial plexus: roots)	Between anterior and middle scalene muscles at level of C6
Supraclavicular (i.e., brachial plexus: trunks/divisions)	Lateral to the clavicular attachment of the SCM
Infraclavicular (i.e., brachial plexus: cords)	Three centimeters caudal to the midpoint of a line between the coracoid process and the medial clavicle
Axillary (i.e., brachial plexus: branches)	At the point of palpation of the axillary artery
Radial nerve	Between the brachioradialis and the biceps tendon
Ulnar nerve	Between the medial epicondyle and olecranon
Median nerve	Medial to the brachial artery at the antecubital fossa

Axillary artery

- Direct continuation of the subclavian artery, it begins at the border of the first rib, coursing laterally until the border of the *teres muscle* where it becomes the brachial artery.

Brachial artery

- The pulsation that is typically felt just *medial to the biceps brachii tendon* at the cubital fossa
- Subsequently bifurcates into the *radial and ulnar arteries* (Figure 1.5)

Upper Extremity Innervation

Brachial plexus

- Originates from a complex network of nerves formed by ventral rami of *C5–T1*
- Provides sensory and motor innervation of the upper extremities. Clinically, the anesthesiologist can provide surgical anesthesia to the upper extremity via blockade of the brachial plexus (see Box 1.1)

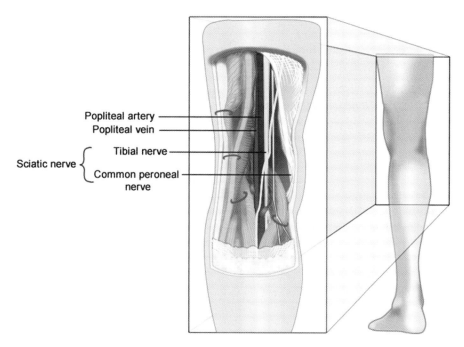

Figure 1.6 Normal anatomical relationships of the major vessels, nerves, bones, and muscles of the popliteal fossa

- ROOTS: After exiting the spinal column, the C5–T1 *roots* split and recombine to form the *superior (C5–C6), middle (C7), and inferior (C8–T1) trunks*, which lie between the anterior and middle scalene muscles.
- TRUNKS: Further split into anterior and posterior divisions
  - *Superior trunk* gives rise to the *suprascapular nerve* which innervates 70 percent of the shoulder joint. Of the brachial plexus blocks, the interscalene block (ISB) is the only one that blocks this nerve. It is also the only block that can be used for shoulder surgery without supplementation.
  - *Roots/trunks* are blocked for the ISB.
  - Due to proximity, the phrenic nerve, stellate ganglion, superficial cervical plexus, recurrent laryngeal nerve, and CN XI are frequently blocked with ISB.
- DIVISIONS: Recombine into the *lateral, medial, and posterior cords*, which are named for their relationship with the *subclavian artery*
  - Level of blockade for supraclavicular block
- CORDS: Split further and recombine to form the terminal *branches*
  - Level of blockade for *infraclavicular block*
- BRANCHES:
  - There are five major terminal branches of the brachial plexus, including:
    - Axillary nerve (C5–C6)
    - Musculocutaneous nerve (C5–C7)
    - Radial nerve (C5–T1)
    - Median nerve (C5–T1)
    - Ulnar nerve (C8–T1)

Intercostobrachial nerve
- Skin over axilla and medial arm is the only part of the arm not innervated by the brachial plexus.
- Intercostobrachial nerve which is derived from T2–T3
- If not blocked separately, can contribute to tourniquet pain (Figure 1.7)

Lower Extremity Vasculature
Small saphenous vein
- Begins posterior to the lateral malleolus and extends proximally on the posterior lower leg until the popliteal fossa, where it drains into the popliteal vein

Popliteal vein
- Lies between the popliteal artery and the tibial nerve at the popliteal fossa (Figure 1.6)
- Continues proximally through the adductor magnus muscle, where it becomes the femoral vein

Great saphenous vein
- Longest vein in the body. Typically found superficially at the dorsum of the foot medial to the medial malleolus
- Commonly cannulated in pediatrics for peripheral venous access
- Used as a landmark to block the saphenous nerve at the ankle. It innervates the medial aspect of the foot
- Courses proximally on the medial surface of the leg before entering the fossa ovalis to empty into the femoral vein on the anterior thigh near the inguinal crease

Femoral artery
- Arises as the direct continuation of the *external iliac artery*
- Lies just lateral to the femoral vein at the inguinal ligament

- Divides into superficial femoral artery and profunda femoris
  - The profunda femoris (deep artery of the thigh) provides vascular supply to the structures of the thigh.
  - The superficial femoral artery courses posteriorly and distally until resurfacing at the popliteal fossa as the popliteal artery.

Popliteal artery
- Divides into two major branches: anterior and posterior tibial arteries
- Anterior tibial artery
  - Terminates as the dorsalis pedis (DP) artery
  - DP pulse can be palpated on the dorsal surface of the foot between the extensor hallicus longus and extensor digitorum longus tendons.
  - DP pulse is a landmark for deep peroneal nerve blockade which innervates the space between the first and second toes.
- Posterior tibial artery (PT)
  - Pulsation can be felt posterior to the medial malleolus at the ankle.
  - PT pulse is a landmark for blockade of the posterior tibial nerve which innervates the plantar aspect of the foot (Figure 1.7).

Lower Extremity Innervation

Lumbar plexus
- Originates from a complex network of nerves formed by ventral rami of T12–L4
- Gives rise to femoral, obturator, lateral femoral cutaneous, ilioinguinal, genitofemoral, and iliohypogastric nerves
- **Femoral nerve** (L2–L4):
  - Found deep into the inguinal ligament lateral to the femoral artery
  - Provides motor innervation to the muscles for knee extension. Blockade of the femoral nerve results in 80 percent reduction in quadriceps strength
  - Sensory innervation anterior and medial thigh via two anterior cutaneous branches
- **Lateral femoral cutaneous nerve (LFCN)** (L2–L3):
  - Provides only cutaneous innervation of the lateral thigh
- **Obturator nerve** (L2–L4):
  - Innervates the adductor muscles
  - Sensory innervation varies within the population:
    - One-third posterior knee, one-third medial thigh, one-third no innervation

Sacral plexus (L4–S4)
- **Sciatic nerve** (L4–S3)
  - Front of the piriformis muscle, traveling distally toward the popliteal fossa
  - Two major branches
    - Tibial nerve
      - Motor function of all the muscles of the posterior compartment of the leg

- Common peroneal nerve
- Supplies the muscles of anterior compartment of leg
  - Blockade or damage results in foot drop

Cutaneous innervation of the distal lower extremity, ankle, and foot is supplied by a combination of five nerves – four derived from the **sciatic nerve** and one derived from the **femoral nerve** (Figure 1.8).

- Sciatic branches (all of these can be blocked at once with a popliteal block)
  - **Tibial nerve**: Provides sensory innervation to the heel and plantar surface of the foot
    - Blocked by injection next to PT pulsation posterior to medial malleolus
  - **Superficial peroneal nerve:** Sensory to the dorsum of the foot
    - Blocked by superficial infiltration of local anesthetic between medial and lateral malleoli
  - **Deep peroneal nerve:** Sensory to the web space between the first and second toes
    - Blocked at the intermalleolar axis by injection posterior to the extensor hallicus longus tendon
    - Blocked at the dorsum of the foot by injecting next to DP pulsation
  - **Sural nerve:** Derived from both the tibial and common peroneal nerves. Provides sensory innervation to the posterior lower leg and lateral ankle
    - Blocked by injection of local anesthetic between lateral malleolus and Achilles tendon
- Femoral branch
  - **Saphenous nerve** provides sensory innervation at the medial lower leg and medial ankle and foot.
    - Blocked by injection medial to medial malleolus next to great saphenous vein

Box 1.2 lists some of the normal anatomical relationships and topographic landmarks associated with nerve blocks of the lower extremities.

Radiological Anatomy

See Figures 1.9–1.11.

Spinal Anatomy, Landmarks, and Dermatomes

Surface Landmarks

Box 1.3 describes some of the clinically relevant surface landmarks, and important key sensory and motor areas of innervation.

Spinal Anatomy

Vascular supply
- Anterior two-third of spinal cord receives its blood supply from a single *anterior spinal artery*, which arises from the vertebral arteries.
  - Receives branches from 6–8 radicular arteries, most important of which is the *artery of Adamkiewicz*, arising most commonly from T9–T12

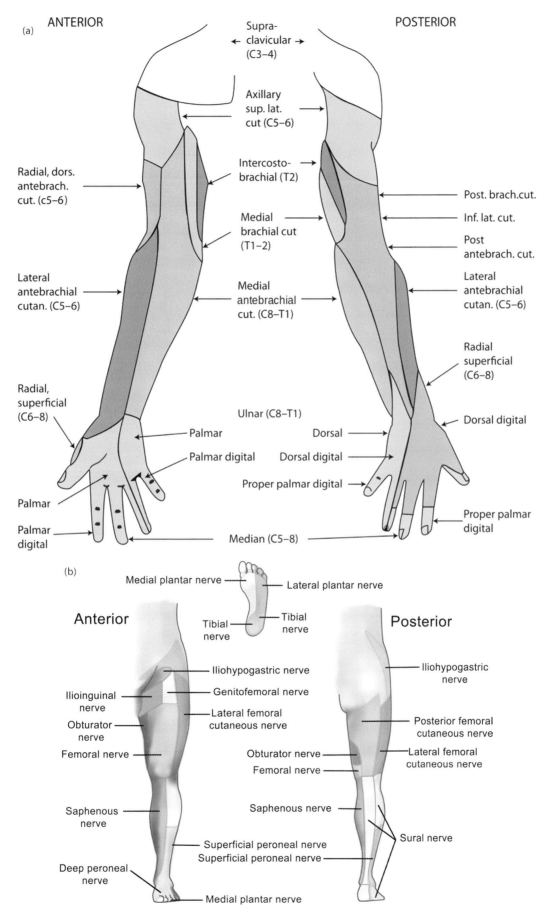

Figure 1.7 Distribution of the major cutaneous nerve branches of the upper and lower extremities

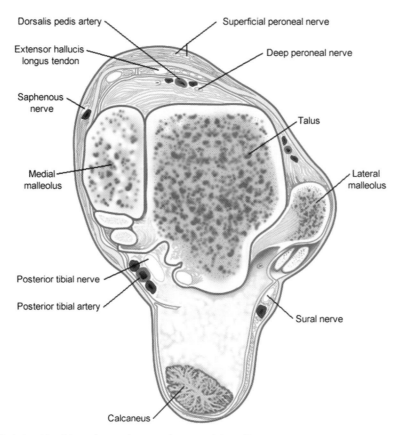

Figure 1.8 Normal anatomical relationship of the major vessels, nerves, bones, and the ankle

Box 1.2 Lower extremity nerve block landmarks	
Femoral nerve	Lateral to the pulsation of femoral artery at the inguinal ligament
Lateral femoral cutaneous nerve	Medial to anterior superior iliac spine
Sciatic nerve	Four centimeters distal to the midpoint of a line between the greater trochanter and posterior superior iliac spine
Saphenous nerve	Anterior to the medial malleolus near the saphenous vein
Superficial peroneal nerve	Anterior to the lateral malleolus
Deep peroneal nerve	Near the pulsation of the dorsalis pedis artery at the ankle
Posterior tibial nerve	Posterior to the pulsation of the posterior tibial artery
Sural nerve	Posterior to the lateral malleolus

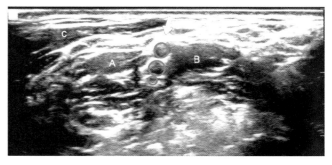

Figure 1.9 Ultrasound image of the brachial plexus at the location for the ISB. At this level, the roots of C5, C6, and C7 appear as hypoechoic circles between (A) the anterior and (B) middle scalene muscles, deep to the (C) SCM muscle.

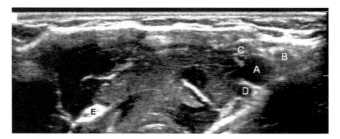

Figure 1.10 Ultrasound image of the brachial plexus at the location for the axillary block. (A) The axillary artery is surrounded by the (B) median, (C) ulnar, and (D) radial nerves. (E) The musculocutaneous nerve is seen laterally within the coracobrachialis muscle.

- o Damage to artery of Adamkiewicz causes *anterior spinal cord syndrome*
  - ▪ Flaccid paralysis of the lower extremities
  - ▪ Bowel and bladder dysfunction
  - ▪ Proprioception and sensation typically spared
    - • Occurs most commonly in emergent repair of dissecting or ruptured thoracic aortic aneurysm (40 percent)

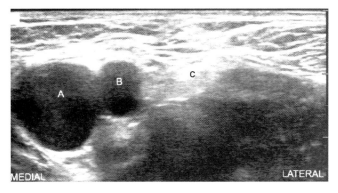

Figure 1.11 Ultrasound image of the inguinal area, depicting the normal relationship between the (A) femoral vein, (B) femoral artery, and (C) femoral nerve. The mnemonic "VAN" can be used to remember the orientation of these structures in the medial to lateral direction.

Box 1.3 Clinically relevant topographic landmarks

Mastoid process	Cervical 1
Thyroid cartilage	Cervical 5
Vertebral prominens	Cervical 7
Suprasternal notch	Thoracic 2–3
Sternal angle	Thoracic 4–5
Inferior angle of the scapula	Thoracic 7
Xyphoid process	Thoracic 9–10
Inferior costal margin	Lumbar 2–3
Iliac crest	Lumbar 4–5
Anterior superior iliac spine	Sacral 1–2
Greater trochanter	Distal coccyx
Symphysis pubic	2.5 cm inferior to distal coccyx

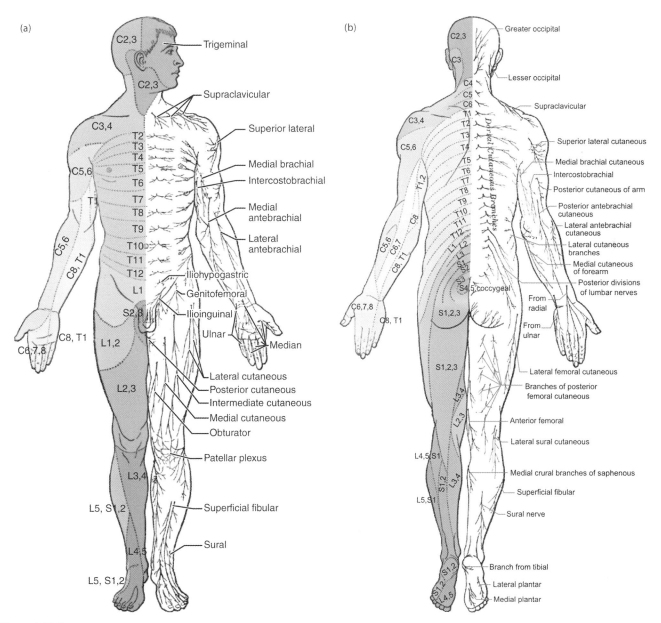

Figure 1.12 Dermatome map

- Posterior one-third of the spinal cord receives its blood supply from two *posterior spinal arteries*.
  - Conversely, *posterior spinal cord syndrome* (very rare) is characterized by loss of sensation and proprioception and spares motor innervation.

Cauda equina
- Nerve roots of the lumbar and sacral plexus that arise following the termination of the spinal cord at the *conus medullaris*

- Conus medullaris terminates at L1–L2 in adults and L3–L4 in infants.
- Damage to this structure can result in *cauda equina syndrome*, which is characterized by pain, and paralysis of the lower extremities, and loss of bowel and bladder function.

Caudal space
- Lowest part of the epidural space
- Dural sac ends at S2 (S3–S4 at birth) where it fuses to filum terminale.
- Sacral hiatus is a defect in the lower part of the posterior wall of the sacrum due to failure of S4/S5 laminae to fuse at midline.
- Roofed by the *sacrococcygeal ligament*, an extension of ligamentum flavum

Dermatome
- Describes the cutaneous sensory innervation of a single nerve root

Myotome
- Describes the muscular innervation of a single nerve root

Radiological Anatomy

See Figure 1.12.

Bibliography

Gray H. *Anatomy of the human body*, 20th ed. 1918. Online edition from Bartleby.com. Published May 2000. www.bartleby.com/br/107/ (Accessed March 2017).

Miller RD, Pardo M, Stoelting RK. *Basics of anesthesia*. Philadelphia, PA: Elsevier/Saunders; 2011.

NYSORA – The New York School of Regional Anesthesia [Internet]. (Accessed March 14, 2017). Available from: www.nysora.com/

Anesthesia Delivery Systems

Morgane Giordano, Bryan Hill, and Jeron Zerillo

Anesthesia Workstation

- Components[1]
  - Anesthesia machine
    - Pressure regulating component
    - Gas mixing component
  - Anesthesia breathing circuit
  - Vaporizers
  - Ventilator
  - Scavenging system
  - Physiological monitors
    - Electrocardiogram
    - Arterial blood pressure measurement
    - Pulse oximetry
    - Temperature
    - Capnograph
    - Inhaled concentrations of oxygen, carbon dioxide, inhaled anesthetics
    - Exhaled concentrations of oxygen, carbon dioxide, inhaled anesthetics
- Alarm systems[3]
  - Apnea and patient circuit disconnect
  - Pulse oximetry and capnograph alarms are audible
- Goals[3]
  - Delivery of oxygen
  - Delivery of controlled concentrations of inhaled anesthetic gases to common gas outlet
  - Removal of carbon dioxide
    - Via carbon dioxide absorbent or scavenging to a waste gas removal limb
- **Fail safe valve**[1]
  - Prevents hypoxic gas mixture delivery if oxygen supply fails
    - Oxygen supply failure decreases pressure in delivery line
    - Protects against lack of oxygen delivery from central source or cylinder
    - Does not prevent against delivery of 100% nitrous oxide if pressure is maintained but oxygen flow is zero
      - Oxygen analyzer needed in this scenario
- **Compressed gases**[3]
  - Most common: oxygen, air, nitrous oxide

- Central supply pipeline with color-coded pressure hose → color-coded wall outlet
  - Oxygen = green
  - Nitrous oxide = blue
  - Air = yellow
  - Diameter index safety system (DISS)
    - Non-interchangeable gas-specific diameter fittings
    - Prevents pipeline misconnection
- Gas delivery from central source requires appropriate pressure (~50 psi)
- Cylinders of compressed gas on machine in case of central supply failure
  - Similarly color-coded
    - Pin index safety system (PISS)
      - Two metal pins in cylinder valve casing that connect via hanger yoke
      - Prevents cylinder misconnection
- Characteristics of compressed gases in E cylinders
  - Oxygen
    - Green
    - Gaseous state
    - 625 L
    - 2,000 psi
  - Air
    - Yellow
    - Gaseous state
    - 625 L
    - 1,800 psi
  - Nitrous oxide
    - Blue
    - Gaseous and liquid state
    - 1,590 L
    - 750 psi
  - Carbon dioxide
    - Gray
    - Gaseous and liquid state
    - 1,590 L
    - 838 psi
- Calculation of E cylinder contents
  - Pressure and volume directly proportional in oxygen and air cylinder

- $P_1 V_1 = P_2 V_2$
- Pressure and volume NOT proportional in nitrous oxide cylinder
  - Pressure begins to decrease after all liquid nitrous oxide is vaporized which is when approximately 75% of nitrous oxide cylinder content has been used.
  - Must weigh cylinder and subtract from tare weight to calculate contents
- **Flowmeters**[1]
  - Measure and control gas flow to common gas inlet
  - Flow
    - Upper limit of bobbin
    - Middle of ball
  - Proportion between flow and pressure affected by
    - Resistance (tube shape)
    - Gas density
    - Gas viscosity
  - Flowmeter → manifold (mixing chamber)
    - Oxygen should be last gas in manifold
    - Decreases chance that proximal leak will decrease concentration of delivered oxygen
    - May still deliver hypoxic gas mixture
  - Manifold → outlet port → vaporizer OR anesthetic breathing system
    - Oxygen flush valve
      - Directly connects high pressure oxygen circuit with low pressure breathing circuit
      - Bypasses flowmeter and manifold
      - May cause barotrauma if utilized during mechanical ventilation

Vaporizers

- Vaporization: conversion of liquid to vapor
- Vaporizer: closed container where vaporization occurs
- Volatile anesthetics: liquid at atmospheric pressure and room temperature
- **Physics of vaporization**[3]
  - Asymmetrical arrangement of intermolecular forces at liquid–oxygen interface for volatile anesthetic in vaporizer
    - Net attractive force keeps molecules in liquid phase
    - Heat energy can be applied so that the molecules can overcome the force to enter the gaseous phase
    - Heat energy required increases as liquid temperature decreases
  - Vaporization stops when there is a liquid–gas equilibrium
  - Molecules in vapor phase collide and create vapor pressure
    - Vapor pressure and temperature are directly proportional
- **Vaporizer classification and design**
  - Classified as

- Variable bypass, flow-over[2]
  - Total fresh gas flow (FGF) is split into two portions
    - One portion enters vaporizer and becomes saturated with volatile anesthetic vapor
      - This is referred to as flow-over which is determined by concentration control dial
    - Second portion travels via bypass chamber of vaporizer
    - Both portions meet at patient outlet of anesthesia machine
- Agent-specific[2]
  - Desflurane vaporizer is unique
    - Electrically heated to 23–25°C
    - Backpressure of 1,500 mmHg
    - Allows for more predicted volatility
- Temperature-controlled[2]
  - Constant vaporizer output over a range of temperatures
  - Controlled by temperature-sensitive bimetallic strip
    - If liquid anesthetic temperature decreases, vapor pressure decreases and increased gas inflow will occur to help raise the pressure
- Vaporizers are often copper or bronze[3]
  - Minimizes heat loss
- Vaporizer tipping[2]
  - Liquid anesthetic from vaporizing chamber enters bypass chamber
    - Causes increased concentration of anesthetic vapor leaving vaporizer
- Vaporizer safety mechanisms[2]
  - Safety interlock on anesthesia machine allows use of only one vaporizer
  - Depression of a release button to turn on vaporizer prevents accidental dial movement
  - Filler port window allows verification of liquid anesthetic levels
  - Anesthetic-specific keyed filler device enables if proper anesthetic is filled into proper vaporizer

Anesthetic Breathing Systems

- Function: deliver oxygen and volatile anesthetics, remove carbon dioxide
- Can be open, semi-open, semi-closed, closed
- **Mapleson breathing systems**[3]
  - Classified into five different semi-open breathing systems (Mapleson A to E)
  - Absence of valves to separate inspired and expired gases
    - Rebreathing when inspiratory flow > FGF
  - Absence of chemical neutralization of carbon dioxide
  - **Mapleson F**[3] = Jackson–Rees modification of Mapleson D

- Uses a reservoir bag and adjustable pressure limiting (APL) valve distal to the reservoir bag
- Must adjust mode of ventilation and APL valve to prevent rebreathing
- Can be used when transporting intubated patients
- Disadvantages include lack of humidity, need for high FGF to prevent rebreathing, possible barotrauma if APL valve is occluded

  o **Bain system**[3]
  - Modification of Mapleson D circuit
  - Fresh gas supply tube runs concentrically within expiratory tubing
  - Exhaled gas vented out the overflow valve near reservoir bag
  - Fresh gas inflow is warmed by the surrounding exhaled gases
  - Easy to scavenge waste via overflow valve
  - Often difficult to recognize problems with inner fresh gas tube such as disconnection

  o **Circle system**[3]
  - Most widely used in the United States
  - Components arranged in circular fashion: fresh gas inlet, unidirectional inspiratory and expiratory valves, inspiratory and expiratory tubing, Y piece connector, APL valve, reservoir bag, carbon dioxide absorbent canister, bag/vent switch, mechanical ventilator
  - Allows for chemical neutralization of carbon dioxide to prevent rebreathing
  - Can be closed, semi-closed, or semi-open depending on fresh gas inflow
  - Semi-closed is most popular, can rebreathe exhaled gases
  - Allows for conservation of body heat and moisture in circuit
  - Increased circuit resistance from unidirectional valves and carbon dioxide absorbent

  o **Closed anesthetic breathing system**[3]
  - Total rebreathing of exhaled gases after carbon dioxide is absorbed
  - Maximizes humidification, economizes use of volatile anesthetics
  - Unable to rapidly change delivered amounts of anesthetic and oxygen
  - Risk of delivering unpredictable concentration of oxygen and unknown amounts of volatile anesthetic.

References

1. Brockwell R. C., Andrews J. J.: Delivery systems for inhaled anesthetics. In Barash P. G., Cullen B. F., Stoetling R. K., editors: *Clinical Anesthesia*. Philadelphia, PA: Lippincott Williams & Wilkins, 2006, pp. 557–94.

2. Brockwell R. C., Andrews J. J.: Inhaled anesthetic delivery systems. In Miller R. D., editor: *Miller's Anesthesia*, 7th edn. Philadelphia, PA: Churchill Livingstone, 2010, pp. 667–718.

3. Roth, P.: Anesthesia delivery systems. In Miller R. D., Pardo M. C., Jr., editors: *Basics of Anesthesia*, 6th edn. Philadelphia, PA: Elsevier Saunders, 2011, pp. 200–20.

Monitoring Methods

Aleksey Maryansky and Tyler Chernin

General Monitors

Blood Pressure Monitoring

Arterial Line[1]

An invasive continuous blood pressure monitoring method.

Indications: Repetitive blood sampling, severe cardiovascular disease with expected hemodynamic instability, titration of vasopressors or antihypertensives, respiratory disturbance requiring persistent arterial blood gas monitoring, inability to obtain blood pressure with a noninvasive cuff[1]

- Arterial cannula transmits mechanical pressure wave through fluid-filled noncompliant tubing to transducer which converts mechanical energy into kinetic energy and is displayed as a waveform on the monitor.[1]
- The arterial waveform is composed of a series of sine waves which are analyzed by Fournier analysis. The arterial pressure system must be able to transmit high-frequency waves in order to obtain a precise arterial blood pressure reading. The natural frequency (or the frequency at which the system oscillates freely) must be set higher (at least 25 Hz but usually 100–200 Hz) than the frequency of any possible sine wave in order to prevent resonance and thus signal deformation.[2]
- Natural frequency can be changed by: changing diameter, density, compliance, or length. *Increasing the length* of the tubing will *decrease natural frequency*.[2]
- The arterial line is "zeroed" to ensure negligible effect by atmospheric pressure on the pressure reading by opening the transducer to air. The arterial line transducer is normally placed at the level of the heart to measure arterial pressure. It can also be placed at the level of the circle of Willis if measuring cerebral perfusion pressure.[1]
- A 10-cm change in the height of the level of the transducer will change the reading by 7.5 mmHg opposite to the direction of change. A change in the level of the arterial cannula is negligible as long as the transducer remains at the same level of measurement.[1]
- An arterial pressure system can be overdampened or underdampened which is due to interference resulting in change in the amplitude of the wave and thus in incorrect blood pressure readings. Dampening can occur due to bubbles, kinks, the addition of stopcocks, and tubing. In an overdampened system, the systolic blood pressure will be underestimated and the diastolic blood pressure will be overestimated. The reverse will occur in an underdampened system. The mean arterial pressure will remain accurate.[1]

Noninvasive Blood Pressure

- By ASA guidelines, blood pressure must be measured at least every 5 minutes in any case where an anesthetic is provided.[3]
- Oscillometric: Internal pressure transducer senses oscillations after cuff is inflated; if no oscillations are sensed, then the cuff deflates and senses again at the next level. Once oscillations are sensed, a microprocessor within the system compares oscillation amplitudes. The *systolic blood pressure* is obtained at the point where *oscillation amplitude* first increases. The *mean arterial pressure* (MAP) is obtained at *the maximum amplitude of oscillations*. The *diastolic blood pressure* is obtained at the point where the *oscillation amplitude* drops off.[4]
- This method is reliable for obtaining MAP and diastolic blood pressure but can underestimate systolic blood pressure.[4]

Pulse Oximetry

Used to continuously monitor a patient's saturation but appreciable pulse must be present to achieve accuracy. The pulse oximeter can thus also measure and display heart rate. In low blood-flow conditions, pulse oximetry may not be reliable. Pulse oximetry correlates predictably with PaO_2.[4]

- The probe detects two wavelengths of light: *red* (660 nm) and *infrared* (940 nm). Oxyhemoglobin absorbs more infrared light and deoxyhemoglobin absorbs more red light. The ratio of infrared to red light determines the SpO_2.[4]
- The pulse oximeter does not differentiate between oxyhemoglobin and other types of hemoglobins such as carboxyhemoglobin and methemoglobin. Therefore, in the presence of one of these conditions, the SpO_2 may not correlate to the PaO_2. In methemoglobinemia the SpO_2 will be displayed as 85% whereas in carboxyhemoglobinemia it may be falsely elevated. In order to clinically differentiate between these hemoglobins, a co-oximeter should be employed instead.[4]
- The pulse oximeter is not a good measure of assessing ventilation, especially if a patient is breathing 100% oxygen as this can significantly prolong apnea time.
- Other entities that can affect pulse oximeter readings are methylene blue, hypothermia, indigo carmine, and nail polish.[4]

Temperature

As per ASA guidelines, temperature should be continuously monitored in any case with anesthesia where clinically significant changes in body temperature are intended, suspected, or anticipated.[4]

- Temperature can be monitored in a variety of locations. Skin temperature can differ depending on where the temperature probe is placed and is not a good reflection of core temperature.[4]
- Esophageal or nasopharyngeal temperatures are most reflective of core temperature but can often only be used under general anesthesia.[4]
- Bladder temperature, as commonly attached to a Foley catheter, is also reflective of core temperature but is dependent on urine flow.[4]

Neuromuscular function

A nerve stimulator monitor is used intraoperatively after muscular blockade.[4]

- The nerve stimulator is commonly placed at the *adductor pollicis (ulnar nerve)* or the *orbicularis oculi (facial nerve)*. Monitoring at the orbicularis oculi during induction allows for faster *intubation* as laryngeal blockade occurs at the same time.[4]
- Nerve stimulators can be qualitative and quantitative:
  - Qualitative: Rely subjectively on tactile or visual analysis of stimulation. Reliable for assessing twitch count and "depth" of paralysis but poor for estimating train-of-four (TOF) ratio. Twitches correspond to the percentage of receptor blockade: four twitches (0–75% blocked), three twitches (75% blocked), two twitches (80% blocked), one twitch (90% blocked), zero twitch (100% blocked).[4]
  - Quantitative: Directly measures and divides the amplitude of the first twitch by the amplitude of the fourth twitch and thus provides the ability to objectively calculate TOF ratio. A TOF ratio > 0.7 classically corresponds with full return of neuromuscular function. A TOF ratio > 0.9 is ideal criteria for extubation and reduces postoperative complications.[4]

Bispectral index (BIS)

A monitor usually placed on the forehead which detects raw EEG data and converts it into a BIS number. It is presumed to be useful in the titration of anesthesia to an appropriate level to try to ensure that the patient is not awake.[4]

- A BIS # of 91–100 correlates with the patient being awake. A BIS # of 61–90 correlates with light anesthesia. A BIS # of 41–60 correlates with acceptable general anesthesia. A BIS # of 1–40 correlates with deep anesthesia and a BIS # of 0 correlates with electrical silence.[4]
- The raw EEG waveform and thus the BIS # are susceptible to artifact from any electrical (i.e. cautery, defibrillator) devices that are close to the BIS monitoring site.[4]

- The BIS # can also become inaccurate due to muscle activity thus the BIS sensor allows you to monitor EMG activity as well. A greater level of EMG is inversely proportional to the accuracy of the BIS #.[4]
- Some anesthetic agents such as ketamine or etomidate may falsely elevate the BIS reading; the former due to an increase in high-frequency EEG activity and the latter due to an increase in high-frequency EMG activity.[4]

Electrocardiogram (ECG)

Critical monitor in the perioperative setting for both diagnosing and monitoring cardiovascular function, including the preoperative setting for risk stratification and guiding the need for more invasive tests.[4]

- Electrical activity emanates from the heart and can be recorded from multiple sites. Leads that are placed on the skin measure electrical potentials. Bipolar leads utilize two electrodes at two different sites to measure the potential difference. Unipolar leads measure the absolute potential difference at one site relative to a control reference site.[4]
- Standard twelve lead ECG: Three bipolar leads (I, II, III), six unipolar leads (V1–V6), and three modified unipolar limb leads (aVR, aVL, aVF).[4]
- P wave: Represents atrial depolarization. Normally proceeds from right to left, so wave is biphasic in V1 and V2 and upright in lateral leads.[4]
- PR interval: Represents conduction through the AV node, bundle branches, bundle of His, and intraventricular conduction systems. Relative delay is due to slow conduction through AV node. Normally 120–200 ms.[4]
- QRS complex: Represents left and right ventricular depolarization. Begins in the septum and spreads toward free walls of the ventricles. The main QRS vector in the frontal plane determines the axis, which is normally −30 to +90. Normal QRS complex lasts 120 ms.[4]
- ST/T wave: Represents ventricular repolarization. Usually begins at epicardial surface and spreads toward endocardium. Normally QRS and T wave both deflect in the same direction. QT interval starts at Q wave and ends at conclusion of T wave and is highly rate-dependent; hence the use of the QTc is corrected for heart rate. Prolonged QTc intervals predispose to malignant ventricular arrhythmias. The ST segment is the most sensitive marker of ischemia on the EKG. ST elevations classically represent transmural ischemia and ST depressions represent subendocardial ischemia, but there is considerable overlap.[4]
- Q waves: When pathologic, they can represent areas of myocardial scarring, usually from prior ischemic events. They more commonly represent a prior transmural infarct and often correlate on the ECG to the specific area involved. V1–V3 usually localize to anteroseptal and apical segments of the left ventricle, V4–V6 to the apical and lateral segments, and II, III, and aVF to the inferior segments.[4]

- Monitoring: Three lead systems utilize RA, LA, LL, and RL (reference) electrodes and represent the simplest form of measuring real-time ECG. This system allows for three bipolar leads (I, II, and III), ideally measures heart rate, R waves, and detects ventricular fibrillation. It is inadequate in the diagnosis and monitoring of more complex arrhythmias and detecting myocardial ischemia. Five lead systems utilize LA, RA, LL, RL electrodes, and one precordial lead (V1 through V6). This allows for leads I, II, III, aVR, aVL, and aVF and is better at detecting left ventricular ischemia in the operating room when leads V3–V5 are chosen (ideal position for detecting the bulk of left ventricular tissue).[4]

Ventilation Monitors

Respirometer – A part of the anesthesia machine that allows for the measurement of tidal volumes and minute volumes. Classically, in the case of the original Wright respirometer, expired gas into a chamber would cause the rotation of a rotor attached to a needle on an indicator dial displaying tidal volume.[4]

Inspiratory force – Negative inspiratory force (NIF) is often measured in anticipation of extubation. Generally, a NIF of more than −25 cm H_2O is required before extubation. NIF corresponds to the negative inspiratory pressure generated by inspiratory musculature during maximal inhalation. This can be performed actively by asking the vented patient to perform maximal inhalation and measuring pressure. It can also be performed passively by steadily increasing the ventilator trigger setting to −25 cm H_2O and checking if the patient is able to trigger breath.[4]

Spirometry – With most modern anesthetic machines, spirometry measures airway flow, volume, compliance, and pressure with each breath. Flow/volume and pressure/volume loops are dynamically displayed. These measurements allow for a more intricate detection of potential problems during the anesthetic as characteristic patterns will be seen. For example, in the case of a leak, the expiratory loop will remain open at the end of exhalation. In obstruction, pressure will be high and volume will be low.[4]

Gas Concentrations

O_2 – Oxygen analyzers are critical to anesthetic practice and are usually located in the inspiratory limb or at the common gas outlet. They exist to ensure that the inspired gas mixture contains an adequate amount of oxygen to prevent hypoxia.[4]

- Exhaled patient oxygen is monitored as well and is useful for assessing whether a patient is adequately pre-oxygenated. These analyzers consist of two chambers, one that samples gas and one that is used as a reference. An electromagnetic field agitates oxygen molecules in the sampling chamber and this is converted into a pressure which is then transduced and essentially displayed as a concentration on the monitor.[4]

CO_2 – Exhaled carbon dioxide monitors allow a practitioner to be able to measure adequate ventilation and avoid

hypercapnia. They are also useful in detection of rebreathing and can be utilized as a surrogate for the presence of cardiac output.[4]

- Changes in $ETCO_2$ can alert a practitioner to acute problems. $ETCO_2$ can be pathologically increased in a variety of scenarios, i.e. hypoventilation, hypermetabolic state, obstructive respiratory disease, insufflation during laparoscopy, or exhausted CO_2 absorbent. In other scenarios, it can be pathologically decreased, i.e. hyperventilation, circuit disconnection or obstruction, pulmonary embolism, and shock/cardiac arrest.[4]

- CO_2 analyzers employ infrared absorption. The more CO_2 present in a sample, the more infrared light can be absorbed. The CO_2 concentration displayed is thus proportional to the amount of infrared light detected by the analyzer to be absorbed. The machine then displays this as both a number and a waveform called a capnogram.[4]

As pictured, a capnogram is divided into four phases:

- The inspiratory baseline (the point at which exhalation begins and is zero in normal patients due to the expired gas at this point coming from respiratory dead space; it is greater than zero in cases of rebreathing and inadequate fresh gas flow).[5]
- Expiratory upstroke (at this point, dead space gas ends and CO_2-containing gas from the alveoli begins to be exhaled). In obstructive lung disease (such as COPD) or an incompetent expiratory valve, this phase is prolonged.[5]
- Plateau phase (only CO_2-containing gas from the alveoli is exhaled at this point). If a patient is spontaneously breathing during mechanical ventilation, a notch called the "curare cleft" can be seen in the middle of the plateau.[5]
- Inhalation (gas is no longer exhaled at this point, so in a normal situation the $ETCO_2$ falls back to zero). During rebreathing (such as in the case of an exhausted CO_2 absorbent), the $ETCO_2$ does not return back to zero at this point (Figure 3.1).[5]

Nitrogen – Many modern anesthetic machines monitor end tidal nitrogen. This can be useful in assessing adequate denitrogenation (pre-oxygenation). An abrupt increase in end-tidal nitrogen has been studied as an early sign of venous air embolism.[6]

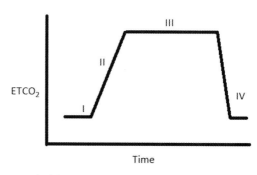

Figure 3.1 End tidal CO_2 capnogram

Volatile anesthetics – Monitoring the concentration of volatile anesthetic delivered to the patient is important to ensure that the patient is at an adequate depth of anesthesia.

- Vapor concentrations are commonly measured by either Raman scattering or mass spectrometry (the most accurate method). In Raman scattering, a laser beam is directed toward a sample of gas in a chamber. When the light from the laser beam comes in contact with a molecule of a gas, the light scatters. The light is then passed through a variety of filters (each individual gas has its own special filter) and into a detector/processing unit. The concentration of the gas is proportional to the number of photons passing through that gas-specific filter.

- In mass spectrometry, a gas sample passes into a low-pressure chamber and then into a high-pressure chamber which results in the ionization of the molecules of gas. Electromagnets separate the ions by mass and charge. The ions are then filtered and processed and a concentration of gas is displayed. Most modern anesthesia machines will convert the concentration into a MAC reading (for each respective gas and sometimes incorporating patient's age).[4]

References

1. Oropello, J. M. et al. Arterial Line Monitoring and Placement. *Critical Care* 2016; 89.

2. Stoker, M. Principle of pressure transducers, resonance, damping and frequency response. *Anaesthesia and Intensive Care Medicine* 2004; 5(11): 371–5.

3. American Society of Anesthesiologists Committee of Origin: Standards and Practice Parameters. Standards for Basic Anesthetic Monitoring. Last amended on October 20, 2010.

4. Barash, P. G. et al. *Clinical Anesthesia*, 7th edition. Philadelphia, PA: Lippincott; 2011.

5. Ortega, R. et al. Monitoring ventilation with capnography. *New England Journal of Medicine* 2012; 367: e27.

6. Sprung, J. et al. End-tidal nitrogen provides an early warning of slow, ongoing, venous air embolism. *Anesthesiology* 1996; 85: 1203–6.

Ventilators, Alarms, and Safety Features

Jonathan A. Paul and Michael D. Lazar

Ventilators

Phase variables[1]: Three main ventilator phase variables make up a ventilator mode.

What is the trigger of breath initiation (i.e. what will cause *start of inhalation*)?

- Time: Initiation of breath after a fixed interval of time after which ventilator delivers a breath such as in controlled mechanical ventilation (MV)
- Flow: Patient inhalation efforts as sensed by flow in the circuit during assisted MV
- Pressure: Patient inhalation efforts as sensed by negative pressure during assisted MV

What is the limit of breath phase (i.e. what is the *quality of inhalation*)?

- Flow limited: There is a set rate of flow and the ventilator will not allow any increase in flow during inspiration.
- Volume limited: There is a set volume and the ventilator will not allow any increase in volume during inspiration.
- Pressure limited: There is a set pressure and the ventilator will not allow any further increase in pressure during inspiration.
- Of note, these variables are fixed if controlled MV and variable if assisted MV.

How long is the cycle of breath transition (i.e. *end of inhalation, beginning of exhalation*)?

- Time cycled: Inspiration and expiration according to the time set by ventilator such as in controlled MV
- Flow cycled: Once the flow decreases, the ventilator allows exhalation such as in pressure support (PS).
- Volume cycled: Once target volume is reached, the ventilator allows exhalation.
- Pressure cycled: Once peak inspiratory pressure is reached, the ventilator allows exhalation.

Modes

Noninvasive ventilation[2]: Noninvasive alternatives to intubation

Continuous positive airway pressure (CPAP)

- Mechanism: CPAP is administered throughout inhalation and exhalation via facemask (although nasal administration is also possible).

- Purpose: CPAP is administered to recruit and stent open alveoli and increase available surface area for gas exchange. It also encourages patency of the upper airway. Commonly used for obstructive sleep apnea (OSA) and respiratory distress syndrome of infancy.

Biphasic Positive Airway Pressure (BiPAP)

- Mechanism: The clinician sets an *inspiratory peak airway pressure* (serving as a form of PS) and an *expiratory peak airway pressure*. The difference between the two is equal to positive end-expiratory pressure (PEEP).
- Purpose: Administered for recruitment and maintenance of airway patency, augmenting tidal volume and eliminating carbon dioxide. May be implemented in an attempt to avoid invasive ventilation for patients with exacerbations of reactive airway disease, pneumonia, or acute heart failure.

Total controlled mechanical ventilation[3]: No patient-initiated breaths. Time triggered, volume or pressure limited, and time cycled.

Volume Control (VC)

- Mechanism: VC delivers constant flow to provide set tidal volume, regardless of characteristics of patient airway.
- Limitations: Opening airway pressure is dependent on patient characteristics, which could result in creation of excessive peak airway pressures (Figure 4.1).

Pressure Control (PC)

- Mechanism: PC delivers set pressure to airway opening. Inhalational flow decreases progressively (see also Figure 4.1), which allows lower peak airway pressures.
- Limitations: In cases of decreased lung compliance, there is a risk of underventilation with variable tidal volumes.

Assisted Mechanical Ventilation

Volume Modes

Assist Control (AC)

- Mechanism: The patient may trigger the ventilator at a set negative pressure or flow threshold; otherwise the ventilator will deliver a breath according to a backup frequency (i.e. time trigger). Each breath is assisted or controlled by

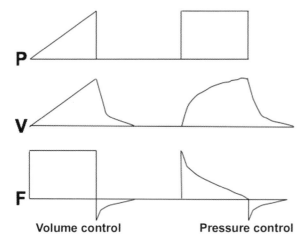

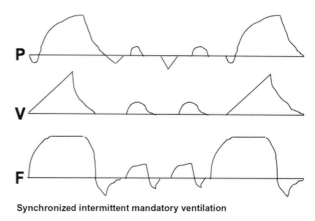

Synchronized intermittent mandatory ventilation

Figure 4.1 Pressure, volume, and flow curves for the two modes of controlled mechanical ventilation: volume control (left) and pressure control (right). P = pressure, V = volume, F = flow.

Figure 4.3 Examples of pressure, volume, and flow curves for synchronized intermittent mandatory ventilation. Note that patient-initiated breaths above the set respiratory rate are not supported by additional positive pressure.

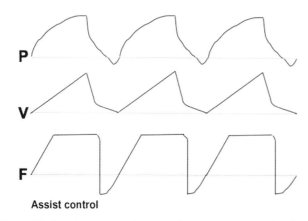

Assist control

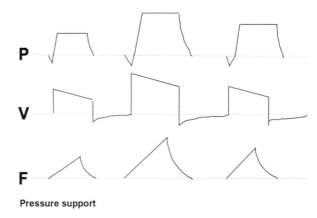

Pressure support

Figure 4.2 Sample pressure, volume, and flow curves representative of assist control ventilation.

Figure 4.4 Pressure, volume, and flow curves illustrating pressure support ventilation.

(unless a combination SIMV–Pressure Support mode is selected). There is evidence that SIMV may reduce cardiac output in certain patient populations and prolong time to extubation during intensive care unit (ICU) weaning attempts.[4,5]

the ventilator and all delivered tidal volumes are *equal*. Pressure, volume, and flow curves are shown in Figure 4.2.

- Limitations: With inadequate expiratory time or excessive respiratory rates, *hyperinflation* may occur. AC is the assisted mode with the most *asynchrony*, as peak inspiratory flows rarely match patient requirements, resulting in *increased work*. Risk of *air trapping* and *respiratory alkalosis*, especially with hyperinflation disease processes (i.e. COPD and asthma) or tachypneic disease processes (i.e. sepsis and hypermetabolic states).[1,3]

Synchronized Intermittent Mandatory Ventilation (SIMV)

- Mechanism: The mandatory ventilation in SIMV refers to a *guaranteed number of breaths* which can be machine- or patient-initiated and which will achieve a *set tidal volume*. This is similar to AC; however, mandatory breaths are synchronized with *spontaneous* efforts. May be volume- or pressure-cycled. During attempts to wean patients from the ventilator, the number of mandatory breaths can be decreased to facilitate an increasing proportion of spontaneous breaths.
- Limitations: Additional patient inspiratory efforts beyond the set rate are not supported, as shown in Figure 4.3

Pressure Modes

Pressure Support

- Mechanism: Triggered by the patient's negative pressure breath, limited by inspiratory pressure, and cycled by inhalational flow rate. PEEP may be added. Useful intraoperatively to supplement spontaneous breathing or during ventilator weaning trials in the ICU to compensate for circuit and endotracheal tube resistance. Decreases work of breathing (WOB). For example, pressure, volume, and flow curves are demonstrated in Figure 4.4.
- Limitations: Clinician must change ventilator settings to achieve desired tidal volumes if there is a change in the mechanical properties of the lungs

Pressure-Regulated Volume Control (PRVC)

- Mechanism: Clinician sets a baseline minute ventilation and the patient may provide a negative pressure or flow

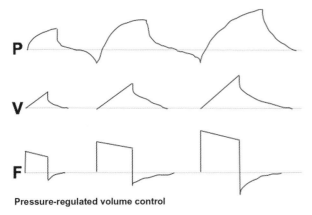

Figure 4.5 Pressure-regulated volume control mode pressure, volume, and flow curves. Note, in particular, the gradual adjustment in pressure is required to achieve the desired tidal volume.

trigger in order to initiate a breath. Uses a closed-loop algorithm to automatically measure the static compliance of the respiratory system and adapt the airway opening pressure to match a target tidal volume on a breath-by-breath basis. Intent is to use minimal pressure to achieve tidal volume and thereby reduce incidence of barotrauma, as illustrated by the progressively increasing pressures in Figure 4.5.[3]

- Limitations: Risk of auto-PEEP

Interactive Modes

Proportional Assisted Ventilation (PAV)

- Mechanism: Uses internal sensors measuring pressure and flow in order to adjust to patient effort. A benefit of PAV, as compared to PSV, is that tidal volumes (as opposed to respiratory rate) can adapt over time to stimuli such as hypercapnia.
- Limitations: Errors in evaluating elastance and resistance may result in inadequate ventilation[4,6]

Neurally Adjusted Ventilatory Assist (NAVA)

- Mechanism: Designed to improve neuroventilatory coupling. Electrodes are placed through a nasal or oral gastric tube into the lower esophagus in order to use sensory information to correlate diaphragmatic movement with ventilator-assisted breaths.[4]
- Limitations: Limited clinical applicability to patients

Ventilator Manipulation Techniques

Positive End-Expiratory Pressure

- Mechanism: Applied at *end-exhalation*, in contrast to CPAP, which is applied throughout inhalation and exhalation. PEEP is intended to expand collapsed alveoli to participate in gas exchange, reduce shunt, and increase functional residual capacity. Up to 10 cm H_2O of PEEP, there is a linear increase in alveolar diameter. PEEP may be increased up to 20 cm H_2O for severe hypoxia secondary to acute respiratory distress syndrome (ARDS).

- Limitations: In the absence of collapsed alveoli available for recruitment, PEEP may result in *hyperinflation* and *increased dead space*. Increased intrathoracic pressure from PEEP may *decrease venous return*, although the clinical significance of this is dependent on patient's characteristics (i.e. volume status) and comorbidities.[5]

Inverse Ratio Ventilation (IRV)

- Mechanism: A form of pressure control ventilation with an increased inspiratory/expiratory ratio, intended to improve oxygenation through reduced peak airway pressures. May be used in refractory cases of ARDS.[4,6]
- Limitations: Mean airway pressures may actually be elevated with resultant *reduction in venous return*. Associated with *risk of auto-PEEP*.

Airway Pressure Release Ventilation (APRV)

- Mechanism: A form of IRV with a very high inspiratory/expiratory ratio and very short expiratory time. Used in ARDS for refractory hypoxia. The prolonged inspiratory phase at high pressure followed by a short expiratory time, during which this pressure is released, creates a gradient that improves exhalation quality. Allows for superimposed spontaneous ventilation.[7]
- Limitations: Concern for hemodynamic compromise due to high inspiration pressures. Requires increased sedation.

Periodic Sigh

- Mechanism: Also described as *periodic hyperinflation*, this consists of an increased tidal volume (approximately 1.5–2 times set tidal volume) delivered approximately once in every 6 to 10 minutes. Goal of the technique is intermittent alveolar recruitment, but PEEP administration has been demonstrated as superior for this purpose.
- Limitations: Avoid with baseline tidal volumes greater than 7 mL/kg or with peak airway pressures greater than 30 cm H_2O.[1,3]

Alternative Ventilation

High Frequency Ventilation

- Mechanism: Unlike the MV modes described earlier, high frequency ventilation uses tidal volumes (1 to 2 mL/kg) that are less than dead space volume. These low volumes are delivered at frequencies of approximately 5 to 15 Hz at high flows and pressures with an oscillatory piston. Mean airway pressures are typically high.
- Limitations: Enough time must occur between breaths to allow passive expiration of carbon dioxide.

Monitoring Parameters

- *Peak pressure*[4]: Peak airway pressure is the highest pressure throughout the respiratory cycle and reflects a combination of all the *resistance* in both physiological (patient) and mechanical (endotracheal tube, circuit, etc.) airways.

- *Plateau pressure*[4]: Plateau pressure is obtained during an inspiratory pause on the ventilator (which eliminates airway resistance) and represents the pressure in the *small airways and alveoli*. Plateau pressure is typically indicative of *lung compliance*, whereas peak pressure is generally proportional to airway resistance. Figure 4.6 depicts peak and plateau pressures on a ventilator pressure curve. With decreased compliance or increased tidal volumes, both plateau and peak pressures should rise.
- *Increased peak and plateau pressure*[4]: Increased tidal volume or decreased compliance (i.e. pneumothorax, abdominal insufflation, Trendelenburg position, pulmonary edema, pleural effusion, ascites)
- *Increased peak, unchanged plateau pressure*[4]: Increased gas flow rate or airway resistance (i.e. bronchospasm, kinked or herniated endotracheal tube, secretions, mucous plugs, foreign body aspiration)
- *Static compliance*[4]: Static compliance (normal 50–100 mL/cm H_2O) = Tidal volume/(plateau pressure – PEEP)
- *Dynamic compliance*[4]: Dynamic compliance (always lower than or equal to static compliance) = Tidal volume/(peak pressure – PEEP)
- *Assisted ventilation monitoring*[4]: Vigilant observation of patient–ventilator interaction is necessary during assisted ventilation.
  - *Asychrony*[4]: May occur secondary to inhalation time discrepancy (i.e. the ventilator is still delivering an inhalational pressure, but the patient has started to exhale), ineffective inspiratory triggering (i.e. ventilator is unable to sense the patient's breath despite adequate effort)
  - *WOB*[4]: Breath-by-breath analysis of patient work is ideal, but a more practical evaluation may be made by computing the work (pressure × volume) of breathing per minute and per liter of minute ventilation. Normal WOB at rest is approximately 0.3–0.6 J/L. Use of any invasive ventilation requires additional work to be exerted by patient in order to trigger the ventilator and overcome the resistance of the circuit and endotracheal tube.

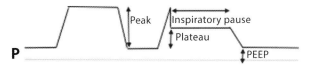

Figure 4.6 Extrapolation of peak and plateau pressure from ventilator pressure curves, which can be used to calculate dynamic and static compliance, respectively. Note that inspiration must be held in order to determine plateau pressure.

Alarms and Safety Features

General Alarm Concepts

- *Design*: Although there is no single organization which regulates alarms pertinent to monitoring for anesthesiology, at the International Standards Organization meeting in 2003, alarm severity was classified into high, medium, and low priorities (Table 4.1).[8,9]
- *Alarm fatigue*[8,10]: Alarm fatigue is a product of the sheer number of alarms encountered, and in particular by excessive false positives, leading to the tendency to ignore meaningful information when it is provided. A significant reduction in false positives can occur by individualizing alarm limits for each patient, although caution must be taken, as limits which are excessively wide can result in false negative data. Innovations in technology have begun to reduce the incidence of false positive alarms (i.e. an EKG monitor automatically switching leads if an electrode is removed or pulse oximeters with algorithms designed to compensate for motion artifact). However, it is the clinician's responsibility to remain vigilant and prevent alarm fatigue from causing inattention to monitor alerts.

Operating Room Safety

- *Alarm sources*: There are a multitude of alarms and alerts within the operating room which can generate background noise. It is the anesthesiologist's responsibility to distinguish these from alarms that are specific to the anesthesia machine and its integrated monitor. Some examples include convection warming devices, electro-cautery equipment, laser devices, and personal communications equipment such as pagers and phones.
- *Line isolation monitor*: Most grounded electrical systems outside of the operating room only require one fault to deliver a potential shock. With the addition of an isolation monitor and transformer, electrical surgery equipment has an added protective layer, as it requires two faults to shock a patient. An alarm will sound if a hazardous amount of current could be transmitted to the patient in the event of a second fault, or the system becoming grounded. The last device or instrument added to the system before the alarm was initiated is typically the culprit and should be removed and analyzed.[3]
- *Air contamination*: The air in operating rooms is changed approximately 12 times per hour. As per National Institute

Table 4.1 Organization of medical monitoring alarm priorities

	High priority	Medium priority	Low priority
Intended response	Immediate action	Prompt action	Awareness
Visual alert	Red, flashing at high frequency	Yellow, flashing at low frequency	Yellow/blue, no flash
Auditory alert	Loud, complex	Loud, monotone	Relatively muted
Examples	Severe hypoxia, malignant dysrhythmia (ventricular tachycardia/fibrillation, asystole)	Hypo-/hypercarbia, Hypo-/hypertension	Temperature probe disconnect

Data obtained from General Requirements, Tests and Guidelines for Alarm Systems in Medical Electrical Equipment and in Medical Electrical Systems (ISO-IEC 60601-1-8).[9]

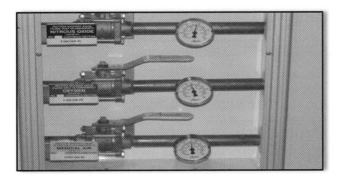

Figure 4.7 Gas-specific shut-off valves, required to be located outside of each operating room to enable control of pipeline supply in the event of emergencies such as fires.

Anesthesia Machine Safety

- *Gas pressures*[8]: First-stage regulators decrease pressures from approximately 85 PSIG inside bulk storage containers to 50 PSIG throughout all pipelines delivering gas into operating rooms and anesthesia machines. Second-stage regulators, located just upstream of flow meters, further reduce gas pressures to 12–16 PSIG in order to reduce the risk of patient barotrauma.
- *Hypoxic mixture avoidance*[10]: Several mechanisms exist in order to prevent delivery of a hypoxic gas mixture to the patient, the most important of which is the *end-tidal oxygen level determined from the circuit's gas-sampling line*. Another features designed to achieve the same goal is the *oxygen analyzer*, a fuel cell located in the inspiratory circuit limb, calibrated to room air but beware, if calibrated at sea level but used at altitude, the reading will be less than 21% because the ambient partial pressure of oxygen is less than 159 mmHg. Fail safe systems are well known to be poorly named, because they are pressure-sensitive (not gas-sensitive) and would not prevent a hypoxic gas mixture in the event of a pipeline switch outside of the operating room. It is worth mentioning that GE-Ohmeda Pressure Sensor Shutoff Valves completely stop the flow of nitrous oxide if oxygen pressure falls below 26 PSIG in the high pressure system. On the contrary, Draeger Oxygen Failure Protection Devices reduce nitrous oxide flows in a stepwise manner in proportion to decreasing oxygen supply pressures. Finally, there is a high-priority Low Oxygen Supply Pressure alarm which is activated if oxygen pressures fall below 30 PSIG in the high pressure system.

for Occupational Safety and Health requirements, volatile anesthetic concentrations must be ≤2 ppm; nitrous oxide must be ≤25 ppm (or ≤50 ppm in dentistry offices or where used without volatile gases).[11] Concentrations are measured with infrared analyzers, which can detect volatiles in ranges from 0 to 30 ppm and nitrous oxide in ranges from 0 to 100 ppm.

- *Gas control*: The gas-specific supply pressures must be displayed in close proximity to operating room clusters. This information is used to convey alarms to gas suppliers automatically so that stores can be replaced before supply pressures fall excessively. In the event of fires or suspected gas delivery errors, there are master shutoff valves for oxygen, air, and nitrous oxide outside each operating room (Figure 4.7).

References

1. Cairo J. M. *Pilbeam's Mechanical Ventilation*, 5th edn. St. Louis, MO: Mosby, 2012.
2. Boldrini R., Fasano L., Nava S. Noninvasive mechanical ventilation. *Curr Opin Crit Care* 2012;18:48–53.
3. Hess D. R., Kacmarek R. M. Ventilator Mode Classification. *Essentials of Mechanical Ventilation*, 3rd edn. (Moyer A., Thomas C., eds.). New York, NY: McGraw-Hill Education, 2014.
4. Miller R. D., Cohen N. H., Eriksson L. I., et al.. *Miller's Anesthesia*. London: Churchill Livingstone, 2015.
5. Goligher E. C., Ferguson N. D., Brochard L. J. Clinical challenges
in mechanical ventilation. *Lancet* 2016;387:1856–66.
6. Marini J. J. Mechanical ventilation: past lessons and the near future. *Crit Care* 2013;17:S1.
7. Daoud E. G. Airway pressure release ventilation. *Ann Thorac Med* 2007;2:176–9.
8. Dorsch J., Dorsch S. *A Practical Approach to Anesthesia Equipment*. Philadelphia, PA: Wolters Kluwer/Lippincott Williams & Wilkins Health, 2011.
9. General Requirements, Tests and Guidelines for Alarm Systems in Medical Electrical Equipment and in Medical Electrical Systems (ISO-IEC
60601-1-8). Geneva, Switzerland: International Standards Organization, 2003.
10. Ehrenworth J., Eisenkraft J., Berry J. *Anesthesia Equipment: Principles and Applications*. Philadelphia, PA: Saunders, 2013.
11. Administration OS and H. Anesthetic Gases: Guidelines for Workplace Exposures. *OSHA Dir Tech Support Emerg Manag*. Available at: www.osha.gov/dts/osta/anestheticgases/ (accessed January 2017).

Defibrillators

Matthew A. Levin

Definition and Types

A defibrillator is a device designed to treat ventricular arrhythmias by delivery of an electrical shock that terminates the arrhythmia and restores a normal cardiac rhythm. Defibrillators can be either externally or internally implanted.

External

External devices consist of electrocardiogram (ECG) leads to sense the rhythm, a battery and capacitor to generate the charge, and paddles/adhesive pads to deliver therapy. There may or may not be a monitor. The paddles/pads can also be used for sensing.[1]

- Manual external defibrillator (Figure 5.1)
  It displays an ECG on a monitor, which the user is required to interpret. The user is also required to choose the amount of energy used and the timing of when to deliver the shock.
- Automated external defibrillator (AED) (Figure 5.2)
  It detects and analyzes the heart's rhythm automatically. If a shockable rhythm is found, the user is prompted to press a button to deliver a shock. There is usually no monitor. Some AEDs are fully automated and will deliver a shock without requiring user intervention. AEDs are now commonly found in airports and other public spaces and are designed to be used by lay persons.

- Wearable defibrillator (Figure 5.3)
  A defibrillator worn by the patient that looks like a vest. Continuously monitors the heart's rhythm, and if a shock is needed, sounds an alarm. If the patient fails to respond, a shock is automatically delivered. Commonly used as a bridge to permanent therapy, or to recovery of heart function.[2,3]

Internal/implantable (Figure 5.4)

An implantable cardioverter defibrillator (ICD) is a type of cardiovascular implantable electronic device (CIED). An ICD consists of *generator* (sometimes called a *can* because of the metal enclosure) containing a battery, capacitor, central processing unit (CPU), and one or more *leads* (wires) that are used to sense arrhythmias. The leads are also used to deliver therapy in the form of an electrical shock that terminates the arrhythmia and restores a normal rhythm. All modern ICDs are also pacemakers. Lead placement can vary as follows:

- Transvenous
  The leads are placed transvenously directly into the right heart. There are usually two leads, one in the right atrium for pacing and the other in the right ventricle for defibrillation. The ventricular lead has two defibrillation coils (Figure 5.1) that are used to deliver a shock.

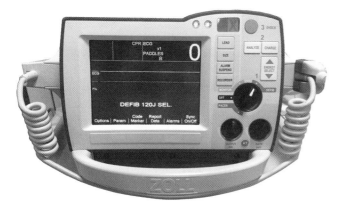

Figure 5.1 An external defibrillator. Note the default energy level of 120 J. Note also the "sync on/off" button. Sync on will deliver a shock timed to the R wave and is used for cardioversion.
Note: The figure was taken and edited by the author himself.

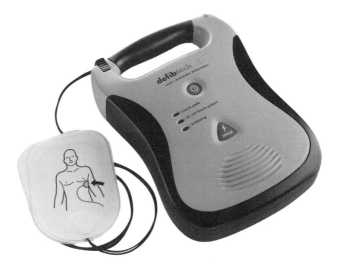

Figure 5.2 An automated external defibrillator. Note the simple interface and lack of a monitor.
Note: The figure was obtained from http://sportcentrumtopfit.nl/wp-content/uploads/2015/03/a940.jpg

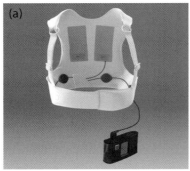
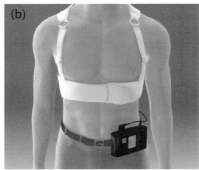

Figure 5.3 LifeVest® model 4000. (a) The vest with connected monitor and defibrillator. Visible are the two back defibrillation electrodes and three (of four) nonadhesive ECG recording electrodes mounted on the elastic belt. (b) The LifeVest on a patient.
Used with permission from Klein et al.[2]

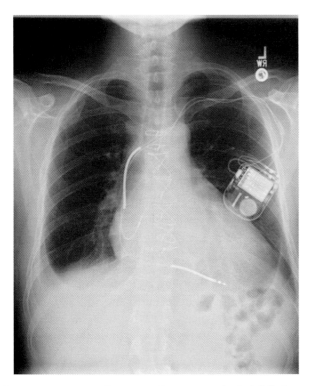

Figure 5.4 Chest X-ray of a patient with an ICD. Note the thick defibrillation coils, one in the superior vena cava and the other in the right ventricle. Also note the thinner pacing lead in the right atrium.
Used with permission from Stone et al.[19]

The generator is located subcutaneously, usually on the left upper chest wall.
- Biventricular leads for cardiac resynchronization therapy (CRT)
  A third lead is placed in the coronary sinus to enable biventricular pacing.
- Epicardial
  The leads are placed directly on the surface of the heart. Generator location is usually the same as above.
- Subcutaneous
  o There is a single lead with two sensing electrodes and a coil tunneled underneath the skin, usually along the right parasternal border. There is no direct vascular access. The generator is located subcutaneously, usually on the left mid-axillary line.
  o Benefits are reduced risk of endocarditis, lead fracture or lead malfunction requiring lead extraction.

Manufacturers and Identification

- External
  There are many manufacturers. Zoll is a commonly seen brand.
- Internal/subcutaneous
  The three major current manufacturers of ICDs are Boston Scientific, Medtronic, and St. Jude Medical. Devices can often be identified by their silhouette on chest X-ray (Figure 5.4).[4]
  An ICD can be distinguished from a pacemaker by the thicker coils on the ventricular lead.

Indications

Indications for External Defibrillation

- Pulseless ventricular tachycardia (VT)
- Ventricular fibrillation (VF)
- Cardiac arrest (excluding asystole or pulseless electrical activity)

Indications for ICD Placement

Indications can be divided into primary and secondary prevention.[5–7]
- Secondary prevention
  For patients who are survivors of cardiac arrest attributable to ventricular fibrillation or unstable ventricular tachycardia.
- Primary prevention
  For patients who are at risk for but have not yet had an episode of sustained VT, VF, or resuscitated cardiac arrest.
- Class I indications include:
  o Left ventricular ejection fraction (LVEF) ≤ 35 percent due to prior MI, ≥40 days post-MI and NYHA Class II or III (symptomatic)

- LVEF ≤ 30 percent due to prior MI, >40 days post-MI (asymptomatic)
- LVEF ≤ 40 percent due to prior MI, with inducible VT/VF on electrophysiologic (EP) study
- LVEF ≤ 35 percent and NYHA Class II or III
- Structural heart disease causing sustained VT
- Syncope of undetermined origin with inducible VT/VF on EP study

Modes/Therapies

Electrode Size and Position

Electrodes can be either self-adhesive pads or handheld paddles.

- Size
  Recommended pad size is 8–12 cm.[8] A larger size is associated with higher success rate because the pad impedance is lower and more current is delivered. Adult size pads can be used on pediatric patients (less than 8 years old or <25 kg) but may misinterpret the rhythm, deliver too much current, or the current delivered may bypass the heart because the pad is larger than the heart.[9] Pediatric size pads and AEDs have been developed. Typical size of a pediatric pad is 4–5 cm.[10,11]
- Position
  Pads should be placed so that the path of electrical current from one pad to the other passes through the heart. There are two accepted positions[8]:
- Antero-apical
  - One pad is placed on the right upper chest wall just to the right of the sternum and just below the clavicle over the 2nd or 3rd intercostal space.
  - The other pad is placed laterally on the left anterior or mid-axillary line at the 5th or 6th interspace, over the cardiac apex.
- Antero-posterior
  - One pad is placed on the back in the left or right infrascapular region.
  - The other pad is placed over the cardiac apex as above, or on the left mid-clavicular line over the precordium.
  - Antero-posterior placement is preferable in patients with an ICD/CIED, to avoid damaging the device.[12,13]

Defibrillation versus Cardioversion

- Cardioversion
  Used when there is an intrinsic cardiac rhythm sensed. Delivery of the shock is timed (synchronized) to coincide with the sensed R wave.
  Use of an unsynchronized shock when there is an intrinsic rhythm can result in an "R on T" phenomenon and trigger Torsades des Pointes (polymorphic VF)
- Defibrillation
  Used when no intrinsic cardiac rhythm is sensed (wide complex VT, VF). Delivery of the shock is unsynchronized and may fall on any part of the cardiac cycle.

Energy and Waveforms for External Defibrillators

The electrical waveform used can be *monophasic* or *biphasic*. The amount of energy delivered depends on the mode.

- Monophasic
  Current flows in only one direction. Only much older devices use a monophasic waveform.
- Biphasic
  Current flows in both directions. Current delivery is more consistent. *All modern devices use a biphasic waveform.*
- Energy requirements
  Depend on the mode and the presence or absence of a pulse. The 2015 ACLS guidelines published by the AHA provides the following recommendations.[14]
- VT with pulse
  - Monophasic – 200 J
  - Biphasic – 100 J
- VT no pulse (pulseless)
  - Monophasic – 360 J
  - Biphasic – 120–200 J
- Atrial fibrillation
  - Monophasic – 200 J
  - Biphasic – 120–200 J
- Atrial flutter
  - Monophasic – 100 J
  - Biphasic – 50–100 J
- Energy levels for an ICD
  The amount of energy delivered by an ICD is much lower, typically less than 30 J.

Perioperative Management

Major Risks

Perioperative management of the patient with a CIED can be challenging.[15,16] The major risk during the perioperative period is that electromagnetic interference (EMI) will disrupt normal device operation. The most common source of EMI in the operating room is *monopolar electrocautery.* Use of monopolar electrocautery below the umbilicus is unlikely to cause interference. Bipolar electrocautery will not cause EMI unless it is applied directly to the device.[17] Some possible effects of EMI are:

- Inhibition of pacemaker function due to oversensing
- Pacemaker-mediated tachycardia[15]
- Delivery of inappropriate therapy (i.e. shock)
- Direct damage to the ICD/CIED

Radio-frequency (RF) energy such as used in surgical sponge counting systems is another source of EMI that may cause CIED malfunction.[18]

- Management strategy (Figure 5.5)
  The Heart Rhythm Society/American Society of Anesthesiologists provides an expert consensus statement on the perioperative management of ICD/CIEDs.

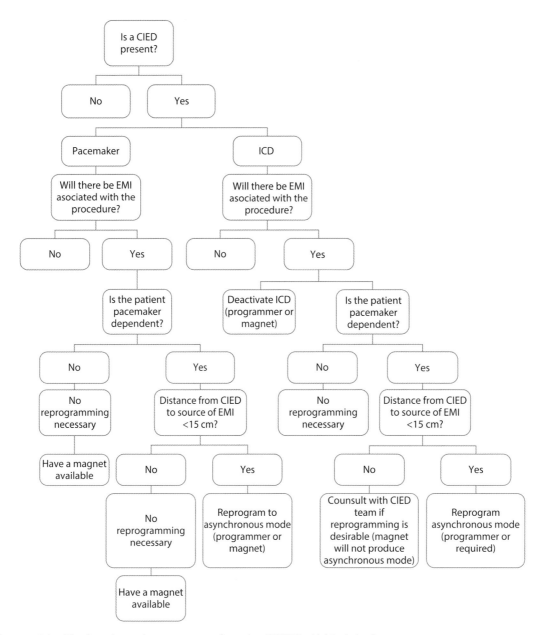

Figure 5.5 Suggested algorithm for perioperative management of a modern ICD/CIED with bipolar lead
Used with permission from Stone et al.[19]

This statement was last updated in 2010.[17] The primary recommendation is to consult with the patient's CIED care team preoperatively to obtain a prescription for the most appropriate management for the specific device and procedure. However, there is a simple algorithm that can be used to guide intraoperative management[19]:

(a) Determine if there will be a source of EMI during the procedure
    If yes, deactivate the CIED by disabling anti-tachycardia therapy using a magnet or programmer.
(b) Determine if the patient is pacemaker-dependent
    If yes, determine if the source of EMI will be ≤15 cm from CIED. The distance should be measured to the closest part of the CIED, including the leads.

If EMI is within 15 cm, reprogram the CIED to an asynchronous pacing mode (requires programmer).

Magnet application

Application of a magnet directly over the CIED/ICD will temporarily suspend VT/VF detection/therapy and prevent inadvertent shock delivery. Detection/therapy will resume when the magnet is removed. It is very important to note that a magnet will *not* affect the pacemaker function of an ICD, i.e. it will *not* place an ICD in an asynchronous pacing mode.

Pros

Easy to use. Can be used sterile in the operative field.

Cons

Some devices may not respond as expected because they can be programmed to ignore the magnet.[17] Also a magnet cannot be used to change the pacemaker mode of an ICD.

Reprogramming

The device can be reprogrammed using a programmer. Programmers are manufacturer-specific.

Pros

The device can be reprogrammed to any mode. An ICD can be placed in an asynchronous pacing mode using a programmer. The device can also be interrogated and a detailed report on the device mode, function and therapy history can be printed for reference.

Cons

Requires a programmer and specialized knowledge/expertise, neither of which may be readily available in the perioperative setting.

Nonoperating Room Locations

The guidelines for management of an ICD in a nonoperating room anesthetizing location are generally the same.

Colonoscopy/Endoscopy

There is no evidence that either procedure interferes with ICD operation. If electrocautery is used, the standard guidelines should be followed.

MRI

The long-standing recommendation is that MRI be avoided in patients with an ICD/CIED, because of concerns for magnetically induced heating of the leads that could result in myocardial injury and/or changes in the lead properties.[20]

Certain devices have been tested to be MRI safe and are labeled "MRI-conditional."

A recent prospective, registry-based study of noncertified devices ("non-MRI conditional") found no device or lead failures among 500 patients who had non-thoracic MRI and had their device reprogrammed appropriately prior to and after the MRI.[20]

References

1. External Defibrillators – What is an External Defibrillator? Center for Devices and Radiological Health. Available from: www.fda.gov/MedicalDevices/ProductsandMedicalProcedures/CardiovascularDevices/ExternalDefibrillators/ucm232088.htm (accessed June 2017)

2. Klein H. U., Goldenberg I., Moss A. J. Risk stratification for implantable cardioverter defibrillator therapy: the role of the wearable cardioverter-defibrillator. *Eur Heart J.* 2013 Aug;34(29):2230–42.

3. Kutyifa V., Moss A. J., Klein H., et al. Use of the wearable cardioverter defibrillator in high-risk cardiac patients. Clinical perspective. *Circulation.* 2015 Oct 27;132(17):1613–9.

4. Jacob S., Shahzad M. A., Maheshwari R., Panaich S. S., Aravindhakshan R. Cardiac rhythm device identification algorithm using X-rays: CaRDIA-X. *Heart Rhythm.* 2011 Jun;8(6):915–22.

5. Epstein A. E., Dimarco J. P., Ellenbogen K. A., et al. ACC/AHA/HRS 2008 Guidelines for device-based therapy of cardiac rhythm abnormalities. *Heart Rhythm.* 2008;5:e1–62.

6. Epstein A. E., DiMarco J. P., Ellenbogen K. A., et al. 2012 ACCF/AHA/HRS focused update incorporated into the ACCF/AHA/HRS 2008 guidelines for device-based therapy of cardiac rhythm abnormalities: a report of the American College of Cardiology Foundation/American Heart Association Task Force on Practice Guidelines and the Heart Rhythm Society. *J Am Coll Cardiol.* 2013;61:e6–75.

7. Russo A. M., Stainback R. F., Bailey S. R., et al. ACCF/HRS/AHA/ASE/HFSA/SCAI/SCCT/SCMR 2013 appropriate use criteria for implantable cardioverter-defibrillators and cardiac resynchronization therapy: a report of the American College of Cardiology Foundation appropriate use criteria task force, Heart Rhythm Society, American Heart Association, American Society of Echocardiography, Heart Failure Society of America, Society for Cardiovascular Angiography and Interventions, Society of Cardiovascular Computed Tomography, and Society for Cardiovascular Magnetic Resonance. *Heart Rhythm.* 2013 Apr;10(4):e11–58.

8. Link M. S., Atkins D. L., Passman R. S., et al. Part 6: Electrical Therapies: Automated External Defibrillators, Defibrillation, Cardioversion, and Pacing: 2010 American Heart Association Guidelines for Cardiopulmonary Resuscitation and Emergency Cardiovascular Care. *Circulation.* 2010 Oct 17;122 (18 Suppl 3):S706–19.

9. Samson R. A., Berg R. A., Bingham R., et al. Use of automated external defibrillators for children: an update: an advisory statement from the pediatric advanced life support task force, International Liaison Committee on Resuscitation. *Circulation.* 2003;107:3250–5.

10. Atkins D. L., Jorgenson D. B. Attenuated pediatric electrode pads for automated external defibrillator use in children. *Resuscitation.* 2005 Jul;66(1):31–7.

11. Atkins D. L., Scott W. A., Blaufox A. D., et al. Sensitivity and specificity of an automated external defibrillator algorithm designed for pediatric patients. *Resuscitation.* 2008 Feb;76(2):168–74.

12. Botto G. L., Politi A., Bonini W., Broffoni T., Bonatti R. External cardioversion of atrial fibrillation: role of paddle position on technical efficacy and energy requirements. *Heart.* 1999 Dec;82(6):726–30.

13. Ambler J. J., Sado D. M., Zideman D. A., Deakin C. D. The incidence and severity of cutaneous burns following external DC cardioversion. *Resuscitation.* 2004 Jun;61(3):281–8.

14. Link M. S., Berkow L. C., Kudenchuk P. J., et al. Part 7: Adult Advanced Cardiovascular Life Support. American Heart Association, Inc. *Circulation.* 2015 Nov 3;132(18 suppl 2):S444–64.

15. Izrailtyan I., Schiller R. J., Katz R. I., Almasry I. O. Perioperative pacemaker-mediated tachycardia in the patient with a dual chamber implantable cardioverter-defibrillator. *Anesth Analg.* 2013 Feb;116(2):307–10.

16. Thompson A., Mahajan A. Perioperative management of cardiovascular implantable electronic devices. *Anesth Analg.* 2013 Feb;116(2):276–7.

17. Crossley G. H., Poole J. E., Rozner M. A., et al. The Heart Rhythm Society (HRS)/American Society of Anesthesiologists (ASA) expert consensus statement on the perioperative management of patients with implantable defibrillators, pacemakers and arrhythmia monitors: facilities and patient management. *Heart Rhythm.* 2011 Jul;8(7):1114–54.

18. Williams M. R., Atkinson D. B., Bezzerides V. J., et al. Pausing with the gauze: inhibition of temporary pacemakers by radiofrequency scan during cardiac surgery. *Anesth Analg.* 2016 Nov;123(5):1143–8.

19. Stone M. E., Salter B., Fischer A. Perioperative management of patients with cardiac implantable electronic devices. *Br J Anaesth.* 2011 Dec;107(Suppl 1):i16–26.

20. Russo R. J., Costa H. S., Silva P. D., et al. Assessing the risks associated with MRI in patients with a pacemaker or defibrillator. *N Engl J Med.* 2017 Feb 23;376(8):755–64.

Electrical, Fire, and Explosion Hazards

Thomas Palaia and Andrew Schwartz

Electrical Considerations

Static Electricity
- Electricity or discharge generated by the movement of electrons across an interface
- Occurs when two distinctly charged items are brought into contact
- Leads to organization of oppositely charged particles on adjacent surfaces
- Magnitude of charge is dependent on material type, contact surface area, and temperature
- Separation of oppositely charged particles leads to a potential difference
- If field strength exceeds a critical level, than there is atmospheric ionization
- Discharge to a less charged object can create a spark which is responsible for most OR (operating room) fires/explosions

Static Electricity as an Ignition Source
- Requires the presence of four elements:
  - Accumulation of static electricity
  - The accumulated static must be insulated from any grounding body
  - The discharged spark must be of adequate ignition energy
  - The spark must occur in an atmosphere containing a fuel source within range[1]

Bonding
- Connection of one conductor to another
- Prevents the accumulation of static charge
- Allows the equalization of charge over the entire conducting system
- Allows an exit of the accumulated charge, eliminating it as an ignition source

Grounding
- Specific type of bonding
- Links conductive material to the ground
- The ground has an unlimited ability to accept electrons
- Any conductive system connected to the ground is devoid of charge
- Prevents the passing of charge within the system to a transient conductor[1]

- Transient conductors include patients and other operating room personnel
- Faulty equipment may provide errant currents to patients

Line Isolation Monitor (LIM)
- OR safety device that will alarm if a faulty ground connection occurs
- Typically alarms with current generation of >2 mA that may be conducted to a patient[1]

Isolation Transformers
- All electrical power sources in the OR are isolated from the ground
- Prevents passage of dangerous current through the patient[1]

Macro and Micro Current Hazards

Macro Shock
- Externally applied current across the surface with high resistance and large spatial distribution (i.e. skin)
- Leads to the disturbance of neural or muscular function
- Current is spread throughout the body/less concentrated impulse
- Requires high energy to be harmful (10–100 mA)
- Degree of injury is affected by resistance of the skin
- Wet/broken skin has 1% the resistance of dry intact skin
- 5–10 mA: sustained muscle contraction and inability to "let go"
- 50–100 mA: mechanical injury
- 100–500 mA: ventricular fibrillation
- >6,000 mA: sustained myocardial contraction and respiratory paralysis[1]

Micro Shock
- Directly applied current concentrated at one point (small spatial distribution)
- Typically applied to the heart
- Acceptable safety limit of 10 μA
- Maximum level of current allowable through catheters or electrodes in contact with heart. Generally caused by leakage current in line-operated equipment
- Since LIM warning occurs at 2 mA, it will not protect against micro shock

Operating Room Fire Considerations

Background

- Unknown incidence (no centralized reporting), but estimated at 500–700 OR fires/year[2]
- ASA Closed Claim Database reports 103 claims for OR fires since 1985
- Eighty-five percent of OR fires occur during the delivery of MAC anesthesia for head, neck, and upper chest surgery
- Fifteen percent of claims were for airway fire mainly occurring during tracheostomy and tonsillectomy
- Electrocautery was the ignition source in 90% of claims

The Fire Triad

- Fire requires a fuel source, an oxidizing agent, and an ignition source
- Fire can be prevented or extinguished by the removal of any of these three critical components[3]

Fuel

- Substance that produces heat from chemical combustion
- Surgical preparation solution (particularly alcohol-based)
- PVC endotracheal tubes; also laryngeal mask airways (LMA) and O_2 masks
- Hair, tissue, patient gowns, linens
- Surgical drapes, sponges/gauze (when dry), packing materials, dressings

Oxidizer

- Oxygen enrichment is the most significant factor contributing to surgical fires
- Facilitates the chemical reaction of combustion
- Nitrous oxide functions equally as well as oxygen at facilitating combustion
- Many items that will not burn in air will readily ignite in the presence of enriched O_2

Ignitions Source

- Current, heat, friction
- Electrocautery is the ignition source in >90% of claims for OR fires[4]
- Other sources: lasers, drills, argon beam, light cables, defibrillator paddles

Risk Factors for Intraoperative Fire

- Procedures involving an ignition source in close proximity to oxidizer-rich environment
- Head and neck procedures
- Ophthalmic procedures
- MAC with supplemental O_2 that involves surgical draping leading to oxygen pooling

OR Fire Prevention

Communication and Education

- Communication between surgeon, anesthesiologist, and OR staff is critical
- Recognition of high-risk procedures
- Preemptive discussion of strategy to mitigate risk for OR fires should be held prior to each case
- ASA practice advisory: Fire safety education is necessary for all OR personnel[5]

Prep Solution

- Alcohol-based prep solution burns easily in room air
- Allow sufficient time for prep solution to completely dry
- Chloraprep is 70% alcohol and is highly flammable
- Chloraprep: 3 minutes to dry on skin and up to 1 hour on hair
- Betadine solution is generally preferred for high-risk procedures
- The large 30 mL chloraprep is contraindicated for head and neck surgery (high fire risk) because of pooling of the solution

MAC for High-Risk Procedures (Head/Neck/Upper Chest)

- Recommend avoidance of open delivery of oxygen (i.e. nasal cannula)
- Always ask, "Is supplemental oxygen really necessary?"
- If supplemental O_2 is required, then use laryngeal mask airway or endotracheal tube
- Securing the airway prevents accumulation of oxygen in surgical field

Special Cases (Supplemental O_2 Required via Open Delivery)

- Surgery that requires the patient be able to communicate
- Carotid artery surgery, neurosurgery, some pacemaker implantations
- Minor surgery when risk of securing airway is more than the risk of open delivery
- Use blended O_2 supply in order to keep supplemental O_2 to a minimum
- Use minimum necessary FiO_2 to maintain acceptable oxyhemoglobin concentration
- Consider the delivery of 5–10 L/min of air under drapes for washout effect
- Alternate surgical tool: scalpel, bipolar, harmonic scalpel
- Open draping techniques

OR Fire Management

- Immediately remove any source of oxygen
- Remove all burning drapes from the patient
- Douse fire and patient with saline
- Use a fire extinguisher to eliminate any remaining fire on drapes once removed

Airway Fire Safety

High-Risk Procedures

- Tonsillectomy
- Tracheostomy
- Laser laryngeal surgery

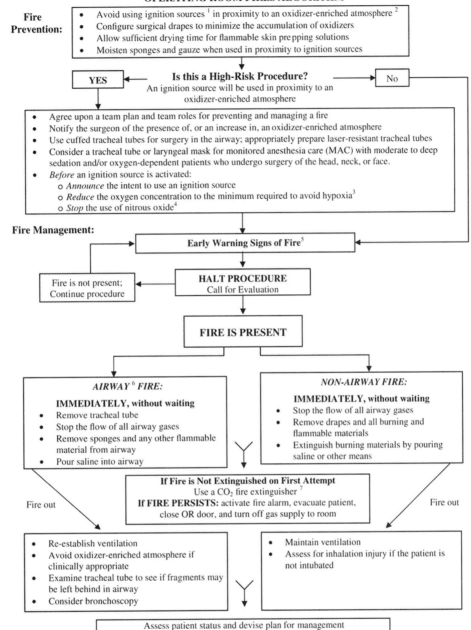

American Society of
Anesthesiologists®

OPERATING ROOM FIRES ALGORITHM

Fire Prevention:
- Avoid using ignition sources [1] in proximity to an oxidizer-enriched atmosphere [2]
- Configure surgical drapes to minimize the accumulation of oxidizers
- Allow sufficient drying time for flammable skin prepping solutions
- Moisten sponges and gauze when used in proximity to ignition sources

Is this a High-Risk Procedure?
An ignition source will be used in proximity to an oxidizer-enriched atmosphere

YES / No

- Agree upon a team plan and team roles for preventing and managing a fire
- Notify the surgeon of the presence of, or an increase in, an oxidizer-enriched atmosphere
- Use cuffed tracheal tubes for surgery in the airway; appropriately prepare laser-resistant tracheal tubes
- Consider a tracheal tube or laryngeal mask for monitored anesthesia care (MAC) with moderate to deep sedation and/or oxygen-dependent patients who undergo surgery of the head, neck, or face.
- *Before* an ignition source is activated:
  - *Announce* the intent to use an ignition source
  - *Reduce* the oxygen concentration to the minimum required to avoid hypoxia [3]
  - *Stop* the use of nitrous oxide [4]

Fire Management:

Early Warning Signs of Fire [5]

HALT PROCEDURE
Call for Evaluation

Fire is not present; Continue procedure

FIRE IS PRESENT

AIRWAY [6] *FIRE:*

IMMEDIATELY, without waiting
- Remove tracheal tube
- Stop the flow of all airway gases
- Remove sponges and any other flammable material from airway
- Pour saline into airway

NON-AIRWAY FIRE:

IMMEDIATELY, without waiting
- Stop the flow of all airway gases
- Remove drapes and all burning and flammable materials
- Extinguish burning materials by pouring saline or other means

If Fire is Not Extinguished on First Attempt
Use a CO_2 fire extinguisher [7]
If FIRE PERSISTS: activate fire alarm, evacuate patient, close OR door, and turn off gas supply to room

Fire out

- Re-establish ventilation
- Avoid oxidizer-enriched atmosphere if clinically appropriate
- Examine tracheal tube to see if fragments may be left behind in airway
- Consider bronchoscopy

- Maintain ventilation
- Assess for inhalation injury if the patient is not intubated

Assess patient status and devise plan for management

---

[1] Ignition sources include but are not limited to electrosurgery or electrocautery units and lasers.

[2] An oxidizer-enriched atmosphere occurs when there is any increase in oxygen concentration above room air level, and/or the presence of any concentration of nitrous oxide.

[3] After minimizing delivered oxygen, wait a period of time (e.g., 1–3 min) before using an ignition source. For oxygen-dependent patients, *reduce* supplemental oxygen delivery to the minimum required to avoid hypoxia. Monitor oxygenation with pulse oximetry, and if feasible, inspired, exhaled, and/or delivered oxygen concentration.

[4] After stopping the delivery of nitrous oxide, wait a period of time (e.g., 1–3 min) before using an ignition source.

[5] Unexpected flash, flame, smoke or heat, unusual sounds (e.g., a "pop," snap, or "foomp") or odors, unexpected movement of drapes, discoloration of drapes or breathing circuit, unexpected patient movement or complaint.

[6] In this algorithm, airway fire refers to a fire in the airway or breathing circuit.

[7] A CO_2 fire extinguisher may be used on the patient if necessary.

Figure 6.1 Operating room fires algorithm
Courtesy of Practice Advisory for the Prevention and Management of Operating Room Fires[5]

Prevention

- Reduction of oxidizer-rich environment as possible
- Eliminate ignition sources as possible (use scalpel or cold ablation)
- Manage fuel sources
- Use cuffed endotracheal tubes

Reduction of FiO_2

- Reduce FiO_2 <30% during high-risk cases[5]
- Recognize the significance of expired gas concentration
- After preoxygenation, will take several minutes of air flow to reduce ETO_2 < 30%[6]
- Questionable evidence on efficacy of suction to reduce oxidizer concentration[5]

Laser Procedure Safety

- Utilize laser-resistant endotracheal tubes
- Utilize a double cuff system in order to prevent O_2 leak in case of single cuff rupture
- Fill ETT cuffs with saline or methylene blue: extinguishes and alerts surgeon
- Open communication: no use of laser until exhaled O_2 < 30%
- Laser airway surgery risk has been lowered considerably secondary to awareness, vigilance, and communication by OR personnel

Airway Fire Management

- Eliminate oxygen source by disconnecting circuit and turning off oxygen flow

- Removal of ETT while attached to oxygen source may result in further fire/injury
- ETT should be removed following disconnection
- Remove ignition source (electrocautery)
- Flood field and oropharynx with saline and suction debris/chemical irritants
- Resecure airway as rapidly as possible
- Endotracheal intubation may prove difficult given the thermal injury; follow ASA difficult airway algorithm
- Consider emergent tracheostomy early on when intubation proves difficult[7]
- Goal is to extinguish fire, maintain oxygenation/ventilation, and manage hemodynamics (Figure 6.1)

Smoke Inhalation Injury Management

- High morbidity and mortality
- Airway edema, mucosal necrosis, inflammation[8]
- Investigate degree of injury with laryngoscopy, bronchoscopy, and endoscopy
- Lavage and debris removal may be warranted
- Inhaled bronchodilation to relieve bronchospasm
- Humidified air may relieve excessive airway drying from thermal injury
- Prophylactic antibiotics and steroids have not been shown to improve outcomes[9]

References

1. R. D. Miller. *Miller's Anesthesia*, 8th edn. Philadelphia, PA: Churchill Livingstone/Elsevier, 2015.
2. P. G. Barash, B. F. Cullen, R. K. Stoelting. Intravenous anesthetics. *Clinical Anesthesia*, 6th edn. Philadelphia, PA: Lippincott Williams & Wilkins, 2009, pp. 185–90.
3. A. M. Barnes, R. A. Frantz. Do oxygen-enriched atmospheres exist beneath surgical drapes and contribute to fire hazard potential in the operating room? *AANA J* 2000;68:153–161.
4. S. P. Mehta, S. M. Bhananker, K. L. Posner, K. B. Domino. Operating room fires: A closed claims analysis. *Anesthesiology* 2013;118:1133–9.
5. J. L. Apfelbaum, R. A. Caplan, S. J. Barker, et al. Practice advisory for the prevention and management of operating room fires: An updated report by the American Society for Anesthesiologists Task Force on Operating Room Fires. *Anesthesiology* 2013;118:271–90.
6. J. H. Eichhorn, J. B. Eisenkraft. Expired oxygen as the unappreciated issue in preventing airway fires: Getting to "never." *Anesth Analg* 2013;117:1042–4.
7. S. Demaria, A. D. Schwartz, V. Narine, S. Yang, A. I. Levine. Management of intraoperative airway fire. *Simul Healthcare* 2011;6:360–3.
8. M. L. Rogers, R. W. Nickalls, E. T. Brackenbury, et al. Airway fire during tracheostomy: Prevention strategies for surgeons and anaesthetists. *Ann R Coll Surg Engl* 2001;83:376–80.
9. S. I. Cha, C. H. Kim, J. H. Lee, et al. Isolated smoke inhalation injuries: Acute respiratory dysfunction, clinical outcomes, and short-term evolution of pulmonary functions with the effects of steroids. *Burns* 2007;33:200–8.

Basic Mathematics and Statistics

Hung-Mo Lin, Hae-Young Kim, and John Michael Williamson

Logarithm

Logarithm is the inverse operation to exponentiation. It is the power to which the base must be raised to produce a given number. For example, as $81 = 3^4$, then $\log_3(81) = 4$. The *logarithm* to base 10 is called the common *logarithm* and the logarithm to base e (≈ 2.72) is called the natural logarithm (ln).

Graph of Simple Equation

The simplest equation for a biological model is of the linear form $y = a + bx$, where the y and x can be described by a linear relationship with slope b and intercept a. The slope represents the amount of change in y for every unit increase in x and is typically the primary interest of analysis (Figure 7.1).

Analysis of Biological Curves

Biological curves are often nonlinear. In medical research, four types of biological curves are often encountered.

Analysis of dose–response curve: A method used to depict the relationship between the dose of a drug administered and its pharmacological response. *ED50* is the abbreviation for the median effective dose, which is the dose required to produce efficacy in half of the population (Figure 7.2).

Analysis of pharmacokinetic modeling: A mathematical modeling technique for predicting the absorption, distribution, metabolism, and excretion of synthetic or natural chemical substances in humans and other animal species.

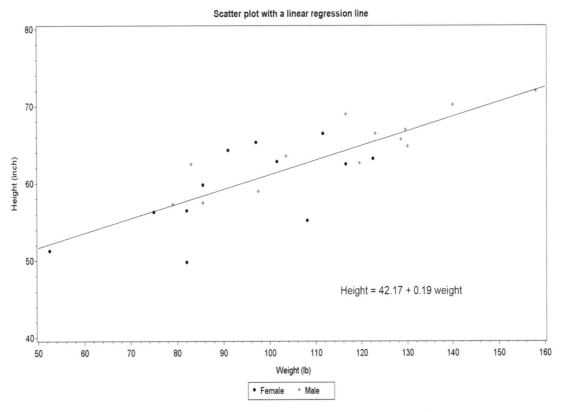

Figure 7.1 Example of a linear equation used to model the relationship between height (in.) and weight (lb) in children aged 11–17

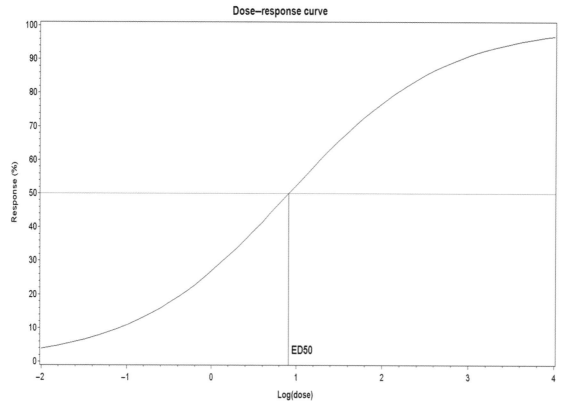

Figure 7.2 Example of a dose–response curve. The y-axis is the percent of response and the x-axis is the amount of dose in logarithmic scale. ED50 is the medium effective dose.

Analysis of growth curves: The modern use of the term *growth curve model* typically refers to statistical methods that allow for the estimation of interindividual variability in intraindividual patterns of change over time.[1] Often the within-person patterns of change are referred to as *growth curves*, or *trajectories*.

Analysis of survival curves: A survival curve is a plot of probability that an individual survives longer than time *t*, or has not experienced the event of interest. In survival analysis, not all individuals continue in the study until the event of interest occurs (they are called *censored*). The Kaplan–Meier survival curve is the most familiar method in medical discipline for depicting the survival probability when some individuals are subject to censored (Figure 7.3).[2]

Sample and Population

Population: A complete set of elements (persons or objects) that possess some common characteristics defined by the sampling criteria established by the researcher.

Sample: The selected elements (people or objects) chosen for participation in a study and are referred to as subjects or participants.

Probability

The proportion of times an event is expected to occur in the long run. Probabilities are numbers between 0 and 1 with 0

corresponding to "never" and 1 corresponding to "always." With probabilistic events, individual occurrences are uncertain, but occurrences over the long term are predictable.[3]

Mean, Median, and Mode

Mean: The arithmetic average. This is the most common measure of central location.[3] To calculate the mean, add up all the values in the data set and divide by the number of observations: $\bar{x} = \frac{1}{n}\sum_{i=1}^{n} x_i$

○ *n* represents the sample size.
○ x_i denotes the value of the *i*th observation in the data set.

Median: The middle value of a distribution and the central value in the order array of the data. To find the median, arrange all the numbers from smallest to greatest.[3]

○ If there are odd number of observations, the middle one is picked. For example, consider the set of numbers: 1, 2, 3, 6, 8, 9, and 10. The median is the fourth number, which is 6.
○ If there are even number of observations, then the median is usually defined to be the mean of the two middle values. For example, in the data set: 1, 2, 3, 4, 5, 6, 8, and 9. The median is the mean of the middle two numbers: that is $(4 + 5) \div 2$, which is 4.5.

Mode: It is the most frequently occurring value in the data set. For example, the following data set has a mode of 7: 4, 7, 7, 7, 8, 8, 9.[3]

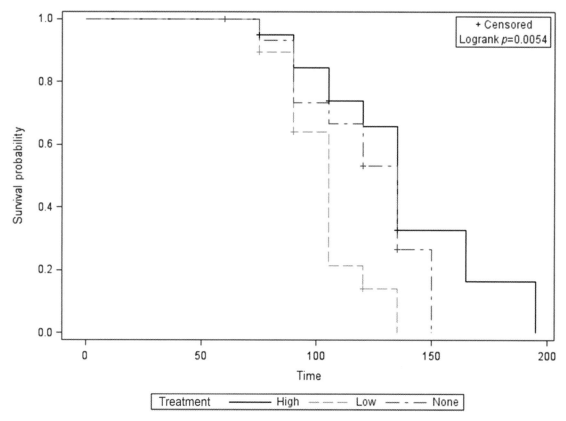

Figure 7.3 Example for a Kaplan–Meier survival curve for three treatment arms with none, low, and high dose. Censoring is indicated by the + symbol.

Standard Deviation and Error

Standard deviation (SD): It is the most common measure of spread. This statistic is based on the average squared distance of values around the data sets mean. It is calculated as follows[3]:

- Determine the deviation of each data point. A deviation is the data point minus its mean: $x_i - \bar{x}$
- Sum the squared deviations. This is the sum of squares (SS): $SS = (x_1 - \bar{x})^2 + (x_2 - \bar{x})^2 + \dots + (x_n - \bar{x})^2$
- Divide the sum of squares by $n - 1$. This is the variance:

$$S^2 = \frac{SS}{n-1}$$

- Take the square root of the variance. This is the standard deviation:

$$S = \sqrt{S^2} = \frac{SS}{n-1}$$

- The percentage of data in one standard deviation above and below the mean is 68% in a bell curve. It is 95% for two standard deviations above and below, and 99% for three standard deviations above and below (Figure 7.4).

Standard error (SE): The standard deviation of the sampling distribution of the sample mean, $\bar{x}$, is often referred to as the standard error of the mean (SEM). SEM is the standard deviation of the sample mean's estimate of a population mean. SEM is usually estimated by the sample estimate of the population standard deviation (sample standard deviation) divided by the square root of the sample size (assuming statistical independence of the values in the sample)[3]:

$$SE_{\bar{x}} = \frac{s}{\sqrt{n}}$$

- s is the sample standard deviation.
- n is the size (number of observations) of the sample.

Types of Data

- Categorical: Values that can be divided into groups or categories.
- Nominal: Values that can be sorted but cannot be placed in an order (i.e. gender, eye color)
- Ordinal: Values that can be counted and placed in order (i.e. residency training year, house number)
- Binary: Data that take only two possible values (i.e. yes or no)
- Numerical: Values that can be measured and placed in order
- Discrete: Values that are a finite whole number (i.e. number of calls a month)
- Continuous: Values that are a number on a spectrum or continuum (i.e. temperature)

35

t-Test

A *t*-test is a statistical examination of one or two population means. The *t*-test is commonly used when the variances of normally distributed variables are unknown. This test is used with *numerical or continuous data*.[3]

- A one-sample *t*-test examines whether one population mean is equal to a specified value. For one-sample *t*-test,
  - The null hypothesis is $H_0 : \mu = \mu_0$, where μ_0 represents the mean under the null hypothesis.
  - The alternative hypothesis is either $H_A : \mu > \mu_0$ (one-sided to the right), $H_A : \mu < \mu_0$ (one-sided to the left), or $H_A : \mu \neq \mu_0$ (two-sided).
  - The one-sample *t*-test statistic is $T = \dfrac{(\bar{x} - \mu_0)}{s/\sqrt{n}}$, where s is the standard deviation.

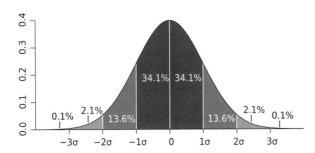

Figure 7.4 Standard Normal Distribution

- With a paired sample, each data value in one sample is matched with a unique one in the second sample (e.g. observations made on the left and right eyes of the same person).
- A two-sample *t*-test examines whether two population means are different.

Chi-Square

The chi-square test is used to test the association between the row (R) and column (C) variables that comprise an R by C contingency table. This test is used with *categorical data*.[3]

- The null hypothesis is H_0 no association between the row and column variables in the source population.
- The alternative hypothesis is H_A: association.

Regression Analysis/Correlation

Regression analysis and correlations are methods used to assess the relationship between explanatory variables (X) and the continuous response variable (Y).[3]

Regression analysis: Linear regression finds the best fitting line for the data using a least squares method. The relationship is described by the linear regression equation $\hat{y} = a + bx$.

Correlation: The Pearson correlation coefficient (r) is used to assess the linear dependence between two variables X and Y (Figure 7.5).

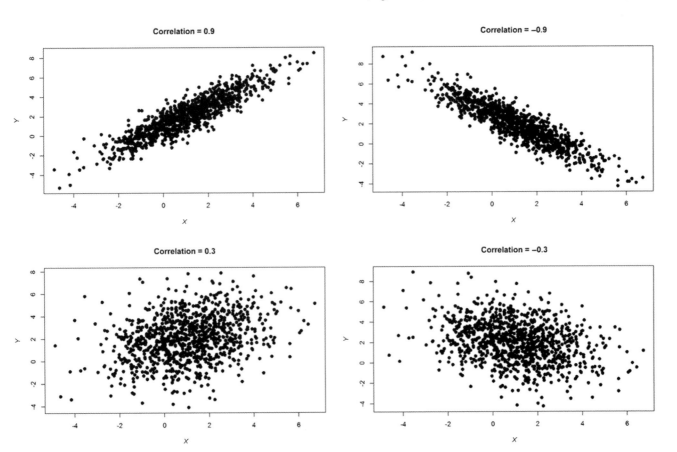

Figure 7.5 Example of the different correlations to assess the relationship between *X* and *Y*.

Table 7.1 Example of a 2 by 2 table for odds ratio and risk ratio

	Disease	No disease	Total
Group 1 (exposed)	a_1	b_1	n_1
Group 2 (nonexposed)	a_2	b_2	n_2

Odds Ratio

The odds ratio (*OR*) is a parameter that measures the relationship between a categorical explanatory variable and a binary response variable. The OR takes on nonnegative values. See below for the example of a 2/2 table. Group 1 can be persons exposed to a certain agent and Group 2 can be the nonexposed persons (Table 7.1).[3]

- The odds ratio of an event is the proportion of disease divided by the proportion of no disease.
- The point estimator for the odds ratio ($\widehat{OR}$) is

$$\frac{Odds\ in\ Group\ 1}{Odds\ in\ Group\ 2} = \frac{a_1/b_1}{a_2/b_2} = \frac{a_1 b_2}{b_1 a_2}.$$

- $OR = 1$ indicates that the exposure is not related to disease. $OR > 1$ indicates that the exposure is positively related to disease. $OR < 1$ indicates that the exposure is negatively related to disease.

Risk Ratio

A risk ratio (*RR*) is a parameter that measures the relationship between a categorical explanatory variable and a binary response variable. The *RR* takes on nonnegative values. See above for the example of a 2/2 table.[3]

- The point estimator for the risk ratio ($\widehat{RR}$) is $\frac{\hat{p}_1}{\hat{p}_2}$, where $\hat{p}_1$

  (a risk of Group 1) = $\frac{a_1}{n_1}$ and $\hat{p}_2$ (a risk of Group 2) = $\frac{a_2}{n_2}$

  are the point estimators of population proportions, p_1 and p_2.
- $RR = 1$ indicates that the risk in exposed is equal to the risk in nonexposed. $RR > 1$ indicates that the risk in exposed is greater than the risk in nonexposed. $RR < 1$ indicates that the risk in exposed is less than the risk in nonexposed.

Analysis of Variance

Analysis of variance (ANOVA) tests the *equality of group means*, not variances. ANOVA can be used for comparison of more than two groups with *numerical or continuous data*.

Power Analysis

The power of a statistical test is its ability to detect an effect if it actually exists. More formally, it is the probability that the test correctly rejects the null hypothesis (H_0) when the alternative hypothesis (H_1) is true. Power calculations are conducted to determine the minimum sample size required so that one can be reasonably confident of detecting an effect of a given size. Power analysis can also be used to calculate the minimum

effect size that is likely to be detected in a study using a specified sample size. Power analysis is usually conducted before the research study and is used for calculating the sample size required to achieve sufficient power (usually 80% or 90%).

Power = 1-beta, where increasing the beta value will decrease the power of the study.

Ways to increase power: Increase the alpha value to lower the chance of false negatives, decrease population variability, increase sample size (most feasible).

Meta-Analysis

Meta-analysis attempts to estimate a common parameter across conceptually similar studies by deriving a pooled estimate that takes into account the error within each study. There are different methods for deriving the weighted average of parameter estimates from the results of the individual studies, although almost always the sample sizes of the smaller studies are taken into account. Meta-analysis has greater statistical power and a more robust point estimate of the parameter than is possible from a single study due to the larger sample size. However, meta-analysis does not inherently correct for bias or flawed study design in the original smaller studies.

Confidence Intervals

A confidence interval (CI) is a range of values that seek to capture the parameter of interest.[3] For example if we are estimating the population mean μ with the sample average $\bar{x}$, then a CI for μ will be $\bar{x} \pm$ a margin of error. For the usual 95% confidence interval, the margin of error is 1.96 times the SEM. A 95% confidence level means that 95% of the intervals obtained from such samples will contain the true parameter, although any particular interval will either contain the true parameter or not. A larger sample size will typically lead to a smaller confidence interval, and thus a better estimate of the population parameter.

Bland–Altman Plot

A Bland–Altman plot is a method of data plotting used in analyzing the agreement between two different *continuous variables*, often different assays or instruments or measurement techniques. The plot lets the viewer note any systematic difference between the paired values (i.e., fixed bias) or possible outliers. The differences between the paired measurements are plotted against the averages of the paired measurements. A horizontal line is drawn at the mean difference allowing the viewer to ascertain any systematic difference between the measurements. Horizontal lines are also drawn at the limits of agreement, the mean difference plus and minus 1.96 times the standard deviation of the differences, allowing the viewer to detect potential outliers.

Types of Error

Type I error (alpha error): Incorrectly rejecting the null hypothesis – false positive
  - Alpha value has been used historically as 0.05, meaning that there is a 5% chance that the incorrect

conclusion is reached. As the alpha value is decreased, there is a less chance of a Type I error but a higher chance of a Type II error resulting in a false negative.

Type II error (beta error): Incorrectly accepting the null hypothesis – false negative

- o Type II error increases with: variability within the population
- o Type II error decreases with: increased difference between control and study sample (i.e. taste test of Coca Cola or Pepsi versus Coca Cola or Sprite), increasing the number of data points

Evaluation of Diagnostic Tests

True positive: TP
True negative: TN

False positive: FP
False negative: FN

Sensitivity: Ability of a test to detect a disease when it is present

- Sensitivity = TP/(TP+FN) = 1 – false negative rate

Specificity: Ability of a test to indicate non-disease when it is not present

- Specificity = TN/(TN+FP) = 1 – false positive rate

Positive predictive value (PPV): Probability that a person with a positive test result actually has the disease

- PPV = TP/(TP+FP)

Negative predictive value (NPV): Probability that a person with a negative test actually does not have the disease[3]

- NPV = TN/(FN+TN)

References

1. P. J. Curran, K. Obeidat, and D. Losardo. Twelve frequently asked questions about growth curve modeling. *J Cogn Dev* 2010; 11(2): 121–36. doi: 10.1080/15248371003699969.

2. J. T. Rich, J.G. Neely, R.C. Paniello, et al. A practical guide to understanding Kaplan–Meier curves. *Otolaryngol Head Neck Surg* 2010; 143(3): 331–6. doi: 10.1016/j.otohns.2010.05.007.

3. B. B. Gerstman. *Basic Biostatistics: Statistics for Public Health Practice,* 2nd edition. Ascend Learning Company, Burlington, MA, 2014.

Chapter 8

General Pharmacology

Shaji Faisal and Ben Toure

Pharmacokinetics vs. Pharmacodynamics

- Pharmacokinetics: The relationship between drug administration and drug concentration at various sites of action throughout the body[1]
  - Involves concepts such as absorption, distribution, metabolism, and excretion
- Pharmacodynamics: The relationship between drug concentration and clinical effect[1]

Potency

- The relationship between amounts of drug required to produce desired clinical effect[1]
  - That is, if drug "A" can produce the same clinical effect as drug "B" at a lower dose, then drug "A" has greater potency relative to drug "B."
  - C_{50} is the concentration at which 50% of the drug is at peak effect.
  - Effective dose$_{50}$ (ED_{50}) is the dose required to produce a desired clinical effect in 50% of individuals.
  - Note: ED_{95} is the average dose required to achieve 95% reduction in maximal twitch response from baseline in 50% of the population. In simpler terms, ED_{95} is the ED_{50} for the desired effect of 95% reduction in train of four twitch height.

Efficacy

- A measure of *the maximum clinical effect* of the drug upon binding to the receptor site irrespective of required drug dosage (Figure 8.1)[1]

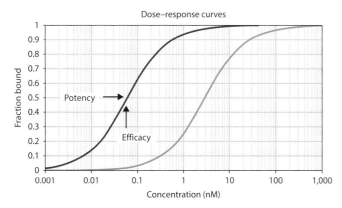

Figure 8.1 Dose–response curve

Absorption

- Process by which a drug moves from the site of administration to the intravascular compartment[1]
  - Oral agents are subject to first pass metabolism. Drugs with high degrees of hepatic metabolism will have decreased bioavailability.
  - Intravenous (IV) drugs completely bypass the process of absorption.

Volume of Distribution

- Volume of distribution (Vd) is the "container size" accounting for the relationship between a given dose of drug and its measured concentration once sufficient time has passed for thorough mixing to occur.[1]
  Vd = Amount of dose/concentration
- Vd within the human body is not a fixed volume. When a drug is administered intravenously, some drug stays in the intravascular space, but most of the drug redistributes to peripheral tissues. The volume of peripheral tissues (i.e. adipose tissue) can add significantly to the overall Vd depending on lipid solubility of the drug.[1]
  - The measured blood concentration of a lipophilic drug (i.e. propofol or thiopental) may be substantially lower than the expected value given the administered IV dose due to peripheral redistribution.

Clearance

- The removal of drug from the intravascular compartment
- Hepatic drug clearance is defined as the plasma volume perfusing the liver that is cleared of the drug per unit time. Three major factors influence hepatic drug clearance[1]:
  - Liver blood flow (Q), which reflects drug delivery to the liver
  - Fraction of drug (f) that exists in the free unbound state vs. protein bound state (not capable of interacting with hepatic enzymes)
  - Hepatic intrinsic enzymatic activity defined as "intrinsic clearance" (Cl_{int}). Intrinsic clearance is the ability of the liver to remove drug in the absence of limitations in hepatic blood flow and protein binding.
- The ratio of the hepatic clearance of a drug to the hepatic blood flow is called the extraction ratio. Extraction ratio can be generally classified as high (>0.7), intermediate

(0.3–0.7), or low (<0.3) according to the fraction of drug removed during one pass through the liver.[1]

- High extraction ratio (>0.7): Hepatic clearance is directly proportional to hepatic blood flow, and clearance is independent of protein binding. These drugs (i.e. propofol, morphine, lidocaine) are rapidly cleared from the plasma after a single liver pass.
- Intermediate extraction ratio (0.3–0.7): Hepatic clearance is dependent on hepatic blood flow, intrinsic hepatic metabolic capacity, and the free drug fraction (i.e. midazolam).
- Low extraction ratio (<0.3): Hepatic clearance is flow independent, and more significantly influenced by the intrinsic hepatic enzymatic capacity and the free drug fraction. An increase in the fraction of unbound drug will increase clearance (i.e. alfentanil).
- If nearly 100% of the drug is extracted by the liver, any decrease in hepatic blood flow due to the vasodilatory effects of anesthetic agents, sepsis, hypovolemia, congestive heart failure, or perioperative bleeding can reduce hepatic drug clearance. However, typically the hepatic metabolic capacity for a drug far exceeds what is required to achieve effective clearance. Thus, moderate changes in hepatic blood flow will have minimal clinical impact.

Context-Sensitive Half-Time

- Time for drug plasma concentration to decline by one-half after a drug infusion has been stopped.
- Continuous infusions of propofol, alfentanil, fentanyl, and remifentanil are used commonly in the clinical setting.
- Propofol has a context-sensitive half-time that varies between 3 minutes for a very short infusion and about 18 minutes for a 12-hour infusion. This small variation in context-sensitive half-time occurs because excretion is rapid compared with redistribution.
  - Fentanyl becomes a long-acting drug with prolonged infusion because it has a large peripheral volume of distribution with rapid redistribution. Remifentanil has a relatively constant and a short context-sensitive half-time as it has a rapid clearance due to plasma ester hydrolysis.[2]

Kinetics

- First-order kinetics: The amount of drug removed is a constant fraction per unit time.[3]
  - Increased concentration of the drug will increase the rate of elimination.
- Zero-order kinetics: A constant amount of drug is eliminated per unit time.[3]
  - Elimination depends on enzymes and membrane transporters which can become saturated. Once these systems are saturated, elimination reaches a maximum level and a constant amount of drug is eliminated per unit time as opposed to a constant fraction. It may

be encountered at high concentrations with aspirin, ethanol, phenytoin, or thiopental.

Hepatic Metabolism

- Oxidation, reduction, hydrolysis, or conjugation of drugs mostly via the cytochrome P450 system.[1]
  - These enzymes are induced by certain drugs (i.e. St. John's wort, rifampin, phenytoin).
  - Other drugs (i.e. erythromycin, cimetidine, amiodarone) or hepatic disease can inhibit these enzymes.
  - The effect of hepatic conjugation is to transform water-insoluble agents into water-soluble agents for subsequent renal excretion.
- All inhalational agents are metabolized to some degree by the liver.[4]
  - Isoflurane is the most commonly used inhalational agent for maintenance of anesthesia in patients with the liver disease due to its minimal degree of hepatic metabolism as compared to sevoflurane and desflurane.

Liver Disease

- Has a significant impact on pharmacokinetics by alterations in protein binding (e.g. decreased synthesis of albumin), altered volume of distribution due to ascites and volume overload, and reduced hepatocellular metabolism of anesthetic agents.[5,6]
- The metabolism of drugs with low hepatic extraction ratios, such as benzodiazepines, is influenced mainly by protein binding and hepatocellular enzyme function. In patients with liver disease, reduced plasma albumin levels result in greater free fractions of drug.[5,6]
  - Highly protein-bound agents (i.e. benzodiazepines) will have an increased Vd, which in conjunction with reduced hepatic metabolism will increase drug half-life.
  - The Vd of water-soluble drugs is often higher in advanced liver disease due to the presence of ascites and volume overload.
- Remifentanil is an ultra-short-acting opioid metabolized by plasma and tissue esterases; its clearance and recovery are independent of liver function.[7]
- Propofol and etomidate have high hepatic extraction ratios. However, clearance of these agents is not significantly prolonged in the setting of cirrhosis. This is perhaps due to extrahepatic sites of metabolism.[8,9]
- Neuromuscular blocking agents, such as vecuronium and rocuronium, are metabolized in the liver and elimination half-lives are prolonged in the setting of liver disease.[10]
- Neuromuscular blocking agents that undergo organ-independent elimination, such as atracurium and cisatracurium, have clinical durations of action unaffected by liver dysfunction. However, renal excretion accounts for approximately 15% of cisatracurium elimination, and renal dysfunction can contribute to the accumulation of the neurotoxic metabolite laudanosine especially when utilizing atracurium.[10]

Renal Disease

- Most anesthetic drugs (i.e. opioids, barbiturates, benzodiazepines, ketamine, and local anesthetics) are lipid-soluble and are nonionized. Their duration of action is not dependent on renal excretion but on hepatic metabolism and/or biotransformation and peripheral redistribution.
- After hepatic metabolism, the majority of drugs are converted to inactive forms and are excreted in urine as water-soluble forms.
- There are several drugs (i.e. muscle relaxants, cholinesterase inhibitors, antibiotics) that are lipid-insoluble or are highly ionized and their duration of action will likely be prolonged in the setting of renal failure.[11]

Extrahepatic Metabolism

- Succinylcholine, mivacurium, esmolol, and remifentanil are metabolized via various plasma enzymes.[12]
- Succinylcholine is a depolarizing neuromuscular blocking agent, metabolized by plasma pseudocholinesterase. Pseudocholinesterase is synthesized by the liver. Severe hepatic disease is associated with decreased pseudocholinesterase levels and prolonged neuromuscular blockade due to succinylcholine.[12]
- Cisatracurium and atracurium exhibit Hofmann elimination, which relies on temperature and pH and is a base-catalyzed nonenzymatic reaction.[13]

Obesity

- Obesity increases the Vd of lipophilic drugs.[14]
- A larger initial loading dose of lipophilic drugs is required in obesity. Decreased maintenance doses of lipophilic drugs are appropriate given the high degree of redistribution of lipophilic drugs from the peripheral compartment to the central plasma compartment over time.[14]
- Substances with high lipophilicity, such as barbiturates and benzodiazepines, have high Vd in obese patients due to a larger peripheral volume of distribution (adipose tissue). Certain lipophilic agents, such as remifentanil, do not demonstrate higher Vd in obese patients due to the rapid enzymatic intravascular metabolism. As such, these drugs should be dosed by ideal body weight and not by total body weight in obese patients. Substances with lower lipophilicity have minimal change in Vd with obesity.[15]
  - Drugs generally dosed on total body weight: succinylcholine, fentanyl, remifentanil
  - Drugs generally dosed on ideal body weight: rocuronium, vecuronium, cisatracurium
  - Drugs generally dosed on lean body weight: profopol
- Desflurane is the inhaled agent of choice in obese patients due to its lower degree of lipid solubility as compared to sevoflurane and isoflurane, providing a more rapid recovery and emergence profile.[15]

References

1. Goodman L., Brunton L., Gilman A., et al. Goodman & Gilman's Pharmacokinetics: The dynamics of drug absorption, distribution, metabolism, and elimination. *The Pharmacological Basis of Therapeutics*, 1st edn. New York: McGraw-Hill Medical; 2011:17–41.
2. Hill S. Pharmacokinetics of drug infusions. *Continuing Education in Anaesthesia, Critical Care & Pain* 2004;4(3):76–80.
3. Roberts F., Freshwater-Turner D. Pharmacokinetics and anaesthesia. *Continuing Education in Anaesthesia, Critical Care & Pain* 2007;7(1):25–9.
4. Carpenter R., Eger E., Johnson B., Unadkat J., Sheiner L. The extent of metabolism of inhaled anesthetics in humans. *Anesthesiology* 1986;65(2):201–5.
5. Gholson C. F., Provenza J. M., Bacon B. R. Hepatologic considerations in patients with parenchymal liver disease undergoing surgery. *American Journal of Gastroenterology* 1990;85:487–96.
6. Verbeeck R. Pharmacokinetics and dosage adjustment in patients with hepatic dysfunction. *European Journal of Clinical Pharmacology* 2008;64(12):1147–61.
7. Tegeder I., Lötsch J., Geisslinger G. Pharmacokinetics of opioids in liver disease. *Clinical Pharmacokinetics* 1999;37:17–40.
8. Servin F., Cockshott I. D., Farinotti R., et al. Pharmacokinetics of propofol infusions in patients with cirrhosis. *British Journal of Anaesthesia* 1990;65(2):177–83.
9. Beem H., Manger F., Boxtel C., Bentem N. Etomidate anaesthesia in patients with cirrhosis of the liver: Pharmacokinetic data. *Anaesthesia* 1983;38(S1):61–2.
10. Craig R., Hunter J. Neuromuscular blocking drugs and their antagonists in patients with organ disease. *Anaesthesia* 2009;64:55–65.
11. Prescott L. Mechanisms of renal excretion of drugs (with special reference to drugs used by anaesthetists). *BJA: British Journal of Anaesthesia* 1972;44(3):246–51.
12. Jensen F., Viby-Mogensen J. Plasma cholinesterase and abnormal reaction to succinylcholine: Twenty years' experience with the Danish Cholinesterase Research Unit. *Acta Anaesthesiologica Scandinavica* 1995;39(2):150–6.
13. Wastila W., Maehr R., Turner G., et al. Comparative pharmacology of cisatracurium (51W89), atracurium, and five isomers in cats. *Anesthesiology* 1996;85(1):169–77.
14. Ingrande J., Lemmens H. Anesthetic pharmacology and the morbidly obese patient. *Current Anesthesiology Reports* 2012;3(1):10–17.
15. Bairamian M. Anesthetic considerations for bariatric surgery. *Survey of Anesthesiology* 2003;47(5):298–9.

Inhaled Anesthetics

Christopher R. Cowart and Himani V. Bhatt

General Pharmacokinetics of Anesthetic Gases and Vapors

There are several important factors that directly affect induction and uptake of inhalational anesthetic agents. Some of these factors (Table 9.1) are modifiable, while others are not. Manipulation of these variables allows for the ability to increase or decrease the rate of induction (Table 9.2).

Effects of intracardiac shunt on induction:

- Right to left (i.e. congenital abnormalities including Tetrology of Fallot, Eisenmenger syndrome):
  - Intravenous anesthetics: rapid induction
  - Inhaled anesthetics: slower induction
    - Insoluble inhaled anesthetic agents affected most
- Left to right (i.e. ventricular septal defect, atrial septal defect):
  - Intravenous anesthetics: limited effect
  - Inhaled anesthetics: limited effect

Table 9.1 Pharmacokinetic factors affecting inhalational induction[1]

Concept	Factors affecting each
Inspired concentration of anesthetic gas (Fi)	Fresh gas flow (FGF) Volume of breathing system Circuit absorption
Alveolar concentration of anesthetic gas (Fa)	Uptake Alveolar ventilation/minute ventilation (MV) Concentration/second gas effect
Uptake	Blood gas solubility Alveolar blood flow/cardiac output Alveolar–venous partial pressure gradient

Table 9.2 Controlling rate of induction

	Speed induction	Slow induction
Gas solubility	Low solubility	High solubility
CO	Low cardiac output	High cardiac output
P–P gradient	Low P–P gradient	High P–P gradient
MV	High MV	Low MV
Fi	High Fi	Low Fi

Physical Properties of Anesthetic Gases

Each of the anesthetic gases has its own unique physical properties that result in different clinical effects. The minimum alveolar concentration (MAC) of each agent is listed in Table 9.3, as are their vapor pressures (Table 9.4) and blood/gas partition coefficients (Table 9.5).

- Nitrous oxide: MAC 105%
  - Odorless – Good for inhalation in awake patients, hence its popularity in dental offices
  - Nitrous oxide is a gas at room temperature (unlike volatile agents) because the critical temperature is greater than the room temperature
  - Very high vapor pressure (much higher than desflurane)[2]
- Desflurane: MAC 6%
  - Boils at room temperature (requires special vaporizer)

Table 9.3 Factors affecting MAC[1–3]

Increase MAC	Decrease MAC
Amphetamines – acute	Amphetamines – chronic
Alcohol – chronic	Alcohol – acute
Cocaine – acute	Pregnancy
Hypernatremia	Hyponatremia
Hyperthermia	Hypothermia
Young age	Old age
Monoamine oxidase inhibitors (MAOIs)	IV Anesthetics
	Local anesthetics
	Lithium

Table 9.4 Vapor pressures[2]

Volatile anesthetics with similar vapor pressures = "HI SE"	
Halothane = 243 mmHg	Sevoflurane = 157 mmHg
Isoflurane = 238 mmHg	Enflurane = 172 mmHg

Table 9.5 Blood/gas partition coefficients of anesthetic gases[2]

	Blood/gas partition coefficient at 37°C
Desflurane	0.45
Nitrous Oxide	0.47
Sevoflurane	0.65
Isoflurane	1.4
Halothane	2.4

- o Very low solubility in blood → rapid induction and emergence (Fa = Fi quicker)
- Sevoflurane: MAC 2%
  - o Halogenated with fluorine
  - o More soluble in blood than desflurane (slower onset)
  - o Non-pungent makes it desirable for inhaled induction[2,3]
- Isoflurane: MAC 1.2%
  - o Pungent odor
- Halothane: MAC 2.3%
  - o Halogenated alkane
  - o Rare use in the United States[2]

Factors Affecting MAC

- *Concentrating effect:* As discussed above, uptake of gases from the alveoli into the blood will slow the rate of induction. This effect can be overcome by increasing the inspired concentration of the gas being delivered. If you deliver a very high concentration of gas to the patient, it will replace whatever amount was taken into the blood, thus increasing the alveolar concentration of that gas with each breath.
- *Second gas effect:* By the same mechanism discussed above, nitrous oxide can be used to increase the concentration of other gases being delivered into the alveoli as well, although probably never to clinically significant levels.

Note: Desflurane is less soluble than nitrous oxide. Despite this, nitrous oxide will still have a faster induction because it can be used at such high concentrations and exert a concentrating effect, which overcomes the small difference in uptake.[2]

Mechanism of Action of Anesthetic Gases

- *Meyer–Overton rule:* Anesthetic gas potency is directly correlated to lipid solubility.[1]
  - o Nitrous
    - ■ NMDA antagonist (Xenon also)
  - o Volatiles
    - ■ Alter neuronal ion channels
    - ■ Particularly the fast synaptic neurotransmitter receptors such as:
      - Nicotinic acetylcholine receptors
      - GABA$_A$
      - Glutamate receptors[2]

Effects on Major Organ Systems

The physiological changes that are seen in each major organ system after administration of anesthetic gases are summarized in Tables 9.6 through 9.8.

Table 9.6 CNS effects of anesthetic gases[2]

	CBF	ICP	CMRO2
Nitrous oxide	↑	↑	↑
Desflurane	↑	↑	↓
Sevoflurane	↑	↑	↓
Isoflurane	↑	↑	↓
Halothane	↑	↑	↓

Table 9.7 Cardiovascular effects of anesthetic gases[2]

	HR	BP	CO	SVR	Contractility	PAP/RAP/CVP
Nitrous oxide	–	–	–	–	↓↓	↑
Desflurane	↑	–/↑	–/↓	↓	–	–
Sevoflurane	–	↓	↓	↓	–/↓	–
Isoflurane	↑	↑	–	↓	–/↓	–
Halothane	–	↓	↓	–	↓↓↓	↑

Table 9.8 Respiratory effects of anesthetic gases[2,3]

	RR	Vt	MV	PCO$_2$	Bronchodilation
Nitrous oxide	↑	↓	–	–	–
Desflurane	↑	↓↓	↓	↑	+
Sevoflurane	↑	↓↓	↓	↑	+++
Isoflurane	↑	↓↓	↓	↑	+
Halothane	↑	↓↓	↓	↑	+++++

Central Nervous System

- Nitrous oxide
  - o Stimulates sympathetic nervous system (SNS)
  - o Increases intracranial pressure (ICP), increases cerebral metabolic rate (CMRO$_2$) → Nitrous is NOT good for Neuro
- Desflurane
  - o Increases CBF and ICP
  - o Decrease in CMRO$_2$ → vasoconstriction → moderates any increases in ICP
- Sevoflurane
  - o Increases CBF and ICP
  - o Decreases CMRO$_2$
- Isoflurane
  - o Increases CBF and ICP > 1 MAC
  - o Silent EEG at 2 MAC
- Halothane
  - o Dilates cerebral vessels → increases cerebral blood flow (CBF), lowers cerebral vascular resistance (CVR), reduces CMRO$_2$
  - o Blunts autoregulation

Cardiovascular System

- Nitrous oxide
  - Directly depresses myocardial contractility but BP, CO, and HR are unchanged or elevated due to SNS stimulation and increased catecholamines (see above)
  - Myocardial depression unmasked in coronary artery disease (CAD) or poor volume status
  - Increases pulmonary vascular resistance (PVR) → increased pulmonary artery (PA) pressures
- Desflurane
  - SVR decreases with increasing dose
  - Rapid rise in desflurane concentration → tachycardia, elevated BP
- Sevoflurane
  - Mild decrease in myocardial function
  - CO drops because of lack of rise in HR
  - QT prolongation more than other volatile agents
- Isoflurane
  - Minimal left ventricular (LV) depression
  - Maintain CO with rise in HR (baroreceptors preserved)
  - Coronary steal from vasodilation (unlikely to be clinically significant)
- Halothane
  - Dose-dependent direct myocardial depression (affects Na^+/Ca^{2+} exchanger and Ca^{2+} utilization in the cell) → increased right atrial pressure (RAP), central venous pressure (CVP), decreases arterial blood pressure (ABP)
  - Decreases coronary blood flow secondary to a drop in ABP; however, supply/demand is maintained because oxygen demand decreases.
  - Blunts reflex tachycardia
  - Sensitizes heart to catecholamines → causes arrhythmias (seen with tricyclic antidepressants [TCAs] and aminophylline)
  - Junctional rhythms are seen as well as bradycardia[1-3]

Pulmonary Function

- All inhaled anesthetics → rapid and shallow breathing with high respiratory rate and low tidal volumes
- Nitrous oxide
  - Hypoxic drive markedly depressed (mediated by carotid bodies) → must watch closely in recovery room
- Desflurane
  - Airway irritant → avoid in asthmatics or hyperreactive airways
- Sevoflurane
  - Sweet smelling
  - Rapid shallow breathing
  - Reverses bronchospasm
- Isoflurane
  - Rapid shallow breathing with drop in MV
  - Good bronchodilator

- Halothane
  - Drop in MV → increased PCO_2
  - Apneic threshold increases (medullary depression)
  - Potent bronchodilator inhibits intracellular Ca mobilization
  - Depresses mucociliary clearance → post-op hypoxia and atelectasis

Neuromuscular Function

- Nitrous oxide
  - Does not cause malignant hyperthermia (MH)
  - No significant muscle relaxation on its own (in contrast to other inhalational anesthetics)
  - Does minimally potentiate relaxation when used with neuromuscular blockers (NMBs)
- Desflurane
  - Dose-dependent decrease in train-of-four (TOF) response and tetany
- Sevoflurane
  - Creates intubating conditions in children after inhalation induction
- Isoflurane
  - Relaxes skeletal muscle
  - Potentiates non-depolarizing NMBs
- Halothane
  - Relaxes skeletal muscle
  - Potentiates NON-depolarizing NMBs
  - Triggers MH[2,3]

Renal Function

- Nitrous oxide
  - Decrease renal blood flow (RBF)
  - Decrease glomerular filtration rate (GFR)/urine output (UOP)
- Desflurane
  - Decrease GFR, RBF, UOP
- Sevoflurane
  - Can metabolize to Compound A → nephrotoxic in rats, never proven in humans
- Isoflurane
  - Decrease GFR, RBF, and UOP
- Halothane
  - Reduces RBF, GFR, and UOP (secondary to drop in ABP and CO)
  - Drop in blood flow > drop in GFR → increased filtration fraction[2,3]

Hepatic Function

- Nitrous oxide
  - Less drop in hepatic blood flow (HBF) compared to other inhalationals
- Desflurane

- No major hepatic effects
- HBF maintained
- Sevoflurane
  - Decreases portal venous flow
  - Increase hepatic artery flow
  - HBF and O_2 delivery are maintained
- Isoflurane
  - Decreased total HBF (both hepatic artery and portal venous flow) but maintained better than halothane
- Halothane
  - Perioperative hepatic dysfunction can be seen with halothane.
  - Drop in HBF is congruent with drop in CO.
  - Halothane hepatitis (rare) – multiple halothane anesthetics at short intervals, middle-aged obese women, and persons with a familial predisposition to halothane toxicity or a personal history of toxicity are considered to be at increased risk.
  - Centrilobular necrosis of hepatic cells[2]

Hematologic and Immune Systems

- Nitrous oxide
  - Bone marrow depression → megaloblastic anemia causing peripheral neuropathy
  - Irreversibly inhibits B12-dependent enzymes (methionine synthetase → myelin, thymidylate synthetase → DNA)
  - May alter immune response to infection → poor chemotaxis and polymorphonucleocyte (PMN) movement[2]

Biotransformation and Toxicity

- Nitrous oxide
  - Avoided in pregnant patients in 1st and 2nd trimesters
  - Thirty-five times more soluble than nitrogen in blood → escapes into closed spaces
  - Hazardous to use in air embolism, pneumothorax, small/large bowel obstruction, pneumocephalus, retinal surgery, tympanic membrane grafting
- Desflurane
  - Minimal metabolism
  - Degraded by desiccated CO_2 absorbents → carbon monoxide production
  - Associated with emergence delirium in pediatrics
- Sevoflurane
  - Broken down to Compound A
  - Clinically significant renal impairment secondary to fluoride ions and/or Compound A has never been proven with sevoflurane in humans
  - Sevoflurane can also break down to hydrogen fluoride → acid burn to respiratory mucosa
- Isoflurane
  - Metabolized to trifluoroacetic acid (TFA), unlikely to cause kidney or liver issues even after prolonged exposure

- Halothane
  - Oxidized in liver by CYP 2EI to TFA which can be inhibited with disulfiram
  - Hepatotoxicity more likely after phenobarbital use and hypoxia[2]

Note: Fluoride production is directly related to the amount of metabolism a gas undergoes, i.e. Sevoflurane produces the most of the fluoride because it undergoes the most extensive metabolism of the anesthetic gas we use today.[2]

Trace Concentrations, Operating Room Pollution, Personnel Hazards

- Nitrous oxide
  - Ozone depleting, greenhouse gas
- Desflurane
  - Carbon monoxide production with desiccated CO_2 absorbents
- Sevoflurane
  - Broken down to Compound A[2]

Volatile Anesthetic Properties from Most to Least Common

Although not commonly tested, enflurane and halothane have been included.

- EEG spike activity: enflurane > sevoflurane > isoflurane = desflurane
- Liver metabolism: halothane (20%) > sevoflurane (2%) > isoflurane (0.2%) > desflurane (0.02%)
- Muscle relaxation: desflurane > sevoflurane > isoflurane > halothane > nitrous oxide
- Hepatic blood flow: sevoflurane > isoflurane > halothane
- Fluoride production: sevoflurane > enflurane > isoflurane > desflurane
- Carbon monoxide production: desflurane > enflurane > isoflurane
  - baralyme > sodalyme, dry > wet
- Respiratory depression: enflurane > desflurane = isoflurane > sevoflurane = halothane > nitrous oxide
- Cerebral blood flow: isoflurane > desflurane > sevoflurane
- Impaired cerebral autoregulation: halothane > isoflurane/desflurane > sevoflurane

Common Volatile Anesthetic Equations

- Amount of liquid volatile used (mL/h) = 3 × FGF rate (L/min) / volume percent of vaporizer
- Vaporizer output (mL) = [carrier gas flow (mL/min) × saturated vapor pressure (SVP)]/(barometric pressure − SVP)
- Percent of volatile delivered = vaporizer output × 100/ (FGF × vaporizer output)

References

1. Bhatt, H., Powell, K. J., and Jean, D. A. (2011). *First Aid for the Anesthesiology Boards*. New York, NY: McGraw-Hill Education LLC.

2. Mackey, D. C., Butterworth, J. F., Mikhail, M. S., Morgan, G. E., and Wasnick, J. D. (2013). *Morgan & Mikhail's Clinical Anesthesiology* (5th edn). New York, NY: McGraw-Hill Education LLC.

3. Miller, R. D. (2010). *Miller's Anesthesia* (7th edn). Philadelphia, PA: Churchill Livingstone/Elsevier.

Chapter 10

Opioids

Christian Estrada, Dion McCall, Anant Parikh, and Vanny Le

Mechanism of Action

Review of Pain Signal Transmission

- A noxious stimulus is detected by nociceptors and transmitted via *A delta or C fibers* to the spinal cord → These first-order neurons have their cell bodies located in the dorsal root ganglion (DRG)[1] → They ascend or descend one or two vertebral segments through *Lissauer's tract* and then synapse with secondary neurons in the *substantia gelatinosa*[2] → The signal propagates via second-order neurons which cross the anterior commissure and ascend the spinal cord via the *contralateral spinothalamic tract* → These second-order neurons synapse in the *thalamus* and third-order neurons carry the signal to the *somatosensory cortex* as well as to other areas including the midbrain and brainstem.

Opioid Receptors

- G-coupled receptors are inhibitory at the cellular level.
- Three classical opioid receptors mu (μ), delta (δ), kappa (κ) exist in peripheral nerves, spinal cord, and brain. Mu (μ) receptors are primarily involved with analgesia.
- Peripheral opioid receptors are synthesized in the DRG and transported to nerve endings.
- Spinal opioids receptors are mostly located in *Rexed lamina I and II of dorsal horn* both pre- and postsynaptically.
- Supraspinal opioids receptors are located throughout the brainstem, thalamus, amygdala, and hypothalamus (Figure 10.1).
- Table 10.1 summarizes the effects of different opioid receptor stimulations.

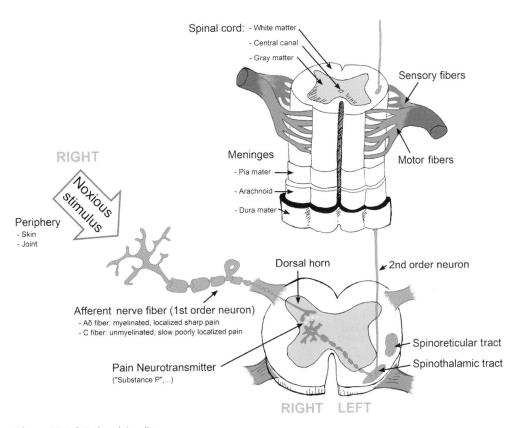

Figure 10.1 Spinal cord signaling

Table 10.1 A summary of the effects of different opioid receptor stimulations

	Mu	Delta	Kappa
Sedation	Yes	No	Yes
Respiratory depression	Yes	No	No
Gastrointestinal effects	Yes	No	Yes
Endogenous ligand	Endorphins	Enkephalins	Dynorphin
Inhibit ADH release	No	No	Yes

- A fourth receptor, *opioid receptor like-1 (ORL1)*, has been discovered along with its endogenous peptide ligand *orphanin*.
  - The role ORL1 plays in modulating pain remains unclear.
  - Preliminary research shows that it may play a role as an anti-opioid (negates analgesic effects of opioids).
  - ORL1 may also be involved in stress, anxiety, substance abuse (opioid and alcohol), anorexia, and possibly neuropathic pain states.[3]

Activation of Opioid Receptors
- Prevents the release of excitatory neurotransmitters, e.g. glutamate, calcitonin gene-related peptide, and substance P.
- Decreases the formation of cAMP, increasing the efflux of K^+ out of the neuron and inhibiting the influx of Ca^{2+} by voltage-dependent Ca^{2+} channels.
- These processes help maintain cell *hyperpolarization* → reducing neuronal depolarization leading to inhibition in the propagation of nociceptive signals.[4]
- Opioids also modulate the transmission of nociceptive stimuli at the level of the brainstem by regulating the ability of the DRG to transmit pain signals. This is achieved by stimulating descending inhibitory pathways from the brainstem to the DRG.[5]

Pharmacodynamics
- Describes the relationship between drug concentration and drug effect

Opioid Categories
- **Natural opioids** – Derived from the seed capsules of the poppy flower
  - Examples: morphine and codeine
- **Semisynthetic opioids** – Drug structure is morphine-based with different functional groups
  - Examples: hydrocodone, hydromorphone, oxycodone, oxymorphone, buprenorphine, and diacetylmorphine (heroin)

- **Fully synthetic opioids**
  - Examples: meperidine, fentanyl, sufentanil and methadone
- **Endogenous opioids** – Synthesized in the brain and spinal cord. They bind with opioid receptors producing analgesia
  - Examples: endorphins and enkephalins

Agonist, Partial Agonist, or Antagonist?
- Agonists are medications that provide a full therapeutic response.
  - Examples: morphine, oxycodone, heroin, methadone, and hydrocodone
- Partial agonists provide less than a full response when fully occupying the receptors.
  - They provide a "ceiling effect," producing significant analgesia while lowering the risk of producing life-threatening respiratory depression as compared to a full agonist.
  - May also decrease the euphoria associated with full agonists thus decreasing the risk of overdose and abuse[6]
  - Example: tramadol
  - Note: If a physically opioid-dependent patient taking a full agonist and were also to take a partial agonist concurrently, the partial agonist would antagonize the full agonist leading to opioid withdrawal symptoms.
- Antagonists are drugs that have a high affinity for receptors without activating them.
  - Examples of opioid receptor antagonists: naloxone and naltrexone
  - Naloxone is used as an antidote to treat opioid overdose because of its fast onset.
  - Methylnaltrexone is a newer medication that has an affinity for antagonizing peripheral mu receptors without affecting analgesia. The chemical structure of methylnaltrexone is a quaternary ammonium cation and it cannot cross the blood–brain barrier. It has been commonly used to treat opioid-induced constipation without a significant decrease in pain relief.[7]
- Buprenorphine
  - Is a mixed agonist–antagonist opioid receptor modulator, a weak partial agonist of the mu and ORL1 receptors, and an antagonist of the kappa and delta receptors
  - Used in the treatment of chronic pain in lower doses and opioid addiction at higher doses
  - Formulation of buprenorphine combined with naloxone (Suboxone©) is available. Buprenorphine treats the opioid addiction while the naloxone deters the abuse of buprenorphine by inducing opioid withdrawal symptoms.

Pharmacokinetics

- Describes how the body impacts the movement of a drug

Opioid Lipophilicity/Hydrophilicity

(Most lipophilic) ↑
Sufentanil
Buprenorphine
Fentanyl
Methadone
Hydromorphone
Hydrocodone
Oxycodone
Morphine
(Most hydrophilic) ↓ Codeine

Neuraxial Opioids (Epidural and Intrathecal)

- Hydrophilic opioids: Delayed onset (30–50 min), longer duration (5–24 hours), extensive CSF spread, site of action primarily spinal.
- Lipophilic opioids: Rapid onset (5–10 minutes), shorter duration (2–4 hours), minimal CSF spread, site of action primarily spinal ± systemic.
- Higher incidence of nausea, vomiting, pruritus, and delayed respiratory depression with hydrophilic opioids. Late respiratory depression due to rostral migration of medication affecting respiratory centers in the brain.

Opioid Dosing Conversion

- Administering intrathecal opioids results in much higher CSF concentrations of opioids compared to epidural and intravenous administration. Onset of analgesia is also fastest with intrathecal injection.
- Morphine: 10 mg IV = 1 mg epidural = 0.1 mg intrathecal (1/10 conversion ratio)
- Hydromorphone: 1 mg IV = 0.2 mg epidural = 0.04 mg intrathecal (1/5 conversion ratio)
- Fentanyl: 100 mcg IV = 25 mcg epidural = 6–7 mcg intrathecal (1/4 conversion ratio)

Metabolism

- Liver is the site of metabolism for most opioids.
- Converted to more water-soluble metabolites in order to be excreted from the body.
- Two main pathways:
  - Phase I metabolism is mediated by the cytochrome P450 system facilitating hydrolysis, oxidation, and reduction reactions.
    - Rate of metabolism of opioids that undergo phase I reactions, such as fentanyl, may be altered if the patient concurrently takes other medications that inhibit or induce the cytochrome P450 system.
  - Phase II reaction involves glucuronidation.

Morphine

- Undergoes phase II metabolism into *morphine-3-glucuronide (M3G)* and *M6G*.

- M6G is a *full mu opioid receptor agonist* and in patients with renal failure, M6G can accumulate in the plasma causing *respiratory depression* and loss of consciousness.[8]
- M3G has been implicated with inducing *hyperalgesia*.

Piperidines

- The piperidine family of opioids which include fentanyl, alfentanil, and sufentanil. They are lipophilic drugs that cross the blood–brain barrier rapidly and are metabolized by phase I reactions.
- Remifentanil is an exception to this group because it is not metabolized by the liver. Instead, it is metabolized in the blood by *nonspecific esterases*.

Codeine

- Codeine is a weak analgesic pro-drug that is biotransformed to morphine.
- About 5–10% of Caucasians are poor metabolizers for codeine and are unable to benefit from analgesia.
- In contrast, patients who rapidly metabolize codeine may experience greater effects such as respiratory depression because of rapid metabolism generating a higher concentration of morphine.

Meperidine

- Meperidine is an older opioid with many side effects including anticholinergic effects due to its structural *similarity to atropine*.
- *Normeperidine* which is one of the metabolites has been implicated with causing *tremors, myoclonus, tachycardia, and seizures.* Patient with *renal or liver disease* are at increased risk for developing these side effects.

Excretion of Opioids

- Ninety percent renal and less than 10% via fecal elimination
- Because many of the metabolites of opioids are active, it is imperative that opioids be used cautiously in the setting of renal insufficiency.
  - Not recommended in renal insufficiency: meperidine, morphine, codeine, hydrocodone, and tramadol due to active metabolites
- Use cautiously and with dose reduction: oxycodone and hydromorphone
- Can be safely used in patients with renal insufficiency: fentanyl, sufentanil, remifentanil, and methadone (no active metabolites)

Opioid Effects on Circulation

- *Nucleus Tract Solitarius* is a part of the brain that processes information from periphery in regards to arterial blood pressure and carbon dioxide concentrations.[9-11]
  - Both mu and delta receptors are located in this region.[11]
  - Stimulation of these receptors results in *hypotension* and *bradycardia*.[11]

- In general, most opioids enhance parasympathetic tone and reduce sympathetic tone.[9]
- Although most opioids cause bradycardia, meperidine causes an increase in heart rate due its atropine like structure.
- Experimental studies on healthy patients and those with cardiac disease have shown that opioids have no direct impact on myocardial relaxation and contractility.[12,13]
  - Often the drugs of choice in cardiac inductions for that reason
- Morphine and meperidine can both lead to *histamine release.*
  - Can have resultant *drop in systemic vascular resistance* and can develop hypotension[14]
  - Can be treated with the use of H_1 and H_2 blockers[14]
- Opioids have been shown to have vasodilatory effects by direct action on vasculature. These mechanisms work independently of their effect on neurogenic centers.[9]
  - A relatively newly discovered opioid receptor subtype, mu-3 receptor, is found on human endothelial cells and may contribute to vasodilation when activated by opioids such as morphine.[9]
  - Studies have also demonstrated that sufentanil has a direct vasodilatory impact on vasculature.[9,15]

Opioid Effects on Respiratory System

- Mu opioid receptor is primarily responsible for respiratory depression.[16–18]
- Although there are opioid receptors found in high concentrations throughout the central and peripheral nervous system, the area that is likely involved in the *ventilatory response to hypercapnia* is the *medullary raphe region.*[16,17,19]
  - Leads to a decrease in respiratory rate
  - Dose–response curve to *carbon dioxide is shifted to the right and downward*, which indicates decreased alveolar ventilation for a given $PaCO_2$.[10]
  - Ultimately leads to an increase in the apneic threshold, which is essentially defined as the highest $PaCO_2$ for which a patient is apneic.[10]
- Opioids are also involved in the regulation of tidal volume, upper airway resistance, and pulmonary compliance.
  - This modulation takes place at the *ventral respiratory group (VRG) neurons*, which are located in the ventrolateral region of the medulla.[21]
  - High-dose opioids cause a decrease in tidal volumes.[21]
- Opioids impact airway reflexes.
  - Investigations into the mechanisms involved in laryngeal and tracheobronchial airway reflexes show that the pathways are centrally mediated.[22,24]
  - It is believed that opioids have a greater impact on inhibiting reflexes in the *lower airway* than they do on upper airway reflexes.[23]
    - This is demonstrated by the use of codeine as an antitussive agent in individuals who have a cough due to lower airway disease.[22]
    - Opioids still have some activity in the upper airway, and this explains their ability to blunt the body's response to laryngoscopy.
- Patients who are opioid naïve are more likely to develop respiratory depression.[21–23]
- Patients on chronic opioids develop a *central tolerance* to opioids, but they *do not* develop a *tolerance to the peripheral effects.*[25]
  - Leads to the development of abnormal breathing patterns during non-REM sleep[25]
  - Mechanism: During non-REM sleep, peripheral carotid chemoreceptors are responsible for detecting hypoxia and maintaining a breath by breath control of the ventilatory pattern.[25,26]
    - Mu receptor activation inhibits the peripheral chemoreceptors control of ventilatory pattern, which may lead to abnormal breathing patterns during non-REM sleep.[27]
- Elderly patients are usually more sensitive to the respiratory depressant effects.[19,20]
- The depressant effects are also more severe when used in conjunction with alcohol, benzodiazepines, and barbiturates.[28]

Opioid Effects on Other Organ Systems

Gastrointestinal

- The enteric nervous system (ENS) is the neural network that dictates activity in the gastrointestinal system.[29,31]
- The ENS integrates information from sensory receptors throughout the GI tract, regulates reflex activities, controls secretory functions, and coordinates peristaltic movements.
- Opioid receptors, particularly mu opioid receptors, are present throughout the ENS, especially in myenteric and submucosal plexuses.[30,31]
- The opioid receptors modulate the activity on the ENS by inhibiting neurotransmitter release from excitatory motor neurons and by stimulating the release of neurotransmitters from inhibitory neurons.[33]
- The net effect results in a constellation of symptoms such as nausea, vomiting, decreased gastric emptying, and inhibited intestinal peristalsis.[31]
- The body releases endogenous opioids, such as dynorphin and enkephalins due to the stresses of surgery, and this contributes to the development of postoperative ileus in a subset of patients.[34]
- Postoperative constipation and ileus is a common side effect of opioid use and is treated by medications such as methylnatrexone and alvimopan, which are peripheral mu opioid receptor antagonists.[32]
- Opioid agonists also impact biliary duct pressure by increasing tone in the sphincter of Oddi in a dose-dependent manner.[35]

Renal

- Studies involved in measuring levels of plasma renin, ADH, and aldosterone during IV infusions of fentanyl, alfentanil, and remifentanil show that renal function is preserved by opioids.[28]
- Intrathecal morphine and sufentanil decrease bladder function in a dose-dependent manner.[36]
  - Intrathecal opioids impact spinal receptors, which cause suppression of detrusor contractility and create a decreased urge to urinate.[37]

Endocrine

- Opioids cause suppression in multiple axes of the endocrine system.[38]
- Somatotropic axis
  - Leads to *increase in GH secretion* in healthy patients[38,39]
  - In patients with chronic opioids, there is evidence of GH deficiency.[38,40]
- Lactotropic axis
  - Morphine administration *increases serum prolactin* in men and in women who are postmenopausal.[41]
  - Mechanism: Inhibition of dopamine release from the median eminence[42]
- Hypothalamic–pituitary–adrenal axis
  - Thought to decrease the pituitary gland's response to corticotropin releasing hormone (CRH) and subsequently cause a decrease of adrenocorticotropic hormone (ACTH) and cortisol in plasma[42]
    - Likely mediated by the kappa opioid receptor[42]
  - Studies have shown a *decrease in adrenal androgen dehydroepiandrosterone sulfate* (DHEAS) during the administration of opioids[43]
- Hypothalamic–pituitary–gonadal axis
  - Several studies have shown that chronic opioid use is associated with *hypogonadism*[38,44]
    - Some of the side effects seen include loss of libido, erectile dysfunction, depression and anxiety, fatigue and hot flashes[38]

Cancer Progression

- Opioids are thought to aid in the process of cancer progression due to their ability to *stimulate angiogenesis*.[45]
  - Can lead to the growth and dissemination of cancer cells[45,46]
  - Mechanism: Activate cyclooxygenase-2 which increases the production of prostaglandin E_2 and subsequently angiogenesis and tumor progression[45]

Side Effects and Toxicity

- CNS: Sedation, decrease cognition, fine motor impairment, decreased REM and slow wave sleep, ventilatory depression, and miosis[9]
  - Metabolites of hydromorphone, morphine, tramadol, and meperidine can produce CNS excitation precipitating myoclonus and seizures[9]

- Endocrine: Modulation of nociception, and inhibition of the pituitary–adrenal axis.[8] Decreases in plasma epinephrine, cortisol, GH, ADH, ACTH, FSH, LH, and glucose; prolactin increases[8]
- Respiratory: Decreased respiratory rate. Tidal volume decreased secondary to a decrease in chemoreceptor input
  - Leads to decreased CO_2 responsiveness and hypercapnia[8]
  - Opioids should be used with caution in obese, elderly, COPD, neuromuscular disease, chronic opioid, and sleep apnea patient populations as their risk of opioid-induced respiratory depression is higher than the general population.
  - Can potentially lead to increases in CVP, ICP, PVR, PCO_2, and oxygen consumption; and decreases in compliance, functional residual capacity, and ventilation[47]
- Gastrointestinal: Increased smooth muscle tone, decreased pyloric tone, and motility
  - Leads to constipation, biliary stasis, and decreased gastric emptying[8]
  - Increases risk of postoperative nausea and vomiting
  - Tolerance is not observed regardless of chronic use[47]
  - Nausea/vomiting: Opioids activate the *chemotactic trigger zone* in the area postrema projecting to the vomiting center in the medulla, and may sensitize vestibular neurons.[9]
  - Opioids should be used judiciously in patient at high risk for postoperative nausea and vomiting (PONV) (i.e. female gender, previous history of PONV, motion sickness, nonsmoker).
- Genitourinary: Parenteral or neuraxial administration increases urethral sphincter tone and bladder tone can lead to urinary retention.
  - Elderly male patients appear to be most sensitive to these effects[9]
- Cardiovascular: Produce favorable cardiovascular effects, secondary to relative hemodynamic stability and dose-dependent sympatholytic effects preventing tachycardia, and decreasing myocardial oxygen demand[9]
  - Excluding the histamine release associated with hydromorphone, morphine, and meperidine
- Pruritus: May occur following parenteral or neuraxial administration
  - Secondary to histamine release triggered by individual opioid agents
  - Evidence suggests that this effect may be mediated through a mechanism other than opioid receptors[48]

Toxicity

- Titration of opioids is challenging due to:
  - Variable individual response to opioids
  - Lack of analgesic ceiling effects coupled with peak central effects which generally occur much later than the onset of analgesic effects and peak plasma concentrations[8]

Table 10.2 Acute opioid toxicity symptoms

Lethargy/coma	Cold, clammy skin
Hypoventilation	Seizure
Hypoxia	Decreased muscle tone
Pin point pupils	Hypotension
Pulmonary edema	Respiratory failure

- ○ Cases of acute opioid toxicity may be the result of suicide attempts, accidental overdose, or clinical overdose[9]
- It is difficult to define the exact opioid dose which is toxic or lethal to human
  - ○ In nontolerant patients, serious toxicity may occur following oral doses of 40–60 mg of methadone.
  - ○ Opioid naïve patients are not likely to die with <120 mg of PO morphine, or have serious toxicity after <30 mg parenteral.[9]
- The line between therapeutic and potentially lethal effects can be crossed without the occurrence of signs and symptoms until 1–2 hours following drug administration.
- Acute opioid toxicity symptoms[9] (Table 10.2)
- Respiratory failure or the sequelae of respiratory depression is the most common cause of death from opioid use.
- Treatment
  - ○ Establishment of an airway, supplemental oxygen, ventilation, and administration of the opioid antagonist naloxone
  - ○ Naloxone should be titrated to arousal, and return of spontaneous ventilation to prevent precipitation of withdrawal symptoms in opioid-dependent patients.
  - ○ The duration of action of naloxone is shorter than the offending opioid, repeated dosing or a continuous infusion is indicated, as premature discontinuation can lead to recurring opioid toxicity symptoms.

Indications and Contraindications

- Opioids are indicated for:
  - ○ Analgesia
  - ○ Acute postoperative pain
  - ○ Chronic postoperative pain
  - ○ Total intravenous anesthesia (TIVA), in combination with hypnotic and amnestic agents
  - ○ Induction of general anesthesia
  - ○ Postoperative shivering
  - ○ A component of a balanced anesthetic technique to blunt the response to laryngoscopy to decrease risk of hemodynamic depression associated with doses required for single agent anesthesia[9]
- Contraindications
  - ○ *Pregnancy*: Animal studies have shown adverse fetal effects of opioids, but no controlled human studies exist. Neonatal withdrawal has been observed with opioid use late in pregnancy,[48] therefore the fetal risk vs. maternal benefit must be considered before administering opioid therapy.

- ○ *Renal and hepatic failure*: The use of opioids in patients with hepatic or renal failure is complicated by inadequate clearance of the parent drug and active metabolite(s)[8,9,47]
  - ▪ Agents with active metabolites such as codeine, morphine, hydrocodone, and meperidine are avoided secondary to increased risk of respiratory depression and also worsening hepatic encephalopathy in patients with hepatic failure.
  - ▪ When opioids are administered to patients with renal or hepatic failure, lower doses and less frequent dosing intervals should be used.
- ○ *Adrenal insufficiency*: Opioids inhibit the pituitary–adrenal axis resulting in decreases in plasma epinephrine, cortisol, GH, ADH, ACTH, FSH, LH, and glucose which may precipitate adrenal insufficiency in at-risk populations or worsen established adrenal insufficiency.[49]
- ○ *Serotonin reuptake inhibitors and MAO inhibitors*: Phenylpiperidine opioids, methadone, meperidine, and tramadol have weak serotonin re-uptake inhibition.[47]
  - ▪ Combining phenylpiperidines with MAOIs or SSRIs can lead to overstimulation of receptors causing *serotonin syndrome*.

Role of Opioids in Postoperative Pain Control

- The goals of postoperative pain management are to relieve suffering, achieve early mobilization after surgery, reduce length of hospital stay, and achieve patient satisfaction.
- Opioids are considered the most effective analgesic for severe acute pain and cancer-related chronic pain.[9] Unlike non-opioids, which exhibit a ceiling analgesic response, opioids demonstrate greater efficacy as the dose is increased.[50]
- Perioperative opioid use is recommended as part of a multimodal regimen.
- In patients without chronic pain, randomized controlled trials suggest adequate postoperative analgesia by a multimodal approach may facilitate the return of GI function, provide cardioprotective effects, reduce pulmonary complications, and decrease length of hospital stay.[9]
- Acute postoperative pain
  - ○ The World Health Organization developed a three-step ladder initially developed for the treatment of cancer pain which has also been extended clinically in the treatment of acute non-cancer pain[49] (Figure 10.2).
- The WHO ladder guidelines suggest the use of non-opioids and adjuvants (NSAIDs, local nerve blocks, antidepressants, electrical stimulation, acupuncture, hypnosis, and behavior modification) prior to starting opioid therapy, excluding the presence of severe pain.
- The American Pain Society Recommendations for Improving the Quality of Acute and Cancer Pain Management suggest that opioids and nonsteroidal anti-inflammatory drugs should be provided in an around-the-clock dosing schedule during the first several days

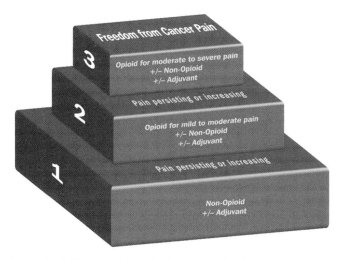

Figure 10.2 World Health Organization cancer pain ladder
www.cancerworld.org/Articles/Issues/30/May-June-2009/Systems--
Services/38/Why-are-cancer-patients-still-suffering-unnecessary-pain.html

after major surgery to prevent and control moderate to severe acute pain.[9,51]

- Non-cancer chronic pain
  - The use of opioids for the treatment of chronic non-cancer pain is controversial.[9]
  - One randomized control study suggests that capacity and quality of life are not improved.[52]
    - The sole use of opioids for chronic nonmalignant pain is not recommended.[9]
- Postoperative pain control in patients with chronic pain
  - Patients with chronic non-cancer and chronic cancer pain may have increased central sensitization or reduced inhibition, and altered sensitivity secondary to long-term exposure to opioids. These factors make postoperative pain control difficult in this population.
  - Chronic pain patients are at increased risk of developing chronic pain after surgery.
  - Accurate history of preoperative opioid medications and doses should be recorded, and medications should be continued during the perioperative period to prevent opioid withdraw.
  - Baseline long-acting drugs, administered at fixed dosing intervals, can decrease fluctuations in plasma drug concentration and lead to better pain control while minimizing side effects.
  - Fast-acting, short-duration opioids are also important for treatment of breakthrough pain in chronic pain patients.
  - A conscious effort must be made to transition majority of the effective daily dose to the long-acting form to decrease the likelihood of *mu opioid receptor desensitization, internalization, and G protein uncoupling* associated with repeated opioid administration.[8]

References

1. McMahon, S. B., Koltzenburg, M., Tracey, I., et al. *Wall and Melzack's Textbook of Pain*, 6th edn. Philadelphia, PA: Elsevier Saunders, 2013, 421.
2. Purves, D., G. J. Augustine, D. Fitzpatrick, et al. *Neuroscience*, 2nd edn. Sunderland: Sinauer Associates; 2001.
3. McMahon, S. B., et al. *Wall and Melzack's Textbook of Pain*, 6th edn. Philadelphia, PA: Elsevier Saunders; 413–4.
4. Chieng B., M. J. Christie. Hyperpolarization by opioids acting on μ-receptors of a sub-population of rat periaqueductal gray neurons in vitro. *British Journal of Pharmacology* 113(1994): 121–8.
5. Dubin, A. E., A. Patapoutian. Nociceptors: The sensors of the pain pathway. *The Journal of Clinical Investigation* 120(11)(2010): 3760–72.
6. Dahan, A., et al. Buprenorphine induces ceiling in respiratory depression but not analgesia. *British Journal of Anaesthesia* 96(2006): 627.
7. Meerveld, B. G.-V., K. M. Standifer. Methylnaltrexone in the treatment of opioid-induced constipation. *Clinical and Experimental Gastroenterology* 1(2008): 49–58.
8. Barash P. G., Cullen, B., Stoelting, R., et al. *Clinical Anesthesia*, 7th edn. Philadelphia, PA: Wolters Kluwer, Lippincott Williams & Wilkins; 2013: 501–22.
9. Miller, R. D., and Erikssonn Li. *Miller's Anesthesia*. Philadelphia, PA: Churchill Livingstone; 2015: 864–914.
10. Morgan, G. E., and M. S. Mikail. *Opioids. Clinical Anesthesiology*. New York, NY: McGraw-Hill, 2011: 192–7.
11. Feldman, P. D., N. Parveen, S. Sezen. Cardiovascular effects of Leu-enkephalin in the nucleus tractus solitarius of the rat. *Brain Research* 709(2)(1996): 331–6.
12. Bolliger, D., Seeberger, M. D., Kasper, J., et al. Remifentanil does not impair left ventricular systolic and diastolic function in young healthy patients. *British Journal of Anaesthesia* (2011): aeq414.
13. Hanouz, J.-L., Yvon, A., Guesne, G., et al. The in vitro effects of remifentanil, sufentanil, fentanyl, and alfentanil on isolated human right atria. *Anesthesia & Analgesia* 93(3)(2001): 543–9.
14. Blunk, J. A., Schmelz, M., Zeck, S., et al. Opioid-induced mast cell activation and vascular responses is not mediated by μ-opioid receptors: An in vivo microdialysis study in human skin. *Anesthesia & Analgesia* 98(2)(2004): 364–70.
15. Ebert, T. J., Ficke, D. J., Arain, S. R., et al. Vasodilation from sufentanil in humans. *Anesthesia & Analgesia* 101(6)(2005): 1677–80.
16. Freye, E., L. Lazx tasch, P. S. Portoghese. The delta receptor is involved in sufentanil-induced respiratory depression – Opioid subreceptors mediate different effects. *European Journal of Anaesthesiology* 9(6)(1992): 457–62.
17. Dahan, A., Sarton, E., Teppema, L., et al. Anesthetic potency and influence of morphine and sevoflurane on respiration in μ opioid receptor knockout mice. *The Journal of the American Society of Anesthesiologists* 94(5)(2001): 824–32.
18. Zhang, Z., Xu, F., Zhang, C., et al. Activation of opioid μ receptors in caudal medullary raphe region inhibits the ventilatory response to hypercapnia in anesthetized rats. *The Journal of the American Society of Anesthesiologists* 107(2)(2007): 288–97.

19. Bernard, D. G., L. Aihua, E. E. Nattie. Evidence for central chemoreception in the midline raphe. *Journal of Applied Physiology* 80(1)(1996): 108–15.

20. Nattie, E. E., Aihua, L. CO_2 dialysis in the medullary raphe of the rat increases ventilation in sleep. *Journal of Applied Physiology* 90(4)(2001): 1247–57.

21. Lalley, P. M. μ-Opioid receptor agonist effects on medullary respiratory neurons in the cat: Evidence for involvement in certain types of ventilatory disturbances. *American Journal of Physiology-Regulatory, Integrative and Comparative Physiology* 285(6)(2003): R1287–304.

22. Erb, T. O., et al. Fentanyl does not reduce the incidence of laryngospasm in children anesthetized with sevoflurane. *The Journal of the American Society of Anesthesiologists* 113(1)(2010): 41–7.

23. Bennett, J. A., et al. Difficult or impossible ventilation after sufentanil-induced anesthesia is caused primarily by vocal cord closure. *The Journal of the American Society of Anesthesiologists* 87(5)(1997): 1070–4.

24. Bolser, D. C. Current and future centrally acting antitussives. *Respiratory Physiology & Neurobiology* 152(3)(2006): 349–55.

25. Walker, J. M., et al. Chronic opioid use is a risk factor for the development of central sleep apnea and ataxic breathing. *Journal of Clinical Sleep Medicine* 3(5)(2007): 455–61.

26. Santiago, T. V., et al. Respiratory consequences of methadone: The Response to Added Resistance to Breathing 1–3. *American Review of Respiratory Disease* 122(4)(1980): 623–8.

27. Santiago, T. V., A. C. Pugliese, N. H. Edelman. Control of breathing during methadone addiction. *The American Journal of Medicine* 62(3)(1977): 347–54.

28. Yuan, C.-S., et al. Methylnaltrexone prevents morphine-induced delay in oral–cecal transit time without affecting analgesia: A double-blind randomized placebo-controlled trial. *Clinical Pharmacology & Therapeutics* 59(4)(1996): 469–75.

29. Viscusi, E. R., et al. Peripherally acting mu-opioid receptor antagonists and postoperative ileus: Mechanisms of action and clinical applicability. *Anesthesia & Analgesia* 108(6)(2009): 1811–22.

30. Kurz, A., D. I. Sessler. Opioid-induced bowel dysfunction. *Drugs* 63(7)(2003): 649–71.

31. Wood, J. D., J. J. Galligan. Function of opioids in the enteric nervous system. *Neurogastroenterology & Motility* 16(s2)(2004): 17–28.

32. Cassel, J. A., J. D. Daubert, and R. N. DeHaven. [3H]Alvimopan binding to the μ opioid receptor: Comparative binding kinetics of opioid antagonists. *European Journal of Pharmacology* 520(1)(2005): 29–36.

33. Sternini, C., et al. The opioid system in the gastrointestinal tract. *Neurogastroenterology & Motility* 16(s2)(2004): 3–16.

34. Meerveld, G.-V., et al. Preclinical studies of opioids and opioid antagonists on gastrointestinal function. *Neurogastroenterology & Motility* 16(s2)(2004): 46–53.

35. Fragen, R. J., et al. The effect of remifentanil on biliary tract drainage into the duodenum. *Anesthesia & Analgesia* 89(6)(1999): 1561.

36. Kamphuis, E. T., et al. The effects of spinal anesthesia with lidocaine and sufentanil on lower urinary tract functions. *Anesthesia & Analgesia* 107(6)(2008): 2073–8.

37. Kuipers, P. W., et al. Intrathecal opioids and lower urinary tract function: A urodynamic evaluation. *The Journal of the American Society of Anesthesiologists* 100(6)(2004): 1497–503.

38. Buss, T., W. Leppert. Opioid-induced endocrinopathy in cancer patients: An underestimated clinical problem. *Advances in Therapy* 31(2)(2014): 153–67.

39. Delitala, G., et al. Opioids stimulate growth hormone (GH) release in man independently of GH-releasing hormone. *The Journal of Clinical Endocrinology & Metabolism* 69(2) (1989): 356–8.

40. Abs, R., et al. Endocrine consequences of long-term intrathecal administration of opioids. *The Journal of Clinical Endocrinology & Metabolism* 85(6) (2000): 2215–22.

41. Hemmings, R., G. Fox, G. Tolis. Effect of morphine on the hypothalamic pituitary axis in postmenopausal women. *Fertility and Sterility* 37(3) (1982): 389–91.

42. Howlett, T. A., L. H. Rees. Endogenous opioid peptides and hypothalamic pituitary function. *Annual Review of Physiology* 48(1)(1986): 527–36.

43. Grossman, A., et al. Different opioid mechanisms are involved in the modulation of ACTH and gonadotrophin release in man. *Neuroendocrinology* 42(4)(1986): 357–60.

44. Daniell, H. W. Hypogonadism in men consuming sustained-action oral opioids. *The Journal of Pain* 3(5) (2002): 377–84.

45. Bovill, J. G. Surgery for cancer: Does anesthesia matter? *Anesthesia & Analgesia* 110(6)(2010): 1524–6.

46. Amano, H., et al. Roles of a prostaglandin E-type receptor, EP3, in upregulation of matrix metalloproteinase-9 and vascular endothelial growth factor during enhancement of tumor metastasis. *Cancer Science* 100(12)(2009): 2318–24.

47. Goodman, L. S., L. L. Brunton, B. Chabner, B. C. Knollmann. *Goodman & Gilman's Pharmacological Basis of Therapeutics.* New York: McGraw-Hill, 2011. Print. Chapter 18, p. 481.

48. Babb, M., G. Koren, A. Einarson. Treating pain during pregnancy. *Canadian Family Physician* 56(1)(2010 Jan): 25, 27.

49. Demarest, S. P., R. S. Gill, R. A. Adler. Opioid endocrinopathy. *Endocrine Practice* 21(2)(2015):190–8.

50. Fishman, S., J. J. Bonica. *Bonica's Management of Pain.* Baltimore, MD: Lippincott Williams & Wilkins, 2015.

51. American Pain Society Recommendations for improving the quality of acute and cancer pain management. *Archives of Internal Medicine* 165(14):1574–80.

52. Williams, J. P., Thompson, J. P., McDonald, J., et al. Human peripheral blood mononuclear cells express nociception/orphanin FQ. But not mu, kappa, delta opioid receptors. *Anesthesia & Analgesia* 105(2007):998–1005.

Chapter 11

Intravenous Anesthetics

Sriniketh Sundar and Christopher Sikorski

Overview

Pharmacodynamics

- Sedative–hypnotic: all intravenous (IV) anesthetics
- Amnestic: benzodiazepines > other IV anesthetics
- Anxiolytic: benzodiazepines > other IV anesthetics
- Anticonvulsant: barbiturates, benzodiazepines, etomidate, propofol
  - Exception: methohexital is epileptogenic
- Analgesic: ketamine, dexmedetomidine
- Antiemetic: propofol

Pharmacokinetics

See Table 11.1.

Comparison of Context-Sensitive Half-Time (CSHT)

See Figure 11.1.

Propofol

Pharmacodynamics[1,2,3]

- Propofol acts via agonism of neuroinhibitory $GABA_A$ receptors, and perhaps via antagonism of NMDA receptors.
- Effects: sedative–hypnotic, amnestic, anxiolytic, anticonvulsant, and antiemetic
  - Antiemetic mechanism of action is unclear (possibly antidopaminergic and/or antiserotonergic activity causing depression of the chemoreceptor trigger zone in the area postrema).

Pharmacokinetics

- Propofol exhibits rapid onset and prompt offset after boluses or brief infusions.
  - It has a relatively short CSHT even after prolonged infusions.
- Undergoes rapid hepatic and extrahepatic metabolism to renally excreted inactive metabolites
  - Propofol clearance exceeds hepatic blood flow.
  - Sites of extrahepatic metabolism: lungs, kidneys.

Cerebrovascular Effects

- Propofol reduces cerebral metabolic rate of oxygen ($CMRO_2$), cerebral blood flow (CBF), and intracranial pressure (ICP).

Cardiovascular Effects

- Induces substantial *hypotension via vasodilation* (both venodilation/↓ preload and arterodilation/↓ afterload) and direct myocardial depression (↓ contractility)
- Inhibits the baroreceptor reflex so the hypotension it induces does not result in tachycardia
  - The lack of reflex tachycardia may account for the more profound hypotension from propofol than from thiopental.

Respiratory Effects

- Propofol causes significant dose-dependent *respiratory depression* through *reduction in minute ventilation* and

Table 11.1 Intravenous anesthetics: dosage, onset, and duration of action

Drug	Induction dose (mg/kg)	Onset (s)	Duration of action (min)
Thiopental	3–5	<30	5–10
Methohexital	1–1.5	<30	5–10
Propofol	1–2.5	15–45	5–10
Etomidate	0.2–0.3	15–45	3–10
Ketamine	1–2	45–60	10–20
Midazolam	0.1–0.3	30–90	10–30
Diazepam	0.3–0.6	45–90	15–30
Lorazepam	0.03–0.1	60–120	60–120

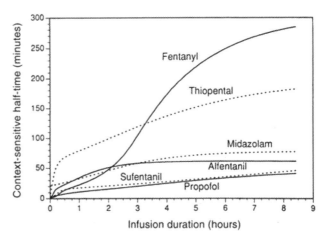

Figure 11.1 Comparison of context-sensitive half-times

suppression of the ventilatory response to hypercarbia and hypoxemia.
- Suppresses airway reflexes and induces bronchodilation

Other Physiological and Adverse Effects
- Pain on injection is common but can be attenuated by injection into larger veins, dilution of propofol, injection of lidocaine before propofol, or premedication with an opioid.
- Prolonged infusion (>48 h) of high-dose propofol (>67 mcg/kg/min) can cause propofol infusion syndrome, particularly in pediatric and critically ill patients.
  - Symptoms: hyperlipidemia, metabolic acidosis, rhabdomyolysis, renal failure, refractory bradycardia, cardiovascular collapse
- Rare anaphylaxis in patients with allergy to eggs or soy
- The propofol emulsion supports bacterial growth. Strict aseptic technique is recommended when drawing up the medication and it should be administered within 12 h after being drawn up.

Indications and Contraindications
- Primarily used for induction of general anesthesia and for sedation for surgeries under local/regional anesthesia, endoscopies, or mechanical ventilation in the ICU
- Total intravenous anesthesia (TIVA) with propofol in lieu of inhalational anesthesia can help prevent postoperative nausea and vomiting (PONV), and subanesthetic boluses/infusion can be used to treat PONV.
- Avoided or used with caution in patients with hemodynamic instability, cardiac disease (i.e., coronary heart disease [CAD], aortic stenosis), or cerebrovascular disease.

Barbiturates: Methohexital, Thiopental

Pharmacodynamics[1,2,3]
- Barbiturates act via *agonism of neuroinhibitory GABA$_A$ receptors*, which increases their chloride conductance and causes neuronal hyperpolarization and inhibition.
  - Lower doses: impede dissociation of GABA from its receptor and hence increase duration of chloride channel opening
  - Higher doses: activate GABA receptor chloride channels directly

- Effects: sedative–hypnotic, amnestic, anticonvulsant, and potentially *hyperalgesic*
  - Exception: methohexital is epileptogenic.

Pharmacokinetics
- Barbiturates exhibit rapid onset and offset after single induction boluses, but delayed offset/awakening with repeated boluses or infusion.
- Undergo *hepatic metabolism* to inactive metabolites that undergo renal or biliary excretion

- Exception: Phenobarbital is mostly renally excreted in unchanged form.
- Barbiturates undergo oxidation as well as desulfurization and N-dealkylation.

Cerebrovascular Effects
- Barbiturates reduce CMRO$_2$, CBF, and ICP.

Cardiovascular Effects
- Induce substantial hypotension via vasodilation and direct myocardial depression with consequent baroreceptor-mediated reflex tachycardia
  - Therefore, avoid or use with caution in patients with hemodynamic instability and/or cardiac disease (e.g., CAD, aortic stenosis).

Respiratory Effects
- Cause significant dose-dependent respiratory depression through reduction in minute ventilation and suppression of the ventilatory response to hypercarbia and hypoxemia
- Suppress airway reflexes (but less effectively than propofol)

Other Physiological and Adverse Effects
- Methohexital may cause coughing, hiccupping, twitching, and tremors.
- Phenobarbital is a strong CYP3A4 inducer.
- Barbiturates promote production of porphyrins (via stimulation of δ-aminolevulinic acid synthetase) and may precipitate *acute intermittent porphyria* in predisposed patients.
- Mixture of barbiturates (which are dissolved in normal saline or water to produce alkaline solution) with acidic solutions (e.g., Ringer's lactate, neuromuscular blockers, midazolam) results in *precipitation and blood vessel occlusion.*
- Extravasation of barbiturates causes local *tissue irritation.*
- If accidentally injected intra-arterially, barbiturates cause *severe painful vasoconstriction* and *tissue ischemia.*
  - Treatment: intra-arterial injection of papaverine or lidocaine, heparinization, and stellate ganglion block (i.e., sympathectomy)

Indications and Contraindications
- Barbiturates are used primarily for induction of general anesthesia.
  - Methohexital may be administered rectally (e.g., pediatric patients).
- Methohexitals epileptogenicity makes it particularly useful for anesthetic induction for electroconvulsive therapy (ECT).
- Thiopental may be used for sedation after traumatic brain injury, reduction of elevated ICP, or neuroprotection from focal cerebral ischemia.

Benzodiazepines: Midazolam, Diazepam, Lorazepam

Pharmacodynamics[1,2,3]

- Benzodiazepines act via *agonism of neuroinhibitory GABA$_A$ receptors*, which increases their chloride conductance and causes neuronal hyperpolarization and inhibition.
  - Specifically, they enhance coupling of GABA with its receptor and hence increase frequency of chloride channel opening.
- Effects: sedative–hypnotic, amnestic, anxiolytic, and anticonvulsant
  - Particularly potent for anxiolysis and anterograde amnesia
  - Greater sensitivity in geriatric patients

Pharmacokinetics

- Benzodiazepines have quick onset but their offset is relatively slow even after a single bolus and is substantially protracted after infusion.
- Undergo hepatic metabolism to renally excreted metabolites
  - Midazolam and diazepam undergo metabolism by *CYP3A4* with *active* metabolites.
    - Dose cautiously in patients with renal impairment or on medications that are CYP3A4 inhibitors
- Lorazepam undergoes conjugation to an inactive metabolite.
- Benzodiazepine metabolism is increased with habitual alcohol consumption, but decreased with cirrhosis.

Cerebrovascular Effects

- Benzodiazepines decrease CMRO$_2$ and CBF, but to a lesser extent than barbiturates and propofol, and have negligible effect on ICP.

Cardiovascular Effects

- Cause relatively modest BP reduction via mild arteriodilation (decrease SVR) without affecting HR or cardiac contractility
  - Hypotensive effect potentiated by coadministration with opioids

Respiratory Effects

- When used alone, benzodiazepines produce relatively minimal, dose-dependent respiratory depression and rarely cause apnea.
  - Hypoventilatory effect potentiated by coadministration with opioids
- Predisposed to upper airway obstruction by reduction of oropharyngeal tone

Other Physiological and Adverse Effects

- Associated with *postoperative delirium* in patients with critical illness, advanced age, and/or dementia
- *Prolonged sedation* from midazolam and diazepam can occur with renal insufficiency or coadministration of CYP3A4 inhibitors (i.e., antifungals, antiretrovirals).
- Diazepam and lorazepam are formulated with propylene glycol, which makes IV injection painful and has the potential for toxicity with prolonged infusions.
  - Propylene glycol toxicity: skin and soft tissue necrosis (from extravasation), hemolysis, dysrhythmias, hypotension, lactic acidosis, seizure, coma, multi-organ failure

Indications and Contraindications

- Benzodiazepines have effective anxiolytic and amnestic properties with minimal respiratory depressant effect. It is typically used for premedication before general or regional anesthesia.
  - Midazolam can be administered IV, IM, or also in PO form (i.e., pediatric patients).
- Used as adjuncts for intraoperative sedation and induction or maintenance of general anesthesia
  - Can reduce the minimum alveolar concentration (MAC) of volatile anesthetics
- Can be used for *treatment of seizure activity* secondary to local anesthetic systemic toxicity (LAST), alcohol withdrawal, or status epilepticus
- Use midazolam and diazepam with caution in the setting of renal impairment due to active, renally excreted metabolites.

Antagonism: Flumazenil

- Flumazenil is a *competitive antagonist* at benzodiazepine GABA$_A$ receptors that is effective at rapidly reversing their sedative effect.
- It may be used for benzodiazepine-related delayed awakening or overt benzodiazepine overdose.
- May have a shorter duration of action than the benzodiazepine so *re-sedation may occur*, requiring redosing
- Unlike naloxone for opioid reversal, flumazenil for benzodiazepine reversal has *negligible cardiovascular effects*.

Dexmedetomidine

Pharmacodynamics[4]

- Dexmedetomidine acts as a highly *selective central α_2-adrenergic receptor agonist* that induces endogenous sleep-promoting pathways.
- Effects: sedative-hypnotic, amnestic, anxiolytic, and analgesic
  - It generates natural sleep patterns and allows easy arousal.
  - Unlike most other IV anesthetics, it also has analgesic and opioid-sparing properties (but less than ketamine).

Pharmacokinetics

- Slower onset and offset of sedation than propofol
- It undergoes hepatic metabolism (both glucuronidation and CYP2A6-mediated metabolism) to renally excreted inactive metabolites.
  - Dose cautiously in patients on medications that are CYP2A6 inhibitors.

Cerebrovascular Effects

- The effects of dexmedetomidine on $CMRO_2$, CBF, and ICP are not well-established.

Cardiovascular Effects

- Infusion of dexmedetomidine may cause bradycardia, vasodilation, and hypotension.
- However, a "loading" bolus may transiently cause either hypotension or hypertension, depending on whether central α_2-mediated vasodilation or peripheral α_2-mediated vasoconstriction predominates.

Respiratory Effects

- Generally preserves respiratory drive; there may be a slight reduction in tidal volumes but the respiratory rate and ventilatory response to hypercarbia are unchanged.

Other Physiological and Adverse Effects

- Prolonged (>24 h) infusion of dexmedetomidine may cause receptor upregulation and consequent *withdrawal if abruptly discontinued* (e.g., hypertension, tachycardia, agitation).

Indications and Contraindications

- Due to its ability to produce *sedation with preservation of respiratory drive,* dexmedetomidine is useful for awake fiber-optic intubation and intraoperative sedation.
- In the critical care setting, dexmedetomidine can be used to provide sedation for mechanically ventilated patients to keep them comfortable yet interactive or easily awakened.
- Due to its analgesic and opioid-sparing effects, dexmedetomidine is a useful anesthetic in patients prone to postoperative hypoventilation/apnea (i.e., obstructive sleep apnea [OSA]).
- Because of its bradycardic and hypotensive effects, dexmedetomidine should be used with caution in patients with baseline bradycardia or hypotension.

Etomidate

Pharmacodynamics[1,2,3]

- Etomidate acts via agonism of neuroinhibitory $GABA_A$ receptors.
  - Lower (clinical) doses: reduces amount of GABA necessary to activate GABA receptors
  - Higher (supraclinical) doses: directly activates GABA receptors without GABA
  - Effects: sedative–hypnotic, anticonvulsant
    - Also possibility of activating epileptic foci on EEG without causing convulsions

Pharmacokinetics

- Exhibits rapid onset and prompt offset after boluses or even prolonged infusions
- *Hydrolyzed* by *hepatic and plasma esterases* to renally excreted inactive metabolites

Cerebrovascular Effects

- Etomidate decreases $CMRO_2$, CBF, and ICP.

Cardiovascular Effects

- Relatively minimal cardiovascular effects (slight decrease in SVR and MAP, negligible increase in HR and CO) and so allows hemodynamic stability on induction
- Will not blunt the sympathetic response to direct laryngoscopy so it should be coadministered with an opioid

Respiratory Effects

- Causes relatively minor dose-dependent respiratory depression and is unlikely to cause apnea when used alone

Other Physiological and Adverse Effects

- Even a single induction dose of etomidate can *induce adrenocortical suppression* for several hours, blocking the normal stress-induced increase in cortisol production, and its use in critically ill patients has been associated with *increased mortality.*
  - Mechanism: *inhibition of 11β-hydroxylase*, which aids in biosynthesis of cortisol
  - Thus, despite its excellent CSHT, etomidate is not used for continuous infusion.
- Formulated with propylene glycol, which makes IV injection painful and has the potential for propylene glycol toxicity with prolonged infusions
- Associated with myoclonic movements, hiccups, and PONV
  - Myoclonic activity is due to subcortical disinhibition as opposed to cortical seizure activity, and may be attenuated by preadministration of benzodiazepine or opioid.

Indications and Contraindications

- Generally reserved for induction of general anesthesia
- Due to its minimal cardiovascular effects, etomidate is advantageous for induction in patients with cardiac disease (e.g., CAD, aortic stenosis) and/or hemodynamic instability.
- Due to its adrenocortical suppression, etomidate should be used with caution for induction in patients who have sepsis, other critical illness, or adrenal insufficiency, and should not be used for continuous infusion.
- Due to its emetogenic effect, etomidate should be avoided in patients who are at high risk for PONV.

Ketamine

Pharmacodynamics[1,2,3]

- Ketamine acts primarily via antagonism of neuroexcitatory *N*-methyl-D-aspartate (NMDA) receptors and, to a lesser extent, via agonism of opioid and monoamine (serotonin, norepinephrine, dopamine) receptors.

- ○ It produces a functional dissociation between the thalamocortical system (depressed) and limbic system (stimulated).
- ○ NMDA receptors are involved in central sensitization.
- Effects: sedative–hypnotic, amnestic, anticonvulsant, and analgesic
  - ○ Ketamine produces *dissociative anesthesia*, a unique cataleptic trance-like state with preservation of brain-stem reflexes, spontaneous breathing, and possibly consciousness but profound analgesia and amnesia.
  - ○ Unlike other IV anesthetics, ketamine has *potent analgesic properties* with potential opioid-sparing effects and inhibits central sensitization.
- Ketamine is a racemic mixture of R(−) and S(+) isomers, the latter of which has 3–4 times more anesthetic and analgesic potency with faster offset and fewer psychomimetic effects.

Pharmacokinetics

- Exhibits rapid onset and prompt offset after boluses or brief infusions
- Undergoes hepatic cytochrome P450 metabolism (CYP3A4, CYP2B6, CYP2C9) to multiple renally excreted metabolites, including the seizure-inducing metabolite *norketamine* (one-third as potent as parent compound)
  - ○ Dose cautiously in patients with renal impairment or on medications that are CYP450 enzyme inhibitors.

Cerebrovascular Effects

- Unlike other IV anesthetics, ketamine increases $CMRO_2$, CBF, and ICP, as well as intraocular pressure (IOP).

Cardiovascular Effects

- Stimulates the sympathetic nervous system and *increases plasma catecholamine* levels, which increases HR, cardiac contractility, CO, and BP
  - ○ Its hyperdynamic effects can be attenuated with benzodiazepines or opioids.
- Has *direct myocardial depressant effects* (normally counteracted and outweighed by its sympathomimetic effects)

Respiratory Effects

- Generally preserves respiratory effort and is unlikely to cause apnea even after induction doses
- Causes *bronchodilation* and preserves upper airway reflexes, though airway protection is not guaranteed

Other Physiological and Adverse Effects

- May cause *psychomimetic emergence reactions*: vivid dreams, extracorporeal experiences, and hallucinations, which may be euphoric or dysphoric
  - ○ Less common in children than in adults
  - ○ Premedication with a benzodiazepine can attenuate this.
- Causes *sialorrhea*, which can potentially provoke laryngospasm in an unprotected airway
  - ○ Premedication with glycopyrrolate can attenuate this.
- May also cause lacrimation, nystagmus, and myoclonic movements

Indications and Contraindications

- Most often used for induction of general anesthesia or as an intraoperative anesthetic adjunct (continuous subanesthetic infusion or intermittent boluses) for *preventative analgesia*
  - ○ It may be given IM (i.e., pediatric patients).
  - ○ It is the best IV anesthetic for induction in patients with active bronchospasm.
  - ○ It is particularly useful for chronic pain patients.
- Due to its analgesic and opioid-sparing effects, ketamine is a useful IV anesthetic in patients prone to postoperative hypoventilation/apnea (i.e., OSA).
- Due to its sympathomimetic effects, ketamine is advantageous in patients with hypovolemia, hemorrhage, septic shock, or cardiac tamponade, but disadvantageous in patients with CAD, uncontrolled HTN, and aneurysms.
- Ketamine infusions are used to treat complex regional pain syndrome (CRPS) and severe depression.
- Due to its direct myocardial depressant effect, ketamine should be used with caution in patients with heart failure or potentially depleted catecholamine reserves.
- Due to its potential to increase CBF and ICP, ketamine should be avoided in the setting of head trauma or cerebral space-occupying lesions.
- Due to its potential to increase IOP, ketamine should be used with caution in patients with open eye injuries.
- Due to its psychomimetic effects, ketamine is contraindicated in schizophrenia.
- Because it exhibits serotonin norepinephrine reuptake inhibitor (SNRI) effects, ketamine should be used cautiously in patients taking SNRIs, or monoamine oxidase inhibitors.

Overview of Pharmacodynamics

- After induction doses
  - ○ Rapid onset is due to *lipophilicity* and relatively *high CBF*.
  - ○ Offset is due to *redistribution* from the brain (highly perfused) to muscle and fat (less perfused).
- Time to offset after discontinuation of infusion depends on the CSHT, which is how long it takes for the plasma level to decrease 50% in relation to the duration of infusion (the "context") once stopped[5,6]:
  - ○ Short CSHT (optimal for infusion):
    - ■ Etomidate (<5 min after 0.5 h, 25 min after 8 h), ketamine (<5 min after 0.5 h, 40 min after 8 h), propofol (<10 min after 0.5 h, 40 min after 8 h)

- o Intermediate CSHT (suboptimal for infusion):
  - Midazolam (25 min after 0.5 h, 75 min after 8 h)
  - o Long CSHT (not recommended for infusion):
    - Thiopental (>60 min after 0.5 h), diazepam (>150 min after 0.5 h)
- In general, IV anesthetics are eliminated via *hepatic metabolism* followed by *renal excretion* of metabolites, which may be inactive (majority) or active (minority).
  - o Active metabolites (dose cautiously in setting of *renal insufficiency*): midazolam, diazepam, ketamine
  - o Inactive metabolites: all other IV anesthetics
- Plasma protein binding (PPB) impedes diffusion across membranes, which opposes its action but also slows its elimination.
  - o Decreased PPB (e.g., due to hepatic or renal disease) may increase IV anesthetic duration of action as well as its elimination.

Hepatic Effects
- Hepatic clearance of IV anesthetic depends on hepatic blood flow and function (i.e., enzymatic activity and protein production).
  - o Reduced hepatic blood flow (e.g., CHF, ↓ CO, ↑ SVR) impairs hepatic clearance.
    - High hepatic extraction ratio: etomidate, ketamine, propofol
    - Intermediate hepatic extraction ratio: methohexital, midazolam
    - Low hepatic extraction ratio: thiopental, diazepam, lorazepam
- Cirrhosis has an unpredictable effect on hepatic clearance because of enzyme hypoactivity.

Cerebrovascular Effects
- Barbiturates, etomidate, and propofol significantly decrease $CMRO_2$, CBF, and ICP.
- Benzodiazepines modestly decrease $CMRO_2$ and CBF without reducing ICP.
- Effects of dexmedetomidine on $CMRO_2$, CBF, and ICP are not well-established.
- Ketamine increases $CMRO_2$, CBF, and ICP.

Cardiovascular Effects
- Hypotension: barbiturates (↓ BP, ↑ HR), dexmedetomidine (↓ BP, ↓ HR), propofol (↓ BP, stable HR)
- Stability: benzodiazepines (stable or mild ↓ BP, stable HR), etomidate (mild ↓ BP, stable HR)
- Hypertension: ketamine (↑ BP, ↑ HR)

Respiratory Effects
- Substantial, dose-dependent respiratory depression: barbiturates, propofol
  - o Transient apnea may occur after induction doses.
- Minimal, dose-dependent respiratory depression: benzodiazepines, dexmedetomidine, etomidate, ketamine (least)
  - o Apnea is unlikely to occur when these agents are used alone.

Other Physiological and Adverse Effects
- Adrenocortical suppression: etomidate
- Bronchodilation: ketamine, propofol
- Epileptogenic activity: methohexital
- Myoclonic activity: etomidate, ketamine
- Painful injection: lorazepam, diazepam, etomidate, propofol
- Porphyrogenic (precipitate acute intermittent porphyria): barbiturates
- Propylene glycol toxicity: lorazepam, diazepam, etomidate
- Psychomimetic effects: ketamine
- Sialorrhea: ketamine

Indications
- Premedication: midazolam
- Sedation: midazolam, dexmedetomidine, ketamine, propofol
- Induction of general anesthesia: barbiturates, etomidate, ketamine, propofol
  - o Etomidate: patients requiring hemodynamic stability (i.e., CAD, cerebrovascular disease, cerebral aneurysms)
  - o Ketamine: patients requiring hemodynamic augmentation (i.e., hypovolemia, hemorrhage, septic shock, cardiac tamponade)
  - o Methohexital: patients undergoing ECT
  - o Propofol, thiopental: patients able to tolerate cardiovascular depression
- TIVA: propofol (primary anesthetic), ketamine (adjunct), midazolam (adjunct)
- Preventative analgesia: ketamine and, to a lesser extent, dexmedetomidine
- PONV, prevention/treatment: propofol

References

1. J. F. Butterworth and D. C. Mackey. Clinical Pharmacology: Intravenous Anesthetics. In: Butterworth J. F., Mackey D. C., and Wasnick J. D., eds. *Morgan & Mikhail's Clinical Anesthesiology*, 5th edn. New York: McGraw Hill, 2013; 175–87.

2. H. Eilers. Intravenous Anesthetics. In: Stoelting R. K. and Miller R. D., eds. *Basics of Anesthesia*, 6th edn.

Philadelphia, PA: Elsevier Saunders, 2011; 99–114.

3. F. Puskas, M. B. Howie, and G. P. Graviee (2013). Induction of Anesthesia. In: Hensley F. A.,

Martin D. E., and Gravlee G. P., eds. *A Practical Approach to Cardiac Anesthesia*, 5th edn. Philadelphia, PA: Lippincott Williams & Wilkins, 2013; 180–91.

4. K. J. Tietze and B. Fuchs. Sedative-Analgesic Medications in Critically Ill Adults: Properties, Dosage Regimens, and Adverse Effects. In: Parson P. E. and Avidan M. eds. *UpToDate*, Waltham, MA. www.uptodate.com/contents/sedative-analgesic-medications-in-critically-ill-adults-properties-dosage-regimens-and-adverse-effects (accessed February 28, 2017).

5. J. Vuyk, E. Sitsen, and M. Reekers. Intravenous Anesthetics. In: Miller R. D., Cohen N. H., Eriksson L. I., et al., eds. *Miller's Anesthesia*, 8th edn. Philadelphia, PA: Elsevier Saunders, 2015; 821–63.

6. P. F. White and M. R. Eng. Intravenous Anesthetics. In: Barash P. G., Cullen B. F., Stoelting R. K., et al., eds. *Clinical Anesthesia*, 7th edn. Philadelphia, PA: Lippincott Williams & Wilkins, 2013; 478–500.

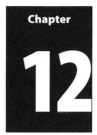

Chapter 12

Local Anesthetics

Christina L. Jeng and Chang H. Park

General Characteristics

Structure

There are three major structural components of local anesthetics (see Figure 12.1)[1]:

1. Lipophilic benzene ring
2. Hydrophilic tertiary amine (responsible for weak base properties)
3. Amide or ester linkage connects above components; determines class of local anesthetic

Amide vs. ester local anesthetics

- Esters (chloroprocaine, tetracaine, procaine, cocaine, benzocaine) are metabolized by pseudocholinesterase in plasma.
- Amides (lidocaine, ropivacaine, bupivacaine, mepivacaine, etidocaine, prilocaine – all have letter "i" before "caine") are metabolized by hepatic microsomal enzymes and are affected by liver dysfunction such as cirrhosis.

Function and mechanism of action

- Local anesthetics are placed in proximity to nerve membranes to produce reversible conduction of blockade. Systemic absorption progressively reduces their effect.
- Uncharged form of local anesthetics readily crosses cell membranes. Charged form of local anesthetics bind to intracellular sodium channels to keep them closed → Prevents increase in permeability of nerve membrane to sodium ions → Slows rate of depolarization. Threshold potential is not reached → Action potential is not propagated.
- Three successive nodes of Ranvier have to be blocked in order to have predictable conduction blockade.

Nerve fibers' susceptibility to blockade

- Order of blockade (fastest to slowest): Autonomic > sensory > motor
- Small diameter nerves more easily blocked than large diameter nerves
- Myelinated nerves more easily blocked than nonmyelinated nerves
- Active nerves more easily blocked than nonactive nerves

See Table 12.1 for characteristics of nerve fibers.

Pharmacological Properties

- Potency: Proportional to lipid solubility
- Speed of onset: Largely dependent on pKa (pH at which 50% of molecules exist in unionized form and 50% in ionized form). Lower pKa = higher percentage in unionized form (because uncharged form of local anesthetics readily cross cell membranes) → faster onset
- Duration of action: Dependent on *protein binding*: higher affinity for protein leads to longer duration
- Termination of action: Diffusion away from site of action. See Table 12.2 for summary.

Ester linkage

Lipophilic benzene ring

Hydrophilic amine group

Amide linkage

Figure 12.1 Structural components of amide and ester local anesthetics

Table 12.1 Characteristics of nerve fibers

Fiber	Myelinated?	Diameter (μm)	Function/comments
Aα	Yes	12–20	Motor
Aβ	Yes	5–15	Tactile, proprioception
Aγ	Yes	3–8	Muscle tone/most susceptible to block by local anesthetic
Aδ	Yes	2–5	Pain, cold temperature, touch
B	Yes	3	Preganglionic sympathetic
C	No	0.3–1.5	Dull pain, warm temperature, touch/least susceptible to block by local anesthetic

Table 12.2 Pharmacologic properties of various local anesthetics

Agent	pKa	Relative potency	Duration (min)	Maximum dose (mg/kg)
Procaine	8.9	1	45–60	12
Chloroprocaine	8.7	2	30–60	12
Tetracaine	8.5	8		3
Lidocaine	7.9	2	60–120	4.5; 7 w/ epinephrine
Mepivacaine	7.6	2	90–180	4.5; 7 w/ epinephrine
Prilocaine	7.9	2	60–120	8
Bupivacaine	8.1	8	240–480	3
Ropivacaine	8.1	6	240–480	3

Agents that prolong duration of local anesthetics[2]

- Epinephrine: (1) Causes local tissue vasoconstriction, (2) limits systemic absorption, (3) keeps contact with nerve fibers, (4) prolongs duration of action. Little effect on onset
- Most common epinephrine dilution – 1:200,000 = 5 mcg/mL
- Other agents: Buprenorphine, clonidine, dexmedetomidine, dexamethasone, tramadol

Systemic absorption of local anesthetics:

Systemic absorption of local anesthetics depends upon various factors, including:

- Site of local anesthetic delivery (from greatest to least systemic absorption): Intravenous > trachea > intercostal > caudal > epidural > brachial plexus > sciatic > spinal > skin infiltration
- Choice of local anesthetic: High degree of tissue binding (e.g., etidocaine, bupivacaine) or large volume of distribution (e.g., prilocaine) will have lower blood levels
- Dose: Higher dose → higher blood levels. 1% solution = 1,000 mg/100 mL = 10 mg/mL
- Addition of vasoconstrictors: Lowers blood level and increases time to peak blood level
- Metabolism: Need absorption and delivery to site of metabolism
- Metabolism: Esters are metabolized by pseudocholinesterase in plasma; amides are metabolized by hepatic microsomal enzymes.
- Excretion: Both ester and amide local anesthetics undergo renal excretion.

Characteristics of Individual Local Anesthetics

Which local anesthetic to use for which anesthetic technique:

- Spinal: Tetracaine (hyperbaric), bupivacaine (isobaric, hyperbaric, hypobaric), mepivacaine (isobaric)

- Epidural: Chloroprocaine, lidocaine, bupivacaine, ropivacaine
- Peripheral nerve blocks: Lidocaine, mepivacaine, bupivacaine, ropivacaine
- Lidocaine – Most common offending agent for transient neurologic symptoms (TNS)
- Chloroprocaine – Undergoes *rapid ester linkage hydrolysis* by pseudocholinesterase. It is used commonly in obstetrics because of its rapid onset and decreased risk of fetal exposure due to rapid metabolism in bloodstream. Chloroprocaine has a fast speed of onset mostly due to its high concentration rather than its pKa.
- Cocaine – Only local anesthetic with vasoconstricting properties. Used as topical anesthetic for ENT procedures. Side effects include tachycardia, hypertension, and dysrhythmias.
- Bupivacaine – Poses the greatest risk for cardiotoxicity. Severe cardiovascular collapse can be seen with toxic doses. Bupivacaine toxicity is more likely to contribute to ventricular arrhythmias and is more resistant to cardiopulmonary resuscitation than lidocaine. The reasons for this are believed to be due to:
  1. stronger binding to resting and inactivated sodium channels
  2. slower disassociation from sodium channels
- Ropivacaine – Is an enantiomer of bupivacaine, but has reduced systemic toxicity than bupivacaine due to increased vasoconstriction and decreased lipid solubility
- EMLA Cream – Eutectic mixture of local anesthetics = lidocaine 2.5% + prilocaine 2.5%
  o EMLA Cream provides dermal anesthesia. It is commonly used for pediatric IV placement.
  o Applied to intact skin and covered with occlusive dressing. Onset takes 45–60 min and reaches peak effect in 2–3 h
  o Precautions and contraindications include: Patients with allergy to amide anesthetics Patients with congenital methemoglobinemia; or infants <1 year old receiving treatment with methemoglobin-inducing agents because prilocaine metabolite *o*-toluidine can cause methemoglobinemia Patients undergoing treatment with class I or class III antiarrhythmic drugs due to potential additive or synergistic cardiotoxic effects

Complications of Local Anesthetics

- *Allergies* – True allergies to local anesthetics are rare. Allergic-type reactions to *para-amino benzoic acid (PABA) metabolite* are more common. PABA is an *ester metabolite* that can cause allergic-type reactions in small percentage of people. Most reactions that appear allergic are more likely due to epinephrine, systemic toxicity, or vasovagal reaction.
  o Signs: Urticaria, flushing, edema, dyspnea, hypoxia, wheezing, hypotension, tachycardia

○ Treatment: Stop suspected offending agent. Epinephrine, intravenous fluids, oxygen, bronchodilators, H_1 and H_2 blockers, steroids.

- *Cauda Equina syndrome (CES) – Neurotoxicity of sacral nerves.* Anesthesia-related causes of CES include maldistribution of local anesthetic, direct needle-induced trauma, or intraneural injection during spinal anesthetic; spinal cord hematoma, ischemia, or infection; and improper patient positioning. Lidocaine is the most common local anesthetic associated with CES, but there are case reports of bupivacaine as the offending agent.
  ○ Signs: Saddle anesthesia, pain, bladder/bowel dysfunction
  ○ Treatment: Immediate MRI; discussion with surgeon regarding possible decompression

- *TNS* – A pain disorder after receiving a spinal anesthetic with local anesthetic, especially lidocaine. Onset typically occurs 12–24 h after surgery. Risk factors include lithotomy position.
  ○ Signs: Pain and dysesthesia in lower back, buttocks, and lower extremities. No neurologic dysfunction is noted, and MRI and other diagnostic modalities are normal.
  ○ Treatment: Symptoms are usually transient. Treatment consists of NSAIDs. Symptoms usually resolve within 3 days and rarely last more than a week.

- *Methemoglobinemia* – Excess of certain local anesthetic agents have been known to oxidize normal hemoglobin to methemoglobin; methemoglobinemia decreases oxygen delivery to tissues. Classic offending agents are prilocaine (hepatically metabolized to *o*-toluidine, which can induce methemoglobinemia) and benzocaine. Lidocaine and tetracaine have been implicated but rare.
  ○ Signs: Fatigue, headache, cyanosis, dyspnea, mental status changes; can progress to dysrhythmias, coma, and death (>50% of total hemoglobin levels). Classically described as chocolate brown appearance of blood. Decreased SaO_2 despite satisfactory PaO_2 (requires co-oximetry for accurate diagnosis and treatment).
  ○ Treatment: Methylene blue (reduces methemoglobin to normal hemoglobin). G6PD-deficient patients treated with ascorbic acid.

- *Local anesthetic systemic toxicity (LAST)*[3]: Toxicity of the central nervous system (CNS) and cardiovascular system (CVS) due to excessive plasma concentrations of local anesthetic. Initial signs of excitation are typically seen and eventually lead to signs of depression with increasing blood levels of local anesthetics for both CVS and CNS.

○ Lightheadedness/dizziness, vertigo, tinnitus, perioral numbness, metallic taste in mouth
○ Slurred speech, changes in mental status, agitation
○ Tonic–clonic seizures
○ Coma and apnea
○ Death
○ Signs of CVS toxicity (note that CVS is more resistant to local anesthetic adverse effects than CNS):
  - Hypertension, tachycardia initially possible – likely due to sympathetic activity and vasoconstriction
  - Bradycardia and hypotension from arteriolar vasodilation
  - ECG changes: PR prolongation and widening of QRS complex
  - Dysrhythmias, complete heart block
  - CVS collapse, death

○ Treatment[3] (as outlined by American Society of Regional Anesthesia's Checklist for Treatment of LAST):
  - Call for help.
  - Secure airway if not already done so and ventilate with 100% oxygen. Hyperventilate to normalize pH and increase oxygenation.
  - Treat seizures with benzodiazepine or barbiturates. Avoid propofol in setting of cardiovascular instability.
  - ACLS: Chest compressions, defibrillation, vasopressors – adjustment of medications and prolonged effort may be required. Since epinephrine can exacerbate dysrhythmias caused by local anesthetics and reduce the efficacy of lipid emulsion therapy, *reduced doses of epinephrine are recommended* (<1 mcg/kg). Also avoid vasopressin, calcium channel blockers, beta blockers, or local anesthetic.

○ Lipid emulsion[4,5] – 20% lipid emulsion bolus of 1.5 mL/kg over 1 min, repeat every 3–5 min as needed. After sinus rhythm is restored, start 20% lipid emulsion at 0.25 mL/kg/min until hemodynamically stable. Recommended upper limit of lipid emulsion is approximately 10 mL/kg over the first 30 min.
  - Proposed mechanisms of lipid emulsion:
    1. Increases clearance of local anesthetic from plasma or tissue to decrease effective plasma concentration (lipid sink)
    2. Reverses the inhibition of myocardial fatty acid oxidation caused by local anesthetic
  - Alert nearest facility having cardiopulmonary bypass capability.

References

1. C. B. Berde and G. R. Strichartz. Local Anesthetics. In: Miller, R., ed. *Miller's Anesthesia*, 8th edn. Philadelphia, PA: Churchill Livingstone/Elsevier; 2015; 1028–54.

2. C. M. Brummett and B. A. Williams. Additives to local anesthetics for peripheral nerve blockade. *Int Anesthesiol Clin* 2011; 49(4): 104–16.

3. J. M. Neal, C. M. Bernards, J. F. Butterworth, et al. ASRA practice advisory on local anesthetic systemic toxicity. *Reg Anesth Pain Med* 2010; 35: 152–61.

4. M. A. Rosenblatt, M. Abel, G. W. Fischer, et al. Successful use of a 20% lipid emulsion to resuscitate a patient after a presumed bupivacaine-related cardiac arrest. *Anesthesiology* 2006; 105(1): 217–18.

5. G. Weinberg, R. Ripper, D. L. Feinstein, et al. Lipid emulsion infusion rescues dogs from bupivacaine-induced cardiac toxicity. *Reg Anesth Pain Med* 2003; 28(3): 198–202.

Chapter 13

Muscle Relaxants

Katherine Loftus and Andrew Goldberg

Depolarizing Muscle Relaxants: Succinylcholine

Mechanism of Action

- Succinylcholine is an acetylcholine (ACh) receptor agonist. Its structure is two linked ACh molecules.
- Binds ACh receptors and generates a prolonged action potential because it is not metabolized as rapidly as ACh.
- Voltage-gated Na^+ channels become inactivated. Cannot reopen until succinylcholine unbinds the acetylcholine receptor (AchR) (Phase I block)
- A prolonged period of end-plate depolarization → conformational changes in AchR that cause Phase II block (mimics a non-depolarizing block)

Pharmacokinetics and Metabolism

See Boxes 13.1 and 13.2.

Prolongation of Action

Can be due to decreased amount or decreased activity of pseudocholinesterase

- Decreased amount (levels must be reduced >75% for significant prolongation of blockade)
  - Decreased production of enzyme in liver
  - Dilution of enzyme seen in pregnancy, cirrhosis, malnutrition
- Decreased activity
  - Atypical pseudocholinesterase prolongs the duration of action of succinylcholine
    - Dibucaine number: Dibucaine is an amino amide local anesthetic. It is capable of inhibiting the plasma cholinesterase enzyme.
    - In normal patients, dibucaine will inhibit 80% of enzyme activity which corresponds to dibucaine

Box 13.2 Metabolism/termination of action of succinylcholine

- Termination of action when succinylcholine molecules diffuse away from neuromuscular junction (NMJ)
- Subsequent rapid metabolism by pseudocholinesterase (also called plasma cholinesterase or butylcholinesterase) in plasma

Table 13.1 Dibucaine number

	Inhibition by dibucaine	Duration of action of succinylcholine
Normal pseudocholinesterase	80%	5–10 min
Heterozygote for atypical pseudocholinesterase	40–60%	20–30 min
Homozygote for atypical pseudocholinesterase	20%	4–8 h

number of 80. Heterozygous atypical pseudocholinesterase corresponds to a dibucaine number between 30 and 65 (Table 13.1).

- Cholinesterase inhibitors
  - Increase the ACh concentration at nerve terminals and intensify depolarization
  - Reduce the hydrolysis of succinylcholine by inhibiting pseudocholinesterase
  - Common example: echothiophate eye drops used for glaucoma (an organophosphate which causes irreversible inhibition of pseudocholinesterase)
  - Edrophonium is an exception. Has no effect on pseudocholinesterase
- Other drugs can also decrease the activity of pseudocholinesterase (Box 13.3)

Box 13.1 Pharmacokinetic properties of succinylcholine

Rapid onset (30–60 s)
Duration of action <10 min
$ED_{95} = 0.3$ mg/kg**
Intubating dose 1.0–1.5 mg/kg IV
Low lipid solubility → small volume of distribution

**ED_{95} = dose that produces 95% twitch suppression in 50% of individuals

Box 13.3 Drugs that decrease pseudocholinesterase activity

Cholinesterase inhibitors	Cyclophosphamide
Esmolol	Metoclopramide
Pancuronium	Oral contraceptives
Phenelzine	

Box 13.4 Conditions causing susceptibility to succinylcholine-induced hyperkalemia

Burns
Crush injury/massive trauma
Spinal cord injury
Stroke
Guillain–Barré syndrome
Severe Parkinson's disease
Prolonged immobilization
Prolonged sepsis
Myopathies (e.g., Duchenne's)

Side Effects
- Bradycardia and nodal rhythms (after a second dose in adults or initial dose in children)
- Fasciculations
- Myalgias
- ↑ Intragastric pressure (but also ↑ lower esophageal sphincter tone so no ↑ aspiration risk)
- ↑ Intraocular pressure
- Masseter muscle rigidity (a marked increase in tone that prevents laryngoscopy and may be a sign of malignant hyperthermia [MH])
- MH trigger
- ↑ Intracranial pressure. Can be attenuated by hyperventilation. Can be prevented with a defasciculating dose of a non-depolarizer (10–15% of usual intubating dose given about 5 min prior to succinylcholine)
- Histamine release (usually no adverse effect beyond a transient rash)
- Hyperkalemia. Typically increases K⁺ by 0.5 mEq/L
  - K⁺ release is much more extensive after denervation injuries (see Box 13.4), which leads to upregulation of extra-junctional ACh receptors.
  - Risk is increased with increased amount of tissue affected.
  - Period of risk starts 48 h after injury and peaks at 7–10 days, unknown duration of risk (at least 60 days).

Absolute contraindications to succinylcholine are listed in Box 13.5.

Which side effects can be prevented by pretreatment with a defasciculating dose of a non-depolarizer?
- Prevents fasciculations, which prevents increased abdominal pressure and ICP
- Decreases incidence of myalgias
- *Does not* prevent increased intraocular pressure

Non-depolarizing Muscle Relaxants
Mechanism of Action
- Competitive antagonists at the ACh receptor
- Bind to ACh receptors but cannot induce necessary conformational change
- Prevent ACh from binding to its receptor and generating an end-plate potential
- Neuromuscular blockade can occur with only one subunit blocked

Box 13.5 Contraindications to succinylcholine
- Hyperkalemia or susceptibility to succinylcholine-induced hyperkalemia
- Susceptibility to MH
- Open eye injuries
- Avoid routine use in children due to risk of undiagnosed myopathies

Pharmacokinetics
- Highly ionized and water soluble due to quaternary ammonium groups, therefore they do not easily cross blood–brain barrier, placenta, or other lipid membranes.
- Classified by chemical structure as benzylisoquinolone or steroidal compounds
- Pharmacokinetic properties of individual drugs are listed in Table 13.2.

Priming Dose
- Administering 10–15% of the intubating dose 5 min before induction. Enough receptors are occupied to speed the onset of paralysis when the full dose is given. Rarely this can cause dyspnea, diplopia, dysphagia, or respiratory compromise.

Potentiation of Blockade
- Neuromuscular blockade can be augmented by a variety of factors (Box 13.6).

Antagonism of Blockade
Cholinesterase inhibitors (neostigmine, pyridostigmine, edrophonium, physostigmine)
- Cause increased levels of ACh at the NMJ. ACh competes with non-depolarizing agents to reestablish normal neuromuscular transmission.
- Ceiling effect: Once acetylcholinesterase is maximally inhibited, additional drug will not further increase block recovery. Therefore, neuromuscular blockade cannot be adequately reversed if high concentrations of muscle relaxant are still present at the NMJ.
- There should be evidence of spontaneous recovery (train-of-four [TOF] count ≥ 2) prior to administration of cholinesterase inhibitors to avoid prolonged recovery times.
- Side effects: Bradycardia that can progress to sinus arrest, bronchospasm, nausea and vomiting, fecal incontinence, salivation, increased bladder tone, miosis
  - Physostigmine can cause diffuse cerebral excitation (the only cholinesterase inhibitor which is a tertiary amine and crosses the blood–brain barrier).

Anticholinergic Drugs (Glycopyrrolate, Atropine, Scopolamine)
- Paired with cholinesterase inhibitors to minimize unwanted muscarinic side effects
- Glycopyrrolate: Given with neostigmine based on similar time to onset of action
  - Quaternary amine. Does not cross blood–brain barrier. No effect on pupils or CNS

Table 13.2 Properties of non-depolarizing muscle relaxants

Drug name and chemical structure	ED⁹⁵ (mg/kg)	Intubating dose (mg/kg)	Onset of action (min)	Duration of action (min)	Metabolism	Side effects and other clinically relevant facts
Atracurium (benzylisoquinolone)	**0.2**	**0.5**	**2.5–3**	**30–45**	**Primarily by nonspecific esterase hydrolysis (NOT pseudocholinesterase) Also by Hofmann elimination in plasma**	• *Laudanosine is a breakdown product of Hofmann elimination that is associated with CNS excitation and seizures. Laudanosine is metabolized by the liver and excreted renally* • *Dose-dependent histamine release* • Can cause hypotension, tachycardia, bronchospasm, or anaphylaxis
Cisatracurium (benzylisoquinolone)	0.05	0.15–0.2	2–3	40–75	Hofmann elimination (this process is slowed in hypothermia)	• Tends to produce less laudanosine than atracurium due to greater potency and therefore lower doses administered • *Not associated with histamine release, no autonomic effects*
Mivacurium (benzylisoquinolone)	0.08	0.15–0.3	0.5–1	15–20	Pseudocholinesterase	• Block can last hours in patients homozygous for atypical pseudocholinesterase • Not available in the United States
Pancuronium (aminosteroid)	0.07	0.08–0.12	2–3	60–120	Primarily by the liver, 40% renal excretion, 10% bile excretion (reduced clearance in renal and liver failure)	• Vagal blockade and sympathetic stimulation (increased catecholamine release and decreased catecholamine reuptake) • Dose-dependent tachycardia and hypertension • Increased likelihood of ventricular arrhythmias in predisposed patients
Vecuronium (aminosteroid)	0.05	0.1–0.2	2–3	45–90	Minimal metabolism by liver, 75% bile excretion, 25% renal excretion (duration of action somewhat prolonged in renal failure)	• No significant cardiovascular effects • Long-term administration in ICU patients can cause prolonged neuromuscular blockade possibly due to accumulation of its active 3-hydroxy metabolite and can lead to polyneuropathy in some patients
Rocuronium (aminosteroid)	0.3	0.6	1.5	35–75	Almost no metabolism by liver. 10% renal excretion. Primarily cleared by bile (duration of action somewhat prolonged in severe hepatic failure)	• No active metabolites. No significant cardiovascular effects • Rapid onset (60–90 s) at higher dose (1.2 mg/kg) makes it a suitable alternative to succinylcholine for rapid sequence inductions

Box 13.6 Factors that potentiate neuromuscular blockade

Volatile agents:	Decrease non-depolarizer dosage requirements by at least 15%. Desflurane > sevoflurane > isoflurane > N_2O
Combinations of nondepolarizers:	Mixtures of structurally similar compounds produce additive effects; mixtures of structurally dissimilar compounds (ex. aminosteroid + benzylisoquinoline) produce synergistic effects
Hypothermia:	Decreases drug metabolism
Extremes of age:	Neonates are more sensitive to non-depolarizers due to immature NMJs (though dosage requirements not significantly changed due to a larger volume of distribution)
	Reduced drug clearance in elderly populations
Electrolyte abnormalities:	Acidosis, hypokalemia, hypocalcemia, hypermagnesemia augment blockade
Drug interactions:	Antibiotics: aminoglycosides (streptomycin, gentamicin, tobramycin), tetracycline, polymixin, clindamycin
	Dantrolene
Calcium channel blockers	Lithium
	High-dose local anesthetics
	Furosemide

Note: Antiepileptic drugs have opposite effect and can increase resistance to non-depolarizers.

- o Does not cross placenta (although neostigmine does). Atropine should be used instead of glycopyrrolate when utilizing neostigmine for neuromuscular reversal in pregnancy.
- Atropine: Given with edrophonium based on more rapid onset of action

Atropine and scopolomine are tertiary amines and cross the blood–brain barrier. Cause mydriasis, disorientation, and delirium.

Sugammadex
- Binds steroidal muscle relaxants and prevents them from being competitive at ACh receptors
- Successful antagonism occurs at all levels of neuromuscular blockade (profound through shallow)
- Reversal is faster than with cholinesterase inhibitors
- If a patient requires paralysis after receiving a sugammadex dose, a nonsteroidal muscle relaxant should be used
- Concerns regarding hypersensitivity and allergic reactions delayed its approval in the United States

Monitoring of Blockade
- Degree of neuromuscular blockade is commonly monitored with TOF stimulation (four supramaximal stimuli at 2 Hz frequency)

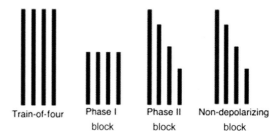

Figure 13.1 Train-of-four evoked responses

- The occurrence of fade indicates a non-depolarizing block or a phase II block with succinylcholine (Figure 13.1)
  - o 1/4 twitches present: 90–95% ACh receptors remain blocked
  - o 2/4 twitches present: 80–90% ACh receptors remain blocked
  - o 3/4 twitches present: 70–80% ACh receptors remain blocked
  - o 4/4 twitches present: 65–75% ACh receptors remain blocked
- Variable sensitivity of muscle groups to muscle relaxants
  - o Diaphragm, muscles of larynx, and facial muscles are most resistant and recover the fastest. Good intubating conditions and surgical conditions associated with loss of eyebrow twitch response
  - o Adductor pollicis and muscles of upper airway patency are more sensitive. Return of twitch response at thumb associated with good extubating conditions

Diseases with altered responses to muscle relaxants (Tables 13.3 and 13.4)

Table 13.3 Response to muscle relaxants in myasthenia gravis and myasthenic syndrome

	Succinylcholine	Non-depolarizers
Myasthenia gravis Antibodies to AchRs on skeletal muscle cause a decreased number of available Ach receptors	Resistance: Exposure to a normal dose may not activate enough ACh receptors to result in perijunctional depolarization	Hypersensitivity (there are less receptors to block, so competitive inhibitors can cause a block at lower doses)
Eaton–Lambert (myasthenic syndrome) Antibodies to calcium channels causing reduced amount of presynaptic ACh release	Hypersensitivity (there are usually increased numbers of postsynaptic ACh receptors)	Hypersensitivity (there is less ACh to compete with, so competitive inhibitors can cause a block at lower doses)

Table 13.4 Diseases with altered responses to non-depolarizing muscle relaxants

Hypersensitivity	Resistance
Myasthenia Gravis	Burns
Eaton–Lambert	Stroke
ALS	Spinal cord injury
Lupus	Prolonged immobility
Familial periodic paralysis	Cerebral palsy
Guillain–Barré syndrome	Tetanus or botulism
Muscular dystrophy	
Myotonia	
Peripheral neuropathies	

References

1. J. F. Butterworth, D. C. Mackey, J. D. Wasnick. *Morgan & Mikhail's Clinical Anesthesiology*, 5th edn. McGraw-Hill Medical, 2013.

2. P. G. Barash, B. F. Cullen, R. K. Stoelting. *Clinical Anesthesia*, 5th edn. Lippincott Williams & Wilkins, 2006.

3. R. D. Miller. *Miller's Anesthesia*, 8th edn. Saunders, 2015.

Chapter 14

Evaluation of the Patient and Preoperative Preparation

Ellen Flanagan

This chapter reviews the role and importance of preoperative assessment and evaluation. Preoperative assessments are performed to prepare patients to undergo anesthesia and surgery while incurring as little risk as possible. The preoperative assessment presents the opportunity to collate patient information available, identify risk, stratify risk, and hopefully mitigate risk by optimization or pre-habilitation. Consideration of the patient's medical risk and the surgical risk in the context of evidence-based guidelines may be used to inform rational decision making when ordering appropriate laboratory and cardiac or pulmonary testing and minimize overuse and underuse of testing. Education regarding what to expect and how to prepare for anesthesia and surgery may reduce the patient and family's anxiety.

Role of preoperative assessment clinic is to have a standardized, evidence-based work up in preparation for anesthesia and surgery. This has been shown to decrease morbidity and mortality.

- Goals of preoperative assessment clinic include:
  - Evidence-based testing
    - Test only when clinically indicated
    - Use national and international guidelines
    - Reduce excessive and unnecessary testing
    - Eliminate testing when there is not a clinical indication
  - Communicating risks to patient and providers
    - Surgeon
    - Anesthesiologist
    - Medicine service
    - Social services, when indicated
  - Ensuring patient optimization
    - Consistent manner of assessment
    - Common systems to optimize
      - Cardiac
      - Pulmonary
      - Anemia
      - Obstructive sleep apnea
      - Smoking cessation
      - Physical reserve
      - Preventive vaccination status
      - Medication management
      - Opioid reduction
      - Treatment of depression or anxiety

- Selective consultation with cardiology, pulmonary, hematology
- Care pathways in place to streamline referrals or facilitate specific optimization goals
- Adequate time between scheduling surgery and surgery to permit optimization efforts (when possible)
- Initiate appropriate medication which may reduce patient risk
  - Statins
  - Beta blockers
  - Minimizing surgical delays and cancellations
    - Reasons for delays and cancellations include:
      - Inadequate preoperative work-up
      - Change in patient's medical condition
      - Failure of patient to arrive on day of surgery
      - Patient's change in desire to proceed to surgery
  - Contribution to the "triple aim" of the Affordable Care Act (ACA):
    - Improve patient experience
    - Improve population health
    - Reduce per capita cost
  - Increased satisfaction for patient and surgeon
    - Facilitating continuity of care from when surgery is scheduled through procedure and discharge
    - Facilitating communication among providers
    - Educating patients
      - Communication regarding patient risks
      - Communication regarding potential opportunities for health improvement and optimization
      - Anesthesia education
        - Preoperative needs
          - Fasting/NPO guidelines
          - Perioperative anticoagulation guidelines
        - Anesthetic technique options

Classification of recommendations:
- Class I: Benefit >>> Risk, no additional studies needed
  - Proceed with procedure/treatment
- Class IIa: Benefit >> Risk, additional studies with focused objectives needed
  - It is reasonable to proceed with procedure/treatment

- Class IIb: Benefit > or = to Risk, additional studies with broad objectives needed
  - It is unreasonable to proceed with procedure/treatment
- Class III: Risk > Benefit, no additional studies needed

  - Do not proceed with procedure/treatment
  Level of evidence:
- Level A: Multiple populations evaluated with general consistency of direction and magnitude of effect with robust evidence to recommend a procedure/treatment
- Level B: Limited population evaluated with a balance of evidence and procedure/treatment is recommended with caution
- Level C: Very limited population evaluated with inadequate evidence and a procedure/treatment is recommended based on consensus opinion.

The level of urgency often dictates the degree of work-up and/or optimization possible.

- Emergent: Threat to life or limb if no surgery <6 h
- Urgent: Life or limb threat if no surgery within 6–24 h
- Time-sensitive: Delay of surgery for >6 weeks will negatively affect outcome
- Elective: Surgery could be delayed up to 1 year without harm
- Surgery performed under emergency conditions proceeds to the operating room with little or no further work-up

  - Need for perioperative invasive monitoring may be increased in emergency surgeries.

The most recent American College of Cardiology (ACC) and American Heart Association (AHA) Guidelines for Perioperative Cardiovascular Evaluation were updated in 2014. For patients with coronary artery disease, the decision to delay surgery for additional work-up can be made based on the following:[1,2,3]

1. If it is an emergency, proceed to surgery.
2. If patient is having acute coronary syndrome (ACS), patient should be referred to or the case should be discussed with a cardiologist for management of ACS prior to surgery.
3. Estimate the risk of having a major adverse cardiac event (MACE) using risk calculators such as the American College of Surgeons National Surgery Quality Improvement Program (NSQIP) or the Revised Cardiac Risk Index (RCRI)
   a. NSQIP risk calculator includes: age, sex, BMI, functional status, ASA score, and variables with patients who have a history of hypertension, diabetes, congestive heart failure (CHF), respiratory comorbidities, etc.
   b. RCRI calculator includes: high risk surgery (i.e. intraperitoneal, intrathoracic, suprainguinal, vascular), history of ischemic heart disease, history of CHF, history of cerebrovascular disease, insulin dependent diabetes, and preoperative creatinine of >2 mg/dL.

4. If MACE risk is <1%, the patient is deemed as low risk and can proceed with surgery.
5. If MACE risk is >1%, their functional capacity needs to be determined.
   a. If metabolic equivalents (METS) >4, proceed with surgery.
   b. If METS <4 or functional capacity cannot be determined, the team needs to determine whether further testing will impact the perioperative management and risk to the patient.
      i. If further testing is recommended, obtain stress test or stress echo.

Other common preoperative management guidelines:
- Electrocardiogram (EKG): Level B evidence, no Class I recommendation for acquiring an EKG
- Echocardiogram: no Class I recommendation
- Balloon angioplasty: Class I recommendation to wait 14 days after a balloon angioplasty before proceeding with noncardiac surgery, 30 days after bare metal stent and 6 months after drug-eluting stent
- Beta-blockers: Class I recommendation to continue beta-blockers in patients on chronic beta-blocker therapy
  - In patients with more than three RCRI risk factors, it is reasonable to start beta-blocker therapy BUT not on the day of the surgery.

American Society of Anesthesiologists (ASA) Physical Status Classification:

1. Normal, healthy patient
2. Patient with mild systemic disease
3. Patient with severe systemic disease but the disease is not a threat to life
4. Patient with severe systemic disease that is a constant threat to life
5. Moribund patient not expected to survive without the surgery
6. Brain dead patient for organ donation.

Risk identification and mitigation is important in determining how best to manage patient and proceed with surgery. It may be necessary to delay surgery for

- Cardiac or pulmonary comorbidities requiring additional information to assess risk of surgery vs. benefit of procedure
- To allow for preoperative risk mitigation and patient optimization

Work-up is necessary in patients with: high-grade Mobitz type II or 3rd degree block, symptomatic ventricular arrhythmias, severe/symptomatic aortic or mitral valve stenosis, pulmonary hypertension, severe respiratory pathology, and stable angina.[4,5]

- Preoperative laboratory testing
  - No tests required in healthy patients undergoing surgery with low risk of complications. However, a urine pregnancy or blood HCG test should be ordered for all child-bearing age women unless they have had a hysterectomy.

- o Order tests based on
  - History
  - Physical exam
  - Medications
  - Type of surgery
- o Do not test based on "someone might want it"
- o Predictive value
  - Normal test values are defined as results that are within two standard deviations of the mean
    - 5% of patients receiving a test will have an abnormal result

- Test results in healthy patients have a low predictive value for disease
- False positives
  - Increase the likelihood of further testing
  - May delay surgery
  - May lead to medico-legal issues when not acted upon
- o May refer to NICE clinical guidelines from the National Institute for Health and Care Excellence in England and Wales (www.nice.org.uk)

References

1. I. Smith, M. Skues, B. Philip. *Miller's Anesthesia,* Eighth edition. W.B. Saunders Co., 2014; chapter-89/ preoperative-assessment 2014 ACC/ AHA Guideline on Perioperative Cardiovascular Evaluation and Management of Patients Undergoing Noncardiac Surgery.
2. L. A. Fleisher, K. E. Fleischmann, A. D. Auerbach, et al. 2014 ACC/ AHA guideline on perioperative cardiovascular evaluation and management of patients undergoing noncardiac surgery: executive summary: a report of the American College of Cardiology/American Heart Association Task Force on Practice Guidelines. *Journal of the American College of Cardiology* Dec 2014, 64 (22), e77–137.
3. S. R. Moonesinghe, M. G. Mythen, P. Das, K. M. Rowan, M. P. W. Grocott. Risk stratification tools for predicting morbidity and mortality in adult patients undergoing major surgery: qualitative systematic review. *Anesthesiology* Oct 2013, 119 (4), 959–81.
4. Committee on Standards and Practice Parameters, J. L. Apfelbaum, R. T. Connis, et al. Practice advisory for preanesthesia evaluation: an updated report by the American Society of Anesthesiologists Task Force on Preanesthesia Evaluation. *Anesthesiology* 2012, 116, 522.
5. Association of Anaesthetists of Great Britain and Ireland. AAGBI safety guideline. Pre-operative assessment and patient preparation. The role of the anaesthetist. January 2010. London. www.aagbi.org/sites/default/ files/preop2010.pdf (accessed on March 2017).

Preparation for General Anesthesia and Premedication

Daniel G. Springer and Theresa A. Gelzinis

Often times, prior to taking a patient to the operating room, premedication is administered to help alleviate anxiety, and pain or to prevent postoperative nausea and vomiting. There are many medications that are utilized for this purpose with the most common being benzodiazepines, including midazolam, diazepam, and lorazepam, opioid medications, including fentanyl, morphine, and hydromorphone, other sedative-hypnotics, such as ketamine and dexmedetomidine, and the antiemetic agents, including ondansetron, aprepitant, and transdermal scopolamine. When administering these medications to patients, it is important to know their mechanism of action, as well as their physiological effects and metabolism, and how they may influence or be influenced by other factors, such as patient comorbidities or other chronic preoperative medications.

Interactions with Chronic Medications and General Anesthetics

Benzodiazepines[1]

- Midazolam 0.5 mg/kg PO or 0.1 mg/kg IV in children has been shown to reduce preoperative anxiety
  - Onset of PO 10 min, peak effect in 20–30 min
  - Onset of IV 1 min, peak effect in 10 min
- Midazolam adult dosing often between 1 and 4 mg as an IV bolus
  - Avoidance of administration in elderly patients (age > 65) given concerns for postoperative delirium and cognitive dysfunction
  - Can administer to an elderly patient on chronic benzodiazepine therapy, but dose reduction may be required
- Combination with other agents, such as the opioids, can lead to significant respiratory depression due to synergism (e.g. fentanyl and midazolam)
- Hepatic metabolism of midazolam and diazepam via CYP3A makes them vulnerable to interactions with agents that induce and inhibit the CYP family of enzymes (see Table 15.1).

Ketamine[3]

- NMDA antagonist (Figure 15.1)
- Premedication dosing
  - Adult
    - 1–2 mg/kg IV

- 4–5 mg/kg IM as single dose
- Geriatric dosing as above
  - Pediatric
    - IV and IM same as adults
    - 6–10 mg/kg PO as single dose
- Often coadministration of a benzodiazepine utilized to reduce the hallucinogenic effects
- Side effects: Increased secretions, hallucinations, nausea/vomiting, and myoclonus

Table 15.1 Significant cytochrome P450 enzymes and their inhibitors, inducers, and substrates

Enzyme	Potent inhibitors	Potent inducers	Substrates
CYP1A2	Amiodarone, cimetidine, ciprofloxacin, fluvoxamine	Carbamazepine, phenobarbital, rifampin, tobacco	Caffeine, clozapine, theophylline
CYP2C9	Amiodarone, fluconazole, fluoxetine, metronidazole, ritonavir, TMP/SMX	Carbamazepine, phenobarbital, phenytoin, rifampin	Carvedilol, celecoxib, glipizide, ibuprofen, irbesartan, losartan
CYP2C19	Fluvoxamine, isoniazid, ritonavir	Carbamazepine, phenytoin, rifampin	Omeprazole, phenobarbital, phenytoin
CYP2D6	Amiodarone, cimetidine, diphenhydramine, fluoxetine, paroxetine, quinidine, ritonavir, terbinafine	No significant inducers	Amitriptyline, carvedilol, codeine, donepezil, haloperidol, metoprolol, paroxetine, risperidone, tramadol
CYP3A4 and CYP3A5	Clarithromycin, diltiazem, erythromycin, grapefruit juice, itraconazole, ketoconazole, nefazodone, ritonavir, telithromycin, verapamil	Carbamazepine, *Hypericum perforatum* (St. John's wort), phenobarbital, phenytoin, rifampin	Alprazolam, amlodipine, atorvastatin, cyclosporine, diazepam, estradiol, simvastatin, sildenafil, verapamil, zolpidem

From Lynch and Price[2]

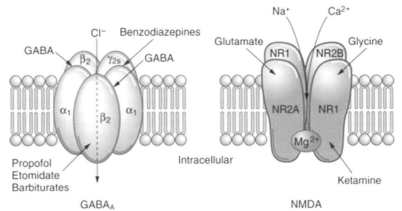

Figure 15.1 GABA, NMDA receptors and the binding sites for common IV anesthetics are similar. Interactions between these agents are likely due to similar binding sites and effects. From *Pharmacology and Physiology for Anesthesia*, Chapter 9: Intravenous Anesthetics: Image of the GABA and NMDA receptors and the binding sites of commonly used IV anesthetic agents. As evidenced by this figure, interactions between these agents are likely due to similar binding sites and effects.

Dexmedetomidine[1]

- Selective alpha-2 agonist with analgesic and sedative effects with minimal amnestic properties
- Premedication dosing
  - Adult and pediatric
    - 0.5–1 mcg/kg bolus
    - Dose reduction in geriatric patients
- Side effects: Bradycardia, hypertension (bolus), hypotension, nausea/vomiting

Fentanyl[4]

- Opioid analgesic mu-receptor agonist
- Premedication dosing
  - Adult
    - 50–100 mcg IV/IM 60 min prior to surgery or 25–50 mcg IV immediately before induction
    - Dose reduction in geriatric patients
  - Pediatric
    - 1–2 mcg/kg IV prior to surgery
- Chronic pain patients may present with transdermal fentanyl patches
- Side effects: Respiratory depression, itching, chest wall rigidity, cough

Concerns with Specific Disease States

Thyroid dysfunction (hypothyroidism and hyperthyroidism)[5]

- Hyperthyroidism
  - Patients with increased metabolism due to elevated thyroid hormone levels
  - May require higher doses of medications to achieve same level of sedation
  - Avoid drugs that stimulate the sympathetic nervous system (e.g. ketamine)
  - Opioid premedication safe in these patients

- Hypothyroidism
  - Patients may be extremely sensitive to any sedative medication.
  - Limit the dose or administration of preoperative sedatives

Uremia[5]

- Extreme levels of urea can lead to sedation and neurologic changes, therefore avoidance of further sedation is advised.

Increased Intracranial Pressure[5]

- Minimize sedative medications as any increase in $PaCO_2$ from hypoventilation may lead to increased cerebral vasodilation, cerebral blood flow, and further increases in ICP

Chronic Steroids[5]

- Will likely require stress-dose of steroids to prevent perioperative hypotension; however no changes to other anesthetic management currently recommended

Obesity[5]

- Often associated with obstructive sleep apnea
- More sensitive to sedatives; use sedatives with caution using lean body weight and titrating to effect
- Can use any of the commonly utilized sedative as long as patient is monitored closely

Obstructive Sleep Apnea[1,5]

- Often avoidance of sedative medications advised given concern for airway obstruction
- Dexmedetomidine can be a useful anxiolytic for the extremely anxious patient as it can preserve respiratory drive better than the other sedatives.

Depression[5]

- May require increased doses of premedication due to alterations in baseline catecholamine balances from antidepressant therapy

- Current antidepressant regimen must be known as there is concern for interactions between antidepressants and anesthetic medications that can lead to serious adverse reaction.[6]
  - Serotonin syndrome: Can occur with the selective serotonin reuptake inhibitors, such as citalopram, fluoxetine, paroxetine, sertraline, and venlafaxine, dexamethorphan, tramadol, and trazodone
    - Management: Stop offending agent, support hemodynamics, control hyperthermia
  - Neuroleptic malignant syndrome: Can occur with the antipsychotic agents haloperidol, perphenazine, riseridone, and thioridazine, the antiemetic agents droperidol, metoclopramide, prochlorperazine, and promethazine, and with the withdrawal of anti-Parkinson medications
    - Management: Stop offending agent, support hemodynamics, control hyperthermia, dantrolene for muscle rigidity or dopamine agonist such as bromocriptine
  - Tardive dyskinesia: Involuntary, repetitive movements occur due to use of high-dose antipsychotics
    - Management: Stop offending agent, support hemodynamics, symptomatic control, medications for treatment include reserpine, ondansetron, donepezil, clonidine, baclofen
- In patients who are taking monoamine oxidase inhibitors (MAOIs), the use of meperidine can result in hyperpyrexia. Due to its mechanism of action, hypotension should be treated with direct acting agents, such as phenylephrine.[6]

Chronic Obstructive Pulmonary Disease (COPD)[5]

- Attempt to minimize sedation given concerns for reduction in respiratory drive leading to development of worsening hypercapnea and hypoxia
- Preinduction anticholinergic and/or beta-agonist inhalers may be useful in preventing perioperative bronchospasm.
- Patients using long-term steroid inhalers or taking oral steroid medications may require intraoperative stress dose steroids.[7]
  - Stress dose steroid recommendations:
    - Non-suppressed hypothalamic pituitary adrenal (HPA) axis: patients taking <5 mg prednisone for <3 weeks or taking <10 mg every other day
      - Continue with routine glucocorticoid regimen
    - Suppressed HPA axis: Patients taking >20 mg prednisone for >3 weeks or have Cushingoid appearance with likely HPA suppression
      - For minor stress procedures: Continue routine glucocorticoid regimen with no extra supplementation
      - For moderate stress procedures (e.g. joint replacement): continue routine glucocorticoid regimen + 50 mg hydrocortisone IV at induction + 25 mg IV q 8 h for 24 h
      - For major stress procedures (e.g. large abdominal cases, open heart surgery): continue routine glucocorticoid regimen + 100 mg hydrocortisone IV at induction + 50 mg IV q 8 h for 24 h
        - Note: Taper dose by half per day to routine maintenance level

Hypertension[5]

- Avoid sedative medications that can increase blood pressure (e.g. ketamine) in the immediate preoperative period
- Depending on antihypertensive agents, patients may have exaggerated blood pressure responses to sedatives.

NPO and Full Stomach Status[8]

- Table 15.2 shows updated guidelines from the American Society of Anesthesiologists published in March 2017.
- Note in Table 15.2 the recommendations for the use of medications to modify gastric pH, volume, and sphincter tone.
- Patients who have violated these NPO guidelines for elective surgery should be postponed until NPO appropriate.
- General endotracheal anesthesia can be used to help minimize the risk of pulmonary aspiration. It is prudent to avoid all anesthetics compromising the airway and laryngeal mask airways.
- Airway management for a patient with full stomach should include a rapid sequence induction (RSI). The utility of cricoid pressure remains controversial but is considered standard of care.
- In addition to NPO status, patients must be evaluated for any underlying medical condition that may lead to decreased gastric emptying or increased gastrointestinal transit time such as diabetes, gastroesophageal reflux disease (GERD), morbid obesity, small bowel obstruction.

Continuation vs. Discontinuation of Chronic Medications

- Anti-hypertensives[6]
  - Beta-blockers: Should be continued in the perioperative period
  - Discontinuation of ACE inhibitors (24–48 h) and angiotensin receptor blocker (ARBs) (24 h) prior to surgery is encouraged to minimize hypotension from vasodilation and effective hypovolemia.
  - Calcium channel blockers can be continued in the perioperative period, especially if the patient has pulmonary hypertension.
  - Diuretics: No consensus on continuation vs. discontinuation
  - Clonidine: Should be continued to avoid rebound hypertension
- Anti-anginals[6]
  - Can be continued into the perioperative period
- Anti-hyperglycemics[6]
  - All PO agents should be held prior to surgery to prevent perioperative hypoglycemia.

Table 15.2 Fasting and Pharmacologic Recommendations

*A. Fasting Recommendations**

Ingested Material	Minimum Fasting Period†
• Clear liquids‡	2h
• Breast milk	4h
• Infant formula	6h
• Nonhuman milk§	6h
• Light meal**	6h
• Fried foods, fatty foods, or meat	Additional fasting time (*e.g.*, 8 or more hours) may be needed

B. Pharmacologic Recommendations

Medication Type and Common Examples	Recommendation
Gastrointestinal stimulants:	
• Metoclopramide	May be used/no routine use
Grastric acid secretion blockers:	
• Climetidine	May be used/no routine use
• Famotidine	May be used/no routine use
• Ranitidine	May be used/no routine use
• Omeprazole	May be used/no routine use
• Lansoprazole	May be used/no routine use
Antacids:	
• Sodium citrate	May be used/no routine use
• Sodium bicarbonate	May be used/no routine use
• Magnesium trisilicate	May be used/no routine use
Antiemetics:	
• Ondansetron	May be used/no routine use
Anticholinergics:	
• Atropine	No use
• Scopolamine	No use
• Glycopyrrolate	No use
Combinations of the medications above:	No routine use

*These recommendations apply to healthy patients who are undergoing elective procedures. They are not intended for women in labor. Following the guidelines does not guarantee complete gastric emptying.
†The fasting periods noted above apply to all ages.
‡Examples of clear liquids include water, fruit juices without pulp, carbonated beverages, clear tea, and black coffee.
§Since nonhuman milk is similar to solids in gastric emptying time, the amount ingested must be considered when determining an appropriate fasting period.
**A light meal typically consists of toast and clear liquids. Meals that include fried or fatty foods or meat may prolong gastric emptying time. Additional fasting time (*e.g.*, 8 or more hours) may be needed in these cases. Both the amount and type of foods ingested must be considered when determining an appropriate fasting period.
Practice Guidelines for Preoperative Fasting and the Use of Pharmacologic Agents to Reduce the Risk of Pulmonary Aspiration: Application to Healthy Patients Undergoing Elective Procedures: An Updated Report by the American Society of Anesthesiologists Committee on Standards and Practice Parameters Anesthesiology 3 2011, Vol.114, 495–511. doi:10.1097/ALN.0b013e3181fcbfd9

- o Long-acting insulin dosages should be reduced prior to patient being made NPO.
- Psychotropic medications[6]
  - o SSRIs/SNRIs: Can be continued into the perioperative period (limited data for SNRIs)
    - o TCAs: Can be continued
    - o Buproprion: No data available
    - o MAOIs: Can be continued
    - o Valproate and lithium: Should be continued, close monitoring of patient on lithium
    - o Antipsychotics: Can be continued but may potentiate effects of sedative/opioids
    - o Antianxiety: Can be continued
    - o Psychostimulants (e.g. methylphenidate): Can safely be discontinued
- Anticoagulants[6,9]
  - o Each has a specific time frame for discontinuation to allow full coagulation
  - o Warfarin: Discontinue 5 days before surgery if deemed appropriate
  - o Dabigatran: Discontinue 2–3 days before surgery
  - o Rivaroxaban: Discontinue 2–3 days before surgery
  - o Apixaban: Discontinue 2–3 days before surgery
  - o Edoxaban: Discontinue 2–3 days before surgery
- Antiplatelet agents[6]
  - o If deemed appropriate based on indication for initiation and type of surgery being performed, these may or may not be discontinued.
  - o Aspirin: Discontinue 7–10 days before surgery
  - o Clopidogrel and ticagrelor: Discontinue at least 5 days before surgery
  - o Prasugrel: Discontinue at least 7 days before surgery

Prophylactic Cardiac Risk Reduction[10]

- All patients should be evaluated for cardiac risk prior to surgery
- Preoperative revascularization
  - o Except in setting of acute coronary syndrome, not recommended as has not been shown to improve outcomes
- Preoperative beta-blockade
  - o Numerous trials have supported the continuation of chronic beta blockade therapy in patients on these agents for specific indications (e.g. prior MI, atrial fibrillation rate control, heart failure, etc.).
    - No outcomes have been shown to be better for one agent over another.
    - No evidence to show that continuation leads to worse outcomes.
  - o Initiation of beta blockade is not recommended for prevention in noncardiac surgery.
- Antiplatelet therapy
  - o Recommendation to hold prophylactic aspirin 5–7 days before surgery and not to initiate an aspirin regimen prior to noncardiac surgery
  - o Other antiplatelet agents as indicated
- Statin therapy
  - o Continuation of statins in the perioperative period encouraged
  - o May initiate statin therapy in patients prior to surgery if indicated

- ACE inhibitors and ARBs
  - Discontinuation for at least 24 h prior to surgery encouraged
  - Initiation in the immediate perioperative period not recommended
  - Chronic therapy may be continued if indicated by clinical conditions.
- Nitrate therapy
  - Prophylactic administration/initiation is not recommended.

Prophylactic Antibiotics[11]
- Goal is prevention of surgical site infections (SSI)
- Antimicrobial agent selection based on cost, safety, pharmacokinetic profile, and antibacterial activity
- Cefazolin is drug of choice for many procedures due to study-proven efficacy and spectrum of coverage.

- Other agents may be chosen based on specific microorganism risks associated with a specific procedure.
- Administration is done parenterally within 60 min prior to skin incision to optimize tissue drug levels.
- Repeat administration timing specific to each antimicrobial drug but generally done when procedure length is greater than 2.5 half-lives of drug and/or blood loss greater than 1,500 mL
- Greatest risk with administration of antimicrobial drugs is allergic reaction.
  - Concern for cross-reactive reaction between penicillin and cephalosporins
    - Safe to administer a cephalosporin as long as no history of reaction to other cephalosporins, and reaction to penicillin is not anaphylaxis
    - There is <2% cross-reactivity between the two classes.

References

1. Hemmings H. C., Egan T. D.: *Pharmacology and Physiology for Anesthesia: Foundations and Clinical Application*. Philadelphia, PA: Elsevier/Saunders, 2013.
2. Lynch T., Price A.: The effect of cytochrome P450 metabolism on drug response, interactions, and adverse effects. *American Family Physician* 2007; 76:391–6.
3. Ketamine: Drug information at www.uptodate.com/contents/ketamine-drug-information (accessed on 03/06/2017).
4. Fentanyl: Drug information at www.uptodate.com/contents/fentanyl-drug-information (accessed on 03/06/2017).
5. Stoelting R. K., Dierdorf S. F.: *Anesthesia and Co-existing Disease*. Philadelphia, PA: Churchill Livingstone, 2002.
6. Muluk V., Cohn S. L., Whinney C.: Perioperative medication management at www.uptodate.com/contents/perioperative-medication-management (accessed on 03/10/2017).
7. Hamrahian A. H., Roman S., Milan S.: The management of the surgical patient taking glucocorticoids at www.uptodate.com/contents/the-management-of-the-surgical-patient-taking-glucocorticoids (accessed on 03/10/2017).
8. Apfelbaum J. L., Agarkar M., Connis R. T., Cote C. J., Nickinovich D. G., Warner M. A.: Practice guidelines for preoperative fasting and the use of pharmacologic agents to reduce the risk of pulmonary aspiration. *Anesthesiology* 2017; 126:376–93.
9. Lip G. Y. H., Douketis J. D.: Perioperative management of patients receiving anticoagulants at www.uptodate.com/contents/perioperative-management-of-patients-receiving-anticoagulants (accessed on 03/10/2017).
10. Devereaux P. J., Cohn S. L., Eagle K. A.: Management of cardiac risk for noncardiac surgery at www.uptodate.com/contents/management-of-cardiac-risk-for-noncardiac-surgery (accessed on 03/08/2017).
11. Anderson D. J., Sexton D. J.: Antimicrobial prophylaxis for prevention of surgical site infection in adults at www.uptodate.com/contents/antimicrobial-prophylaxis-for-prevention-of-surgical-site-infection-in-adults (accessed on 03/09/2017).

Chapter 16

Regional Anesthesia

Poonam Pai and Ali Shariat

Preparation for Regional Blocks

- **Sedation:** Provide anxiolytic and analgesic with short-acting benzodiazepine and opioid during performance of the block, while maintaining meaningful communication with the patient.
- **Monitoring:** Place standard ASA monitors including pulse oximetry, noninvasive blood pressure, electrocardiography and end tidal CO_2 should be available. The thermometer may be placed in the operating room.
- **Patient position:** Position patient comfortably with maximizing block site exposure. Operator should stand in a position comfortable for ultrasound use and needle placement.
- **Equipment:** Ultrasound, block needle (+ catheter kit if continuous block), sterile prep, ultrasound gel, probe cover, local anesthetic (LA) syringes, sedation, +/− nerve stimulator

Neuraxial Anesthesia

- **Position:** Sitting, lateral decubitus, prone
- **Indications:** Anesthesia and/or analgesia for procedures involving the lower limbs, lower abdomen, pelvis, and perineum
- **Contraindications:** Patient refusal, infection at site of injection, sepsis, refractory hypovolemia, coagulopathy, increased intracranial pressure, true allergy to local anesthetics

Technique (Midline):

- Spinal anesthesia: LA placement in *subarachnoid space*
  - Needle trajectory from posterior to anterior: Skin → subcutaneous tissue → supraspinous ligament → interspinous ligament → ligamentum flavum → dura mater → arachnoid mater → subarachnoid space
- Epidural anesthesia: LA placement in *epidural space*
  - Needle trajectory: Skin → subcutaneous tissue → supraspinous ligament → interspinous ligament → ligamentum flavum → epidural space
- Caudal anesthesia: LA placement in *sacral portion of epidural space*
  - Needle trajectory: Skin → subcutaneous tissue → sacrococcygeal ligament → caudal space

- Combined spinal epidural (CSE): Combination of spinal and epidural
  - Spinal provides rapid onset of predictable block and epidural catheter provides possibility for long-lasting analgesia with dose titration.

Factors Influencing Block Height

- Spinal:
  - Baricity of LA solution
  - Position of the patient during and immediately after LA injection
  - Dose and volume of LA
  - Site of injection
  - Other factors: Age, cerebrospinal fluid (CSF) volume, spine curvature, intra-abdominal pressure, needle direction, height
- Epidural:
  - Dose (volume × concentration) of LA
  - Site of injection (i.e., lumbar vs. sacral)
  - Other factors: age, height

Factors Influencing Duration

- Epinephrine: Increases duration by decreasing systemic absorption
- Alpha-2 agonist: Hyperpolarization at the ventral horn of spinal cord
  - Side effects of neuraxial clonidine: Hypotension, bradycardia, dry mouth, and sedation

Factors Influencing Onset of Action

- Bicarbonate: Increases non-ionized form of the drug, allowing it to penetrate nerve cell membranes and speed the process of intraneural diffusion

Termination of Action

- Blood flow to spinal cord: Elimination is by vascular absorption through subarachnoid and epidural blood vessels.

Physiological Effects

- Cardiovascular: Sympathectomy induces hemodynamic changes with extent of changes determined by block height.
  - Block below T4: Sympathetic fibers from T5 to L1 maintain vasomotor tone. Arterial and venodilation lead to ↓ SVR. Increased venous pooling leads to ↓

venous return, ↓ right atrial pressure, and ↓ cardiac output. Initial ↑ HR due to hypotension.
- Block above T4: Blockade of cardiac accelerator fibers (T1–T4). Results in ↓ cardiac contractility, ↓ BP, and ↓ HR.
- Differential blockade: Sympathetic (temperature, autonomic system via C fibers) → sensory (pain, light touch via A delta fibers) → motor (motor, proprioception via A alpha fibers)
- Renal: Urinary retention can occur if detrusor function of the bladder is affected.
- Pulmonary: If high spread then ↓ vital capacity
- Gastrointestinal: Parasympathetic effects include ↑ gut peristalsis, ↑ secretions, sphincters relax, bowel constriction, slight reduction of hepatic blood flow. Nausea and vomiting risk increased with hypotension and concomitant opioid administration.

Test dose: A small test dose of LA with epinephrine (3 mL of lidocaine 1.5% with epinephrine 1:200,000) is injected into the epidural catheter to reduce the risk of keeping a catheter in place that is intravascular or intrathecal.
- Positive test dose: Increase in HR by 20% or greater, tinnitus, dysguesia, perioral numbness/tingling indicates intravascular injection. Significant motor block within 5 minutes of administering test dose indicates intrathecal injection.

Complications
- Epidural/spinal hematoma:
  - Presentation: Motor and sensory deficits, possible bowel/bladder incontinence
  - Risk factors: Coagulopathy, traumatic needle insertion, increased age, and female gender, insertion/removal of epidural catheter (Table 16.1)
  - Treatment: Magnetic resonance image (MRI) should be obtained as soon as possible followed by immediate surgical decompression, if necessary.
- Epidural abscess:
  - Relatively uncommon. Risk factors include prolonged indwelling epidural catheter and immunocompromised patients.
  - Presentation: Fever, severe back pain, radicular pain, motor/sensory deficits, and paraplegia/paralysis. Delay in diagnosis and treatment leads to poor recovery
  - Organisms: *Staphylococcus aureus, Staphylococcus epidermidis*
  - Prevention: Sterile techniques, bacterial micropore filter usage, epidural catheter removal within 4 days, minimal catheter manipulations
  - Treatment: Antibiotics, surgical decompression
- Post-dural puncture headache (PDPH):
  - Mechanism: Results from loss of CSF through dural puncture thereby lowering CSF pressure causing traction on cranial nerves and roots
  - Presentation: Bilateral, fronto-occipital, or retro-orbital headache relieved by lying flat, worsened by upright posture. Cranial nerve signs include diplopia, tinnitus, nystagmus, and hearing loss
  - Onset: 12–72 hours
    - Duration: Typically 5 days with a range of 1–12 days
  - Risk factors: Young, female, pregnancy, use of Quincke needle, cutting, and/or large-bore needle. Obesity is protective
  - Treatment: Conservative treatment first with bed rest, oral and IV hydration, oral or intravenous caffeine, and analgesics. Invasive treatment with epidural blood patch with 15–20 mL of autologous blood in severe cases
- Transient neurologic symptoms (TNS):
  - Presentation: Back pain with radiation to legs without sensory/motor deficits
  - Risk factors: Spinal anesthesia with lidocaine 5%, lithotomy position, obesity, young female, ambulatory surgery
  - Treatment: Spontaneous resolution usually within 10 days
- Total/high spinal:
  - Mechanism: Occurs when local anesthetic spreads high enough to block entire spinal cord and possibly even brainstem. Cervical roots and cardioaccelerator fibers are affected.
  - Presentation: ↓ BP and ↓ HR due to cephalad spread of local anesthetic. ↓ expiratory reserve volume (ERV), ↓ peak expiratory flow, ↓ maximum minute ventilation, apnea, and unconsciousness
  - Treatment: Airway management with intubation and 100% oxygen. Hemodynamic support with fluids and vasopressors
- Bezold–Jarisch reflex:
  - Mechanism: Cardioinhibitory reflex secondary to parasympathetic discharge due to noxious stimuli as sensed by chemo- and mechano-receptors within the left ventricle
  - Presentation: ↓ BP, ↓ HR, coronary artery dilation and cardiovascular collapse
- Cauda equina syndrome:
  - Mechanism: Disk herniation, disk stenosis, spinal lesion, spinal infection leading to compression and/or injury of nerve roots from L1–5, S1–5
  - Presentation: Bowel and bladder incontinence, patchy sensory deficits, pain and paresis of the lower extremities
  - Treatment: Urgent MRI followed by surgical decompression, if necessary
- Adhesive arachnoiditis:
  - Mechanism: Introduction of intrathecal irritant into subarachnoid space leading to inflammation and scarring of the subarachnoid space with collagen deposition and nerve root adherence. Collagen deposits encapsulate spinal nerves resulting in nerve root atrophy as a result of the interruption of blood supply.

Table 16.1 ASRA recommendations for anticoagulants

Anticoagulant (AC)	$t_{1/2}$	Anticoagulant type	Duration from last AC dose to catheter manipulation or needle puncture	Duration from catheter manipulation or needle puncture to AC dosing
IV Heparin	1.5–2 hours	Pro-anti thrombin III	2–4 hours/PTT	1–2 hours nontraumatic, 6–12 hours if traumatic
Heparin SQ <10,000 units BID dosing	1.5–2 hours	Pro-anti thrombin III	None	No restriction
Enoxaparin (Lovenox) 0.5 mg/kg daily	3–6 hours	Anti-Xa	12 hours	2 hours
Enoxaparin 0.5 mg/kg BID	3–6 hours	Anti-Xa	12 hours	Not recommended with catheter, initiate 2–4 hours after removal
Enoxaparin >0.5 mg/kg BID therapeutic	3–6 hours	Anti-Xa	24 hours	Not recommended with catheter, initiate 10–12 hours after removal
Warfarin (Coumadin)	20–60 hours	Vitamin K-dependent inhibition of factors	INR<1.5, 5 days	INR < 1.5
Aspirin	6 hours	Anti-platelet	None	No restrictions
Clopidogrel (Plavix)	6–8 hours	Irreversible platelet aggregation inhibitor	5–7 days	Not recommended with catheter, initiate >2 hours after removal
Ticlopidine (Ticlid)	4–5 days	Irreversible platelet aggregation inhibitor	14 days	Not recommended with catheter, initiate >2 hours after removal
Prasugrel (Effient)	7–8 hours	Irreversible platelet aggregation inhibitor	7–10 days	6 hours
Ticagrelor (Brilinta)	7–8.5 hours	ADP reversible receptor blocker	5–7 days	6 hours
Abciximab (ReoPro)	0.5 hour	Gp IIb–IIIa inhibitor	48 hours	Not recommended with catheter, initiate >2 hours after removal
Eptifibatide (Integrilin)	1–2.5 hours	Gp IIb–IIIa inhibitor	8 hours	Not recommended with catheter, initiate >2 hours after removal
Tirofiban (Aggrastat)	2 hours	Gp IIb–IIIa inhibitor	8 hours	Not recommended with catheter, initiate >2 hours after removal
Bivalurudin, Lepirudin	0.5–3 hours	Thrombin inhibitor	Not recommended – insufficient data	Not recommended – insufficient data
Argatroban	35–40 minutes	Thrombin inhibitor	Not recommended – insufficient data	Not recommended – insufficient data
Dabigatran (Pradaxa)	12–15 hours	Thrombin inhibitor	5 days	6 hours
Fondaparinux (Arixtra)	17–21 hours	Anti-Xa	3–4 days	Not recommended with catheter, initiate >12 hours after removal
Rivaroxaban (Xarelto)	5–9 hours	Anti-Xa	3 days	6 hours
Apixaban (Eliqis)	10–15 hours	Anti-Xa	3–5 days	6 hours

- o Presentation: Back pain that increases on exertion, bilateral leg pain, hyporeflexia, decreased truncal range of motion, sensory abnormalities, and urinary sphincter dysfunction. Neurologic symptoms may progress to permanent disability.
- o Risk factors: Trauma, infections, surgery, contaminants, tumors, or subarachnoid administration of medications
- o Treatment: Physical therapy and opioid analgesics +/− antidepressants

Local Anesthetic Systemic Toxicity (LAST)

- Symptoms: Tinnitus, perioral numbness, blurred vision, muscle twitching, syncope, seizures, bradycardia, junctional rhythms, ventricular fibrillation, cardiac arrest

- Mechanism: LA blocks the fast sodium channels in the Purkinje fibers and ventricles leading to decreased rate of depolarization.
- Treatment: 100% oxygen, hyperventilation, benzodiazepines, propofol, succinylcholine followed by tracheal intubation. Epinephrine and intralipid 20% therapy – 1.5 mL/kg IV bolus, with 0.25 mL/kg/minute infusion for at least 10 minutes after attaining circulatory stability

IV Regional Anesthesia/"Bier Block"

- Technique: Double pneumatic tourniquet placed on extremity → Intravenous catheter placed in dorsal portion of hand → With hand/forearm elevated, it is exsanguinated with elastic bandage → proximal cuff is inflated to 250 mmHg → bandage is removed → 10–15 mL of 1–2%

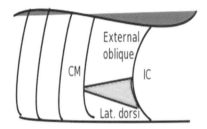

Figure 16.1 Lumbar triangle of Petit: iliac crest (IC) and costal margin (CM)

lidocaine given via IV → distal cuff is inflated. The surgical procedure begins and the proximal cuff is deflated very slowly to avoid sudden flush of anesthetic into systemic circulation.

- Agents: Lidocaine is most commonly used; mepiv-acaine, prilocaine, 2-chloroprocaine have also been used. Bupivacaine is not used due to the higher risk for cardiotoxicity.
- **Contraindications**: Crush injury, cellulitis, compound fractures, peripheral vascular disease, A–V shunts, sickle cell disease
- **Complications**: LAST, hematoma, ecchymosis, neurologic complications

Transversus Abdominis Plane (TAP) Blocks

- Technique: A single entry point, three muscle layers visualized at the mid-axillary line: external oblique (EO), internal oblique (IO), and transversus abdominis (TA). Local anesthetic is deposited in the plane between the IO and TA muscles (Figures 16.1 and 16.2).

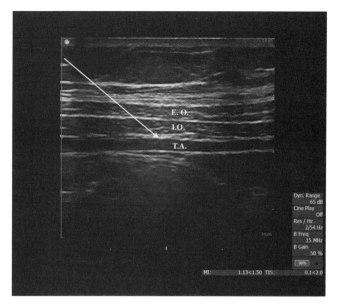

Figure 16.2 Transversus abdominis block: EO – external oblique, IO – internal oblique, TA – transversus abdominis

- Nerves: Anterior rami of T6–T12, ilioinguinal and ilio-hypogastric nerves of L1
- Innervation: Abdominal skin, muscles, and parietal perito-neum will be blocked. Dull visceral pain will not be blocked.
- Indications: Lower abdominal surgeries involving T6 to L1 distribution such as an appendectomy, hernia repair, abdominal hysterectomy, cesarean section, open prostatec-tomy. Bilateral blocks are performed for midline incisions.
- Complications: LAST, visceral injury to bowel, liver, spleen, kidney, or femoral nerve.

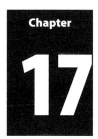

Chapter

17

General Anesthesia

Petrus Paulus Steyn and Jeffrey Derham

- Definition: A complex drug-induced state of unconsciousness, amnesia, analgesia, and immobility. In addition, general anesthesia can cause significant physiological changes, most notably cardiovascular and respiratory depression.[1,2,3]
- The depth of anesthesia is the probability of unresponsiveness in the face of a stimulus with a given strength. In other words, the deeper the anesthetic, the stronger the stimulation needed to elicit a particular response.
- *The presence of an endotracheal tube does not define general anesthesia.* General anesthesia is clinically differentiated from sedation by the following parameters:[4,5]
  - *Responsiveness:* Unarousable even with painful stimulation
  - *Airway:* May require intervention to keep open. Pharyngeal muscle tone decreases under anesthesia and may lead to upper airway obstruction.
  - *Spontaneous ventilation:* Frequently inadequate, thus requiring some form of positive pressure ventilation.
  - *Cardiovascular function:* Possible impairment depending on disease state, function.
- The four stages of ether anesthesia:[4,6]
  1. **Induction**: Awake but cortical processing impaired. Euphoria and/or disinhibition may be present. The threshold of pain perception decreases.
  2. **Delirium:** Loss of consciousness. Eyelid reflex disappears but other reflexes intact. Noxious stimulation can lead to agitated movements, hypertension, tachycardia, vomiting, and laryngospasm. Breath holding and gaze divergence may occur. At the conclusion of this stage, respirations are regular and muscle tone diminishes.
  3. **Surgical anesthesia:** Central gaze, pupillary reflexes diminished, respirations regular, airway muscle tone diminished. At this stage, somatic movement and deleterious autonomic responses do not occur with noxious stimulation.
  4. **Respiratory paralysis/overdose:** Shallow, insufficient breathing, hypotension, and eventual circulatory collapse
- In modern anesthesia practice, these stages are rarely seen with rapid induction with modern agents. However, they are still relevant with mask inductions and emergence from volatile agent maintenance. Also relevant is the fact that in most clinical settings the estimation of the depth of anesthesia depends on patient outputs, such as somatic movement and hemodynamic responses, which serve as

surrogate markers. Unfortunately, these are often unreliable. The use of *bispectral index* (BIS) monitoring can be a helpful estimation of anesthetic depth. BIS is a processed electroencephalogram (EEG) parameter used to monitor the depth of anesthesia.[4,5,7]

- Techniques for general anesthesia:[2,5]
  - **Inhalational** – accomplished using a potent volatile agent with or without nitrous oxide. Historically the first technique. Most common agents are isoflurane, sevoflurane, and desflurane. These agents are "complete" anesthetics in the sense that they achieve amnesia, analgesia, and immobility. However, the dose required to achieve these goals as a single agent is often not tolerated hemodynamically. MAC is the minimum alveolar concentration of volatile anesthetic at which 50% of patients will not move in response to skin incision. The end-tidal concentration of agent is used as a surrogate for brain concentrations and thus MAC levels.
  - **Total intravenous anesthesia (TIVA)** – combination of hypnotic (e.g. propofol) and opioid with or without a paralytic agent. Clinical situations where TIVA may be necessary include malignant hyperthermia, the presence of neuromonitoring utilizing evoked potentials, and where ventilation is often interrupted, as in bronchoscopy. One potential disadvantage is the lack of an end-tidal anesthetic "monitor" to gauge depth of anesthesia possibly leaving the patient more susceptible to light anesthesia and awareness.
  - **Combined** mixture of techniques using a lower concentration of volatile agents with IV analgesics (e.g. opioids, ketamine) with muscle relaxation. Relies on the synergistic interactions between the agents that decrease the likelihood of medication toxicity. Intravenous medications are synergistic with each other and with volatile agents. The MACs of different volatile anesthetics, on the other hand, are additive.
- *Intraoperative awareness with recall* is the consequence of inadequate anesthesia depth. Incidence is estimated at 0.1–0.2%. Awareness with recall often occurs with inadequate depth of anesthesia in the setting of hemodynamic instability. Risk factors include:[4]
  - Cardiac surgery
  - Trauma surgery
  - Cesarean section
  - Airway endoscopy surgery

- Pediatric surgery
  - Difficult airway
  - Chronic alcohol, opioid, or amphetamine abuse
- Anesthetic plan for induction and maintenance of general anesthesia[5]
  - Must take into account a myriad of considerations including airway assessment, patient physiology/comorbidities, and surgical needs/manipulations.
  - Any anesthetic plan must consider three basic management decisions:
    - *The need for an awake intubation* – Does the administration of general anesthesia pose an unacceptable risk to the airway?
    - *The need for a percutaneous (surgical) airway* – Is ventilation and/or intubation via noninvasive means not possible? Notable examples include severe facial trauma or burns.
    - *The need to maintain spontaneous ventilation* – Pontibus ne perreni tua (do not burn your bridges). Spontaneous ventilation is a security blanket and avoids the very dangerous cannot ventilate/cannot intubate clinical scenario.
  - These previous three strategies are safer than the most common induction plans utilizing muscle relaxants, but they have the cost of increased time and effort. Management decision depends heavily on the airway evaluation (see below).
  - The increasing availability of sugammadax, a cyclodextrin synthesized to antagonize rocuronium, may allow for the more liberal use of muscle relaxants.
- Airway evaluation[8,9]
  - History
    - Old anesthesia records may be helpful but do not guarantee correlation.
    - Appreciation of concomitant disease states that could potentially impact the airway (e.g. rheumatoid arthritis, anterior mediastinal mass, etc.). Imaging studies can be helpful.
  - Physical exam – Effective mask ventilation requires a proper mask/tissue seal as well as sufficient pressure to overcome upper airway resistance. Noninvasive endotracheal intubation requires an unobstructed path from the nasal/oral cavities to the trachea. Gross pathology of the face, neck, and pharynx (facial trauma/burns, neck masses, tonsillar abscesses, etc.) are usually obvious from the history and physical. More important and challenging is identifying potential difficulty in apparently "normal" patients.
    - Predictive factors for difficult facemask ventilation (in order of significance)
      1. Presence of beard (poor seal)
      2. Body mass index > 26 kg/m^2 (airway resistance)
      3. Edentulous (poor seal)
      4. Age >55 years (combination of factors)
      5. History of snoring (airway resistance)
    - Other criteria that suggest difficulty:
      1. History of difficult mask ventilation
      2. History of obstructive sleep apnea (airway resistance)
      3. Macroglossia (airway resistance)
      4. Poor atlanto-occipital extension (airway resistance)
      5. Limited mandibular protrusion (airway resistance)
    - Risk factors for difficult intubation
      1. History of difficult intubation
      2. Poor atlanto-occipital extension
      3. Limited mouth opening: Inter-incisor distance <3 cm (or two finger breadths)
      4. Overbite/increased length of maxillary incisors – Decreases the effective inter-incisor distance and hinders oral/laryngeal alignment
      5. Thyromental distance less than 6 cm (three finger-breadths) in length
      6. Short neck
      7. Limited mandibular protrusion (inability of mandibular incisors to touch vermillion)
      8. Mallampati/Samsoon classification of III or IV
    - Mallampati/Samsoon classification: Based on visible structures when patient opens mouth. A measure of relative tongue size for a given oral cavity
      - Class I: Soft palate, fauces, uvula, and tonsillar pillars are visible.
      - Class II: The soft palate, fauces, and uvular are visible.
      - Class III: The soft palate and base of the uvula are visible.
      - Class IV: The soft palate is not visible.
    - Each of the above risk factors by itself has a very poor sensitivity/specificity for difficulty in ventilation and intubation. Thus, in many cases, the difficult airway will be unanticipated. The more risk factors present, the higher the probability for difficulty. Roughly 15% of difficult intubations will be difficult mask ventilations.
- General anesthesia induction techniques[2,10,11]
  - Preparation and optimization – Whatever the anesthetic plan, one should adhere to the following principles of endotracheal intubation:
    - Inform the patient of the plan
    - Coordinate availability of assistance if necessary
    - Aside from the primary technique, a series of backup plans and all equipment necessary should be in place and immediately available
    - Optimize patient positioning
      - Sniffing position: Cervical neck flexion with atlanto-occipital extension. Normal atlanto-occipital extension is 35°. Goal is to align the oral/pharyngeal, and laryngeal axes so the

laryngoscopist has a straight line of site to the larynx. Best position for most techniques.

- Head-elevated laryngoscopy position (HELP) –Helpful for obese patients. Sniffing position plus alignment of the external auditory meatus with the sternal notch. Most often achieved via a pile of blankets underneath the shoulders and upper back (ramp) or with reverse Trendelenburg

- Preoxygenate: Meaning 3 minutes of 100% oxygen or four full vital capacity breaths in 30 seconds.
- Ensure that supplemental oxygen can be delivered throughout the process.
- Minimize intubation attempts and thus airway trauma. Often the best look is the first look.
- Tracheal intubation confirmation:
  - Chest rise
  - End-tidal carbon dioxide monitor
  - Breath sounds
  - Chest X-ray
  - Direct laryngoscopy

- ○ **Inhalational induction**
  - Mask induction with a volatile agent at high flow and concentration
  - Sevoflurane most commonly used secondary to low blood-gas partition coefficient and lack of pungency
  - High levels of end-tidal gas needed for laryngoscopy and intubation. Supplementation with topical lidocaine can be helpful.
  - Requires good facemask technique
  - Advantages
    - Spontaneous ventilation maintained. Potential alternative to awake intubation for uncooperative patient
    - Depth of anesthesia titrated slowly. Respiratory and cardiovascular depression occurs more gradually.
    - Excellent alternative if preoperative intravenous access unattainable (e.g. pediatric patients)
  - Disadvantages
    - Longer time required to secure airway. Not optimal for aspiration risk
    - Longer time spent in stage 2 with higher risk of laryngospasm. Antisialogogue can be helpful.
    - Intubating conditions may be suboptimal without the use of muscle relaxants

- ○ **Intravenous induction**
  - Most often accompanied with hypnotic (i.e. propofol, etomidate, midazolam) for amnesia/ unconsciousness, opioid (i.e. fentanyl) to blunt the hemodynamic effects of laryngoscopy, and muscle relaxant (i.e. rocuronium, succinylcholine)

- Advantages
  - Rapid induction that bypasses the dangerous reflexes of stage 2 anesthesia
  - Optimal intubating conditions that minimize airway trauma
  - Technique of choice in setting of aspiration risk and anticipated complicated airway (rapid sequence induction (RSI) technique)
- Disadvantages
  - Spontaneous ventilation lost (even without the use of muscle relaxants) leaving the potential cannot ventilate/cannot intubate scenario
  - Hemodynamic instability secondary to the sudden onset of hypnotics and narcotics

- ○ **Awake intubation with local anesthesia**[8,12,13,14,15]
  - Successful 80–100% of the time
  - Safe technique for the difficult ventilation/intubation or for potentially difficult intubation with aspiration risk
  - Requires patient cooperation and blockade of sensory nerves of airway:
    - Trigeminal (V) – sensory innervation to the nasal mucosa and nasal cavity
    - Glossopharyngeal (IX) – sensory innervation to posterior third of tongue, pharynx, and superior side of epiglottis
    - Vagal branches (X):
      - ○ Superior laryngeal nerve internal branch – sensory to epiglottis, base of tongue, and supraglottic mucosa up to the false cords
      - ○ Recurrent laryngeal nerve – sensory to the subglottic mucosa including the trachea and motor innervation to the muscles of the larynx except the cricothyroid muscle
  - Local anesthesia can be accomplished via a variety of techniques:
    - Nebulizers/aerosol techniques will cover entire airway but often needs supplementation with other techniques.
    - Topical sprays and gels will cover the nose, mouth, and pharynx
    - Superior laryngeal nerve blocks through the thyrohyoid membrane
    - "Spray as you go" topicalizes the larynx and proximal trachea. Can be facilitated by an epidural catheter threaded through the working channel of a flexible fiberoptic scope. This technique may elicit copious coughing from the patient.
    - Transtracheal injection through cricothyroid membrane – tracheal topicalization
    - Lidocaine 4% for topicalization and 2% for nerve blocks are typically used for efficacy and safety profile

- Anti-sialogogue (e.g. glycopyrrolate) is helpful for visualization and to mitigate dilution of the topicalized anesthetic.
- Sedation (i.e. midazolam, fentanyl, dexmedetomidine) is helpful but can potentially compromise airway
- Intubation accomplished via a variety of techniques and devices (i.e. rigid direct/indirect laryngoscopes, retrograde wire technique, blind techniques, flexible fiberoptic laryngoscope, see below).

o Techniques and devices for unanticipated difficult ventilation (ASA difficult airway algorithm)
  - Oral or nasopharyngeal airways: serve to displace the tongue anteriorly
  - Two-handed/two-person mask ventilation: improves facemask seal and reduces airway resistance
  - Proceed with endotracheal intubation: since a majority of patients do not feel difficulty both to ventilate and to intubate
  - Insertion of supraglottic airway: can serve as a conduit for endotracheal intubation
  - Ventilating rigid bronchoscope
  - Intratracheal jet stylet
  - Cricothyroid puncture and transtracheal jet ventilation: risks barotrauma if air trapped in lungs

o Techniques and devices for intubation
  - No single device or technique perfect for every scenario/patient. Several technique attempts may be necessary in the "easy to ventilate but cannot intubate" situation.
  - **Direct visualization** – requires line of sight from the maxillary teeth to the larynx. Most commonly employed technique. Accomplished with rigid laryngoscopes:
    - Macintosh-curved blade with distal end placed in the vallecula. Accomplishes laryngeal exposure via tension on the hypoepiglottic ligament. Epiglottis "flips up" to expose the cords. The blade's curvature secures tongue anteriorly and creates space in the oral cavity for endotracheal tube manipulation and placement. Chief disadvantage is its reliance on indirect exposure via tension on the ligament. "Floppy epiglottis" refers to insufficient traction to lift the tissue.
    - Miller-straight blade with distal end placed on posterior surface of the epiglottis. This direct elevation exposes the larynx more reliably than the Macintosh does and the view is often superior. Disadvantages include the potential of traumatizing the larynx as the blade's tip is narrow as well as impedance of tube passage given the straight blade's profile.
  - **Indirect visualization** – relies on the transmission of optical information from the distal to proximal

ends of the device. Attainment of optimal sniffing position is not as important. A major limitation of any indirect technique is camera soiling from blood and/or secretions.
- Video laryngoscopy (e.g. Glidescope)
  o Rigid, plastic laryngoscope that provides indirect visualization via a fog-resistant distal-end camera
  o Blade angle more acute, thus improving views in anterior airways
  o Good view does not guarantee successful intubation. Small mouths and oral cavities may hinder or preclude tube maneuverability into the larynx. Oral/pharyngeal trauma can occur "off camera."
- Flexible fiberoptic laryngoscope
  o Nasal or oral approach
  o Flexibility and greater freedom of movement as compared to rigid laryngoscopes give it superior versatility. Tolerated especially well in the awake technique because it does not forcibly displace pharyngeal structures
  o Sniffing position is not necessary. In an asleep patient, better to have cervical spine extended and head flat, thus making it a good choice in cervical spine instability. Assistant may need to pull tongue anteriorly in the asleep patient to expose larynx.
  o Once trachea is entered, loaded endotracheal tube can pass over the scope.
  o Visual confirmation of endotracheal tube position in the trachea
  o Can be used in combination with other devices such as a LMA or retrograde wire to secure airway
- **Blind techniques** – rarely used with the advent of indirect techniques
  - Blind nasal intubation
    o Awake or asleep/spontaneously breathing technique
    o Nasal mucosa treated with topical lidocaine and vasoconstrictor (usually phenylephrine). The tube is pushed through the nares and guided toward the airway by listening to the distal end of the tube for breath sounds.
    o Alternatively, the tube can be connected to a breathing circuit and expired carbon dioxide levels can be used.
    o While oral passage is also possible, the nasal route tends better to align the tube with the larynx.
- **Retrograde wire**
  - More invasive technique involving needle through cricothyroid membrane with cephalad

passage of wire until it exits the mouth. The endotracheal tube is then passed over the wire and into the airway.

- To facilitate passage of the tube, the wire can be threaded through one of the ports of a flexible fiberoptic scope. Some kits have a catheter that fits over the wire and can function as a stylet to pass the tube.
- Particularly appropriate in the setting of airway bleeding, poor mouth opening, or cervical neck immobility
- Contraindicated in presence of the following:
  o Cricothyroid membrane cannot be identified
  o Coagulopathy
  o Anterior neck lesion (i.e. tumors, abscess)
  ▪ **Transillumination (light wand)**
- Any device that uses light at the tip as a guide to intubation
- Light is transmitted through the skin and the position of the trachea is approximated by centering the light at midline.
- With tracheal intubation, the transmitted light remains localized. With esophageal intubation, the light is dimmed and more diffuse.
- A proven technique in the setting of difficult airway, although it requires a steep learning curve.
- Does not work well if patient is not paralyzed or cricoid pressure is used.
- Like all blind techniques, damage to the larynx is higher than with direct visualization.
- Surgical airway
  o A surgical airway is indicated in the event of a true "can't intubate, can't ventilate scenario" where all non-invasive options have been exhausted.
  o The options include:
  1. Needle cricothyrotomy
  2. Jet ventilation with a transtracheal catheter
  3. Surgical cricothyrotomy
     - Surgical cricothyrotomy involves an incision through the cricothyroid membrane where a breathing tube can be inserted.
     - Newer cricothyrotomy kits employ a Seldinger catheter, wire, and dilator technique.
     - A catheter attached to syringe is inserted through the cricothyroid membrane, while pulling back, when air is aspirated, the syringe is removed and a guidewire is passed through the catheter into the trachea, a dilator is then passed over the guidewire removed and finally the tube/introducer is inserted over the guidewire into the trachea.
     - Contraindications include
       a. Airway trauma rendering access across the cricothyroid membrane futile
       b. Age less than 10 as their smaller airways increase the risk of laryngeal trauma

- Alternatives and adjuncts
  o Supraglottic airway devices
  1. Serve as an intermediate between face mask ventilation and endotracheal intubation
  2. Can be used as conduits for endobronchial intubation and are often used for both spontaneously and mechanically ventilated patients during general anesthesia
  3. Supraglottic devices can all be attached to a respiratory circuit or breathing bag.
  4. They all have a sealing device that redirects air to the glottis and occlude the esophagus in varying degrees.
  5. They do not offer the same protection against aspiration of stomach content as cuffed endotracheal tubes do.
  6. Options include:
     - Laryngeal mask airway (LMA)
     - Esophageal–tracheal combitube
     - King laryngeal tube
- Laryngeal mask airway
  o Often used for elective cases in fasting patients
  o It can be a rescue device as described in the difficult airway algorithm.
  o It can be used as a planned intubating conduit in difficult airways.
  o It can also be used in CPR situations if the patient is unresponsive with no gag.
  o There are various LMA designs on the market:
  1. I-Gel – uses a heat-activated gel-like non-inflating cuff that molds to the individual's hypopharyngeal anatomy once placed.
  2. ProSEAL – allows for passage of a gastric tube
  3. Fastrach – intubating LMA is designed for use as an intubating conduit
  o Contraindicated:
  1. Morbidly obese
  2. Patients where peak inspiratory pressures during ventilation will exceed 20 cm H_2O (e.g., restrictive airway disease)
  3. Individuals at higher risk of aspiration such as gestation more than 14 weeks, hiatal hernias, gastroparesis, and others
  4. A relative contraindication is pharyngeal pathology.
  o Advantages over a face mask include
  1. Better seal in heavily bearded patients
  2. A lower incidence of facial nerve and eye trauma
  3. An allowance for hands-free operation
  o Advantages over endotracheal tubes include
  1. Less laryngo- and bronchospasm (especially in setting of URI)
  2. Ease of placement less dependent on patient positioning
  o Disadvantages include

1. Increased risk of airway trauma
2. Need for deeper anesthetic depth
3. Note that obstruction after insertion is common because of a pushed-down epiglottis or laryngospasm
4. A sore throat is a common complaint in the PACU following LMA use.
5. Hypoglossal, recurrent laryngeal and lingual nerve injuries are possible.
6. Limitations in positive pressure ventilation and the risk of gastric insufflation, and a lack of airway security that discourages its use in prone and jack-knife positions.

- Endobronchial intubation[2]
  - There are four absolute indications for one lung ventilation
    1. Protective isolation, confining bleeding or infection to one lung
    2. Control of ventilation distribution in settings like bronchopleural fistula, giant cyst or bullae at risk of rupture, and trauma/lung transplant with major bronchial disruption
    3. Unilateral lung lavage
    4. Video-assisted thoracoscopic surgery (VATS)
  - Three techniques can be used
    1. Placement of a double lumen tube (DLT)
    2. Use of a single-lumen tube in conjunction with a bronchial blocker
    3. Inserting a single-lumen tube into a mainstem bronchus
  - DLT
    1. DLTs all share the following trademarks: Longer bronchial lumen that fits in the left or right bronchus, a tracheal and bronchial cuff, and a pre-formed curve.
    2. DLT is sized by height.
    3. The most commonly used sizes are 35, 37, 39, and 41 F.
    4. Bronchial anatomy dictates the differences between a right-and left-sided DLT.
    5. Left-sided bronchial tube is used for the most surgical situations since the left upper lobe orifice is 5 cm from the carina. This anatomy allows plenty of room to position the blocker optimally.
    6. The right-sided DLT has a proximal portal allowing for ventilation through the very proximal right upper lobe orifice (usually just 1–2.5 cm from the carina).
    7. Although more difficult to place, right-sided DLTs should be considered for:
       - Left-sided lung transplantation or pneumonectomy
       - When left main bronchus anatomy is distorted by tumor or compression from outside by a mass or thoracic aortic aneurysm

8. Malpositioning errors during and after intubation are common.
   - Tracheal intubation is usually accomplished under direct visualization with a Macintosh 3 blade.
   - Upon passage of the bronchial end through the vocal cords, the tube is located 90° counter-clockwise (left-sided tube) or clockwise (right-sided tube). However, this technique does not insure proper bronchial entry.
   - If the tube is inserted too deep, the carina could obstruct the tracheal orifice causing obstruction and poor ventilation if the tracheal side is ventilating.
   - *Underinsertion* can also occur and you will hear no breath sounds and see no $ETCO_2$ when the tracheal lumen is used as the endobronchial cuff is in the trachea.
9. A flexible fiberoptic scope is invaluable in troubleshooting situations of malpositioning.
   - A useful landmark is the right upper lobe, which is unique in that it has three take-off branches.
10. *Advantages*
    - Excellent lung isolation with the ability to quickly ventilate either or both lungs
    - Rapid lung deflation
    - Ability to suction either lung
11. *Disadvantages*
    - Tube's size and stiffness: difficulty with intubation and tracheal/bronchial trauma
    - Must be often switched out with single-lumen tubes for the ICU if the patient is to remain intubated.

- Bronchial blockers
  1. Passed through a single-lumen endotracheal tube and can be used to selectively block off one bronchial orifice at a time.
  2. It has a high-volume low-pressure spherical shaped cuff and an inner lumen diameter of 1.4 mm.
  3. Once the patient is intubated, bilateral breath sounds heard and the endotracheal tube secured, the bronchial blocker is initially placed blindly.
  4. However the blocker must be positioned, advanced, and inflated under direct visualization.
  5. *Advantages* over a DLT
     - Ease of placement
     - Lower incidence of trauma
     - No need to reintubate at the conclusion of the case
  6. *Disadvantages*
     - Blocker does not block the lung as reliably as a DLT
     - More subject to displacing into the trachea during surgical manipulation

- This leads to inability to ventilate or poor lung isolation.
  - In addition, the blocked off lung collapses much more slowly than when a DLT is used because the lumen of the blocker is much smaller.
  - The smaller lumen also makes suctioning of secretions difficult.
- Intubation and tube change adjuncts[12,13,16,17]
  - Bougies (Eschmann tracheal tube introducer)
    1. 24 in. (60 cm) in length, typically 15 Fr (5 mm diameter) with a coude tip
    2. There is a 10 Fr pediatric version for tubes as small as 4–6 mm.
    3. Some have a central lumen with a port for ventilation and is good option for endotracheal tube exchange. It is made of braided polyester with a resin coating. This allows it to be both flexible and stiff at body temperature.
    4. The bougie is useful in a situation where laryngeal visualization is poor but an approximate location can be ascertained (as in incomplete lifting of the epiglottis).
    5. The bougie is passed through the glottis and functions as a guide for the endotracheal tube loaded over it.
    6. The bougie is stiff enough to cause serious damage or even perforate the trachea; attempt to place a bougie under direct vision with a laryngoscope rather than blindly.
    7. A rare, but real complication is that the bougie damages the trachea at the carina causing bilateral tension pneumothorax. This may be hard to diagnose as the breath sounds, though poor, can be equal and classical tracheal shift does not happen.
    8. It is *not* recommended for routine use in exchanging endotracheal tubes.
    9. For endotracheal tube exchange, a standard tube exchanger should be used. They tend to be softer and more flexible.
  - Soft and rigid tube change catheter
    1. Most soft and rigid tube change devices have lumens that are hollow and will allow insufflation or jetting of oxygen if necessary.
    2. The same caution exists for advancing a tube whose cuff is above the cords.
    3. Examples include the Cook airway exchange catheter and the Aintree intubation catheter.
    4. As the name suggests, it is used for replacement/exchange of a DLT, or an endotracheal tube/tracheostomy tube, when one is already in place.
    5. Tube change catheters are long, flexible, with length markings and round tips.
    6. They have a hollow central lumen with holes at each end and a connector that can attach to an Ambubag.
    7. *Cook airway exchange catheter* comes in 5, 10, 15 F with varying lengths.
    8. Use the biggest size feasible. Smaller sizes are prone to kinking, slipping out into the esophagus, or have so much given that the tip of the "railroaded" ETT gets stuck against the arytenoid cartilage; if this happens rotate the ETT tube, its bevel should allow it to slide over the arytenoid cartilage.
    9. Make sure the exchange catheter is lubricated before it is passed through the existing tube into the airway. Oxygen insufflation can be performed until the new ETT is placed.
    10. The old ETT is removed and the new tube is railroaded over the catheter as a guide.
    11. It is highly suggested that a laryngoscope or videolaryngoscope be used to optimize the view of the larynx or ensure that the exchange catheter is not dislodged. It also displaces soft tissues that might resist passage of the new tube.
- Endotracheal tube types
  - Endotracheal tubes are the most familiar elements of anesthesiology practice.
  - Endotracheal tubes maintain airway patency, permit oxygenation and ventilation, allow for suctioning of secretions, lower the risk of aspiration of gastric contents/oropharyngeal secretions, and facilitate the use of inhalation anesthetics.
  - Endotracheal tubes are made of polyvinylchloride (PVC) and are of single use. They have a number of characteristic features and many variations of these designs exist.
  - Endotracheal tubes have a left-facing bevel at the tip and a Murphy eye.
  - The Murphy's eye provides an alternate gas passage should occlusion of the tip occur.
  - The PVC does not absorb x-rays. For this reason most PVC tubes contain a radio-opaque line, which makes them visible on chest radiographs.
  - The bevel is left-facing rather than right-facing to allow the endotracheal tube tip an easier pass through the vocal chords.
  - Endotracheal tubes are placed in the right-hand side in a right-to-left direction toward the larynx.
  - Most endotracheal tubes used today have *low pressure–high volume* type cuffs. This design has comparatively large volume and allows for large contact area between cuff and trachea at lower pressures.
    1. The problem is that this balloon-like cuff can make folds when inflated, creating little tracks through which gastric/oropharyngeal fluid can flow into the trachea. Thus they have a higher risk of aspiration.
  - In contrast, *high pressure–low volume* cuffs are thought to provide better protection against aspiration. Because of their much smaller cuff–trachea contact area and higher inflation pressures used, cuff folds

are less likely to develop, at the expense of more likely tracheal mucosal ischemia.

- ○ "Laser tube":
  1. Has a cuff design that is of high pressure–low volume.
  2. Laser tubes are made of PVC, which is highly flammable in the presence of laser light and oxygen.
  3. The thoracic surgeon may employ a laser to ablate granulation tissue or web that causes airway narrowing in the lung.
  4. The laser tube's PVC core is wrapped in an inner metallic foil and an outer non-reflective core.
  5. The cuff is most vulnerable as it is not protected.
  6. In order to detect when the laser punctures the cuff, the pilot balloon is filled with blue dye granules that dissolves when filled with water.
  7. This blue dye will leak into the trachea so that it will be noticed in the airways during bronchoscopy.
- ○ Nasal–oral endotracheal RAE tubes
  1. Also known as RAE tubes after Ring, Adair, and Elwyn, its inventors.
  2. The RAE tubes facilitate oral and some facial, ophthalmologic surgery by moving the outer part of the endobronchial tube out of the way.
  3. It has a preformed bend and the point of greatest angle is indicated by a little black bar.
  4. RAE endotracheal tubes are the same in all other aspects as standard endotracheal tubes
  5. They have the same left-facing bevel at the tip, a Murphy eye, low-pressure–high-volume cuff, and length/diameter markings on its side.
  6. The "south-facing" tube's connector is facing the patient's feet and the "north-facing" tube (or nasal RAE) has a connector facing toward the head of the patient.
  7. Disadvantage
     - Preformed shape limits insertion depth, the bend naturally sits best at the lower lip or nostril.
     - An alternative would be to use an armored tube that can be bent out of the surgeon's way without kinking.
- ○ Armored tubes
  1. Just look like standard ET tubes, but as the name suggests it is armored or reinforced tubes with an embedded metal wire coil in its wall
  2. It still has a typical left-facing bevel tip and Murphy eye.
  3. It does not have a radio-opaque line as the tubes contain metal.
  4. The armored tubes lack a fixed bend and a stylet will be necessary to ensure successful intubation.

  5. Disadvantage
     - Metal coil has memory and it will not expand once a patient bites into it.
     - It is important to use a bite block to prevent this complication.
     - Armored endotracheal tubes are classified as MR-conditional (considered generally safe in MRI environment, with no real heating in the magnetic field).
     - Of note, no endotracheal tube is designated as MRI-safe, because of the metal spring in the pilot balloon.
- ○ Microlaryngoscopy tubes (MLT)
  1. Adult length endotracheal tubes with pediatric-sized diameter, long but thin.
  2. The microlaryngoscopic tube is also designed with an "adult" size cuff.
  3. They come in three sizes: 4, 5, and 6 mm.
  4. They are used for laryngeal surgery.
  5. The smaller diameter allows a better view of, for example, the vocal cords.
  6. The smaller diameter of these tubes means higher resistance to gas flows, which translates to higher airway pressures for a given tidal volume.
  7. Lower I:E ratios may be needed to allow for complete expiration.
- Standards for basic anesthetic monitoring
  Standard I
  - The "Showing up" mandate: trained anesthesia personnel must be present at all times throughout the delivery of a general, regional, or MAC anesthetic.
  Standard II
  Continuous evaluation of oxygenation, ventilation, circulation, and temperature throughout the case

Oxygenation
- Inhaled gas oxygen analyzer: When anesthesia machine used
- Pulse oximetry: All anesthetics

Ventilation
- Qualitative end-tidal CO_2 (GA without ETT/LMA)
- Quantitative end-tidal CO_2 (ET tube/LMA)
- Disconnect alarm: when anesthesia machine used

Circulation
- Electrocardiography
- Blood pressure
- Pulse oximetry

Temperature
- Temperature probe when clinically significant changes in temperature are expected.

References

1. American Society of Anesthesiologists Committee of Quality Management and Departmental Administration. Continuum of Depth of Sedation: Definition of General Anesthesia and Levels of Sedation/Analgesia. Last amended by the ASA House of Delegates on October 15, 2014. www.asahq.org/quality-and-practice-management/standards-and-guidelines

2. Mackey, D. C., Butterworth, J. F., Mikhail, M. S., Morgan, G. E., Wasnick, J. D. *Morgan & Mikhail's Clinical Anesthesiology*, 5th edn. New York, NY: McGraw-Hill Education LLC.

3. *Clinical Anesthesia Barash*, 7th edn. http://aam.ucsf.edu/article

4. K. Gelb, K. Leslie, D. Stanski, and S. Shafer. Monitoring the depth of anesthesia. In Miller R. D., et al. *Miller's Anesthesia*, 7th edn. Philadelphia, PA: Elsevier Saunders, 2010; 1229–65.

5. S. Forman, R. Yang. Administration of general anesthesia. In Dunn P. F., et al. *Clinical Anesthesia Procedures of the Massachusetts General Hospital*, 7th edn. Philadelphia, PA: Lippincott Williams & Wilkins, 2007; 228–32.

6. J. Savarese. Upcoming improvements in relaxation & reversal. In: Morgan G. E., Mikhail M. S., Murray M. J., eds. *Clinical Anesthesiology*, 4th edn. New York, NY: McGraw-Hill, 2006; 217.

7. American Society of Anesthesiologists Committee of Standards and Practice Parameters. Standards for Basic Anesthetic Monitors. Last amended by the ASA House of Delegates on October 28, 2015. www.asahq.org/quality-and-practice-management/standards-and-guidelines

8. A. Reed. The difficult airway. In: Reed A. P., Yudkowitz F. S., eds. *Clinical Cases in Anesthesia*. Philadelphia, PA: Elsevier Churchill Livingstone, 2005; 247–60.

9. American Society of Anesthesiologists Task Force on Management of the Difficult Airway. Practice Guidelines for Management of the Difficult Airway. *Anesthesiology*. 2013; 118(2); 1–20.

10. J. Henderson. Airway management in the adult. In: Miller R. D., et al. *Miller's Anesthesia*, 7th edn. Philadelphia, PA: Elsevier Churchill Livingstone, 2010; 1573–610.

11. G. Gavel, R. Walker. Laryngospasm in anesthesia, *British Journal of Anaesthesia*, 2014; 14(2):47–51.

12. Fibreoptic guided tracheal intubation through SAD using Aintree intubation catheter (DAS Guideline). *Anaesthesia*, 1996; 51:1123–1126.

13. M. Turk, D. Gravenstein. Aintree Intubation Catheter Technique in Unanticipated Difficult Intubation. Retrieved January 28, 2015, from University of Florida Department of Anesthesiology, Center for Simulation, Advanced Learning and Technology, Virtual. 2007.

14. W. H. Ring, J. C. Adair, R. A. Elwyn. A new pediatric endotracheal tube. *Anesthesia Analgesia*. 1975; 54:273–4. www.mrisafety.com

15. Johannes-Gutenberg-Universität, Mainz. The micro laryngeal tube – a new tube for direct laryngoscopy in the ENT field anaesthesist. *Anaesthesist*, 1989 Mar; 38(3):144–6.

16. Anesthesia machine web site: http://vam.anest.ufl.edu/airwaydevice/aintree/index.html

17. J. P. Nolan, M. E. Wilson. Endotracheal intubation in patients with potential cervical spine injuries: an indication for the gum elastic-bougie. *Anaesthesia*. 1993; 49:630–3.

Chapter 18

Monitored Anesthesia Care and Sedation

Ethan Bryson

Levels of Sedation

Monitored anesthesia care (MAC) is defined as "a specific anesthesia service in which an anesthesiologist has been requested to participate in the care of a patient undergoing a diagnostic or therapeutic procedure."[1] MAC can be as simple as the placement and observance of standard American Society of Anesthesiologists (ASA) monitors during a procedure without sedation or intervention, the administration of anxiolytics, or the administration of anesthetics which bring the patient to a deeper level of sedation. Sedation is defined as a continuum of states and often during the course of an anesthetic the depth of sedation will fluctuate, depending on the level of stimulation or anesthetic concentration.

Levels of sedation are defined by the patient's physical state and degree of responsiveness, not on the dose or type of medication administered[2]:

- Minimal sedation
  1. Responds appropriately to verbal stimulus
  2. Spontaneous respirations
  3. No airway or cardiovascular compromise
- Moderate sedation
  1. Responds appropriately to either verbal or tactile stimulation
  2. Adequate respirations
  3. No airway or cardiovascular interventions required
- Deep sedation
  1. No response to verbal or tactile stimulation, responds only to painful stimulus
  2. Respirations may be inadequate
  3. Airway interventions may be required (jaw thrust, chin lift, oral airway)
  4. Cardiovascular interventions not required
- General anesthesia
  1. No response, even to painful stimulus
  2. Respirations may be inadequate
  3. Airway interventions may be required (laryngeal mask airway [LMA] or endotracheal tube [ETT] insertion)
  4. Cardiovascular function may be impaired

Techniques

There are many different techniques which are used to produce anxiolysis, analgesia, and anesthesia. Any one of these alone may bring a patient to more than one depth of anesthesia depending upon the characteristics of the patient and the dose of the medication used. In general, the intended level of sedation can be reached by the following[3,4]:

- Minimal sedation
  ○ Administration of a single intravenous (IV) anxiolytic (e.g. midazolam)
  ○ Peripheral nerve blocks without sedation
  ○ Local or topical anesthesia
  ○ Administration of less than 50% nitrous oxide (N_2O) in oxygen with no other sedative or analgesic medications by any route
  ○ A single, oral sedative or analgesic medication administered in doses appropriate for the unsupervised treatment of insomnia, anxiety, or pain.
- Moderate sedation
  ○ Administration of more than one IV agent (e.g. midazolam and fentanyl) at doses appropriate to maintain response to verbal or tactile stimulation
  ○ Administration of IV agents via infusion (e.g. propofol or dexmedetomidine) at doses appropriate to maintain response to verbal or tactile stimulation
- Deep sedation
  ○ Administration of multiple IV agents (e.g. midazolam, fentanyl, ketamine, propofol, "Ketofol," dexmedetomidine) or a single agent at doses appropriate to blunt the response to painful stimulus while maintaining spontaneous respirations, with or without intervention.

Risks and Complications

Since the depth of sedation fluctuates during the procedure depending on the level and intensity of stimulation as balanced by the concentration of medications provided, anyone who administers these medications must be properly trained to "rescue" the patient from an unanticipated, deeper level of sedation including agitation, loss of spontaneous respirations, and hemodynamic instability.[5,6]

- Unanticipated response to sedation
  ○ Some patients may become agitated, require more anesthesia than anticipated, or quickly pass from a state of light sedation into a much deeper plane depending on a number of factors including:
    ▪ Comorbid conditions which alter the physiological response to anesthesia (e.g. extremes of age,

chronic obstructive pulmonary disease [COPD], morbid obesity, etc.)

- Medications which increase or decrease tolerance to anesthetics (e.g. chronic benzodiazepine use, antidepressants, etc.)
- Airway anatomy leading to obstruction with resulting hypoxia or hypercarbia
- Loss of patent airway or loss of respiratory drive
  - With sedation, the muscles of the pharynx are relaxed and lead to either partial or full airway obstruction which can result in hypoxia or hypercarbia despite respiratory effort. Rescue maneuvers may include:
    - Head-tilt
    - Chin-lift
    - Jaw-thrust
    - Insertion of an airway device (e.g. oral airway, nasal trumpet, LMA, ETT)
  - When respiratory drive itself is blunted or compromised, rescue maneuvers may include the administration of reversal agents (e.g. naloxone, flumazenil)
- Cardiovascular compromise
  - Relaxation of the vasculature often accompanies deeper levels of sedation and may require cardiovascular support. Rescue interventions may include:
    - Administration of fluids
    - Administration of vasopressors (e.g. phenylephrine, ephedrine)
    - Basic or advanced cardiovascular life support techniques (Basic Life Support [BLS], Advanced Cardiovascular Life Support [ACLS])

ASA Guidelines for Sedation and Sedation Guidelines for Non-Anesthesiologists

ASA Guidelines for Sedation refer to medication provided for procedures performed in a variety of settings, including hospitals, freestanding clinics, physician, dental, and other offices.[2]

- The medical history of every patient should be reviewed with a focus on items which could possibly alter the response to anesthetic agents including:
  - Cardiovascular, pulmonary, or neurologic abnormalities
  - Prior adverse events with anesthesia
  - Current medications
  - Allergies to medications or anesthetic agents
  - Time of last oral intake
  - History of tobacco, alcohol, or substance use or abuse
- A focused physical examination should be performed.
  - Pre-procedure vital signs should be determined.
  - Auscultation of the heart and lungs should be performed.
  - An airway evaluation to determine the potential for obstruction under anesthesia is essential.
- In patients with certain underlying medical conditions (e.g. end-stage renal disease requiring hemodialysis, COPD requiring oxygen therapy) pre-procedure laboratory testing should be performed if there is an increased likelihood that the results of such tests will affect patient management or alter the choice of anesthetic.

ASA Guidelines for sedation when anesthesia is administered by practitioners who are not specialists in anesthesiology:

- These guidelines do not apply to patients receiving general anesthesia or major conduction anesthesia (e.g. spinal or epidural/caudal block).
- When anesthesia is administered, the operating practitioner or another licensed physician should have specific training in sedation, anesthesia, and rescue techniques appropriate to the type of sedation or anesthesia being provided.

References

1. American Society of Anesthesiologists Committee of Origin: Quality Management and Departmental Administration. Continuum of depth of sedation: definition of general anesthesia and levels of sedation/analgesia (Approved by the ASA House of Delegates on October 13, 1999, and last amended on October 15, 2014).
2. American Society of Anesthesiologists Task Force on Sedation and Analgesia by Non-Anesthesiologists. Practice Guidelines for Sedation and Analgesia by Non-Anesthesiologists: An updated report. *Anesthesiology* 2002; 96:1004–17.
3. American Dental Association. *Guidelines for the Use of General Anesthesia and Sedation by Dentists.* Adopted by the ADA house of delegates October 2016.
4. Das S., Ghosh S. Monitored anesthesia care: An overview. *J Anaesthesiol Clin Pharmacol.* 2015; 31(1):27–9.
5. Bhananker S. M., Posner K. L., Cheney F. W., et al. Injury and liability associated with monitored anesthesia care: A closed claims analysis. *Anesthesiology.* 2006; 104(2):228–34.
6. Agostoni M., Fanti L., Gemma M., et al. Adverse events during monitored anesthesia care for GI endoscopy: An 8-year experience. *Gastrointest Endosc.* 2011; 74(2):266–75.

Chapter 19

Intravenous Fluid Therapy

Stefan A. Ianchulev and Charles P. Plant

Water, Electrolytes, Glucose Requirement, Disposition

Total body water	Plasma volume	Plasma content		
60–70% body weight	~3 L	Inorganic ions	Albumin	Small molecules

- Endothelial function: selective permeability
  - Starling's equation underscores the important forces (hydrostatic and oncotic) affecting fluid distribution between capillary and interstitial space (see Figure 19.1):

$$J_v = K_f [(P_c - P_i) - \sigma (\pi_c - \pi_i)]$$

J_v = net filtration or net fluid movement

K_f = filtration coefficient

P_c and P_i = the hydrostatic pressures in the capillaries and interstitial space respectively

σ = reflection coefficient

π_c and π_i = capillary and interstitial oncotic pressure, respectively

- Na$^+$, K$^+$, Cl$^-$ ions: ATP-dependent process maintains a gradient across the membrane.
  - Albumin and other larger molecules remain intravascularly due to endothelial properties.
- Natural driving force and thus fluid movement is from capillary to interstitial space, where the excess fluid is cleared by the lymphatics.
- Endothelial function disruption possibly due to surgery, inflammatory process, and direct injury leads to:
  - Changes in the interstitial fluid composition
  - Reduces the oncotic pressure difference leading to further extravasation of fluid and resulting in tissue edema
  - Compromises local perfusion and accumulation of toxic byproducts causing a vicious cycle of worsening edema
- Perioperative fluid therapy goals:
  - Maintain the intravascular compartment volume to assure adequate delivery of oxygen and nutrients to the organs while maintaining good clearance of metabolic byproducts

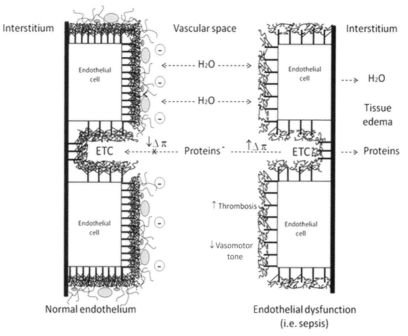

Figure 19.1 Glycocalyx characteristics in normal endothelium (left) and during endothelial dysfunction (right). ETC, endothelial cleft. Chelazzi, C., Villa, G., Mancinelli, P., et al. *Crit Care* 2015, 19:26. DOI: 10.1186/s13054-015-0741-z.

- Ideal resuscitation fluid:
  - Should produce predictable and sustainable increase in the intravascular volume
  - Resemble closely the composition of extracellular fluid
  - Be easily metabolized and freely excreted, be devoid of metabolic or systemic effects
  - Be inexpensive[1]

Resuscitation Fluids

- *Crystalloids*
  - Balanced solutions: Ionic solution and osmolality close to plasma
  - Approximately 20% remains in the intravascular compartment.
  - Crystalloid buffers: Sodium bicarbonate, lactate, acetate, gluconate, and malate
    - Sodium bicarbonate is not suited for long-term storage.
    - Excess administration of buffer-containing solutions causes alkalemia, hyperlactatemia, and hypotonicity.[1]
  - Resuscitation with normal saline can cause hyperchloremic acidosis.
  - Hypertonic saline in traumatic brain-injured patients did not show any short- or long-term improvement of survival.[1]
- Plasma volume expansion rule:
  Plasma volume expansion = volume infused/volume of distribution
- *Colloids*: Dissolved large molecular weight substances
  - *Naturally occurring colloids*: Albumin
    - Produced from fractionation of blood, which is then heat-treated to prevent transmission of infections and then suspended in saline
    - Exists as 4–5% and 20%
  - *Semisynthetic colloids*:
    - Gelatins – Bovine collagen derivatives. Some preparations can contain Ca^{2+} or other inorganic ions.
    - Dextrans – Biosynthesized sucrose derivatives, best described by their molecular weight (dextran 40–40,000 Da, dextran 70–70,000 Da)
    - Hetastarches – Derivatives of amylopectine. They are divided into high molecular weight, medium molecular weight, and low molecular weight and are dissolved in normal saline or balanced solutions.
    - Effects of semisynthetic colloids:
      - Improved viscosity due to hemodilutional effect
      - Red cell aggregation increased by large molecular colloids but decreased by medium and low molecular colloids
      - All colloids affect renal function

Table 19.1 Characteristics of common crystalloid solutions compared to human plasma

	Plasma	0.9% saline	Ringer's lactate	Plasma-Lyte 148°
Sodium (mmol/l)	136–145	154	130	140
Potassium (mmol/l)	3.5–5.0		4	5
Magnesium (mmol/l)	0.8–1.0			1.5
Calcium (mmol/l)	2.2–2.6		3	
Chloride (mmol/l)	98–106	154	109	98
Acetate (mmol/l)				27
Gluconate (mmol/l)				23
Lactate (mmol/l)			28	
Malate (mmol/l)				
eSID (mEq/l)	42		28	50
Theoretical osmolarity (mosmol/l)	291	308	273	295
Actual or measured osmolality[a] (mosmol/kg H_2O)	287	286	256	271
pH	7.35–7.45	4.5–7	5.0–7	4–8

[a]Freezing point depression.
Plasma-Lyte 148 manufactured by Baxter Healthcare, Toongabie, NSW; Australia Ringer's Lactate manufactured by Baxter Healthcare, Deerfield, IL, USA; Hartmann's solution manufactured by Baxter Healthcare, Toongabie, NSW; Australia Ionosteril manufactured by Fresenius Medical Care, Schweinfurt, Germany; Sterofundin ISO manufactured by B. Braun Melsungen AG, Melsungen, Germany, *Crit Care* 2016, 20:59. DOI: 10.1186/s13054-016-1217-5.

- Gelatins have higher incidence of allergic reactions
- No mortality benefit shown in CHEST study with HES 6%[2] (Table 19.1)

Fluid Requirements and Fluid Deficit Calculations

- **Maintenance rule:**
  - 4-2-1 rule:
    - 4 ml/kg first 10 kg
    - 2 ml/kg second 10 kg
    - 1 ml/kg – remainder of the weight
- **Fasting fluid deficit:**
  - Number of hours × maintenance fluid requirement = fluid deficit
    - Replacement administered over the first 3 hours

- Current enhanced recovery after surgery (ERAS) protocols recommend carbohydrate drinks up until 2 hours before surgery.
  - These patients may not have such significant deficit compared to those who fasted 6 hours or more.
- **Insensible losses**
  - Losses due to dehumidification of breathing air, sweating, large exposed intracavitary areas, etc.
  - In the past, those losses were estimated to be as large as 12 ml/kg/h in major abdominal or thoracic surgeries.
  - Presently it is thought that the insensible losses do not exceed 2 ml/kg/h.
- **Blood loss:**
  - Best substitute for lost blood is whole blood.
    - Difficult to come by and associated with infectious and immunological problems
  - Replacement of minor blood losses with crystalloids or colloids is acceptable substitute.
  - Hematocrit decreases to 21% can be well tolerated by some patients.
  - Lower hematocrit can be associated with good outcome if O_2 demand is decreased.
  - *Recommendations*:
    - Substitute individual components – red cells (PRBC), plasma (FFP, Cryo), platelets, recombinant clotting factors
    - Major trauma: 1:1:1 ratio of PRBC:FFP:platelets
- **Perioperative fluid management**
  - Goal-directed therapy (GDT): Protocolized fluid administration based on continuous assessment of fluid deficit. Need for invasive or noninvasive continuous assessment devices
    - Arterial line contour assessment – Calibrated and noncalibrated devices. Dependent on tidal volumes of 8 ml/kg IBW
    - Swan–Ganz catheters for continuous cardiac output – Currently out of favor due to complications, invasiveness, and user familiarity
    - Tissue perfusion model – Gastric tonometry, laser Doppler flowmetry, microdialysis catheters, transcutaneous oxygen saturation measurements, and tissue pH monitors

- Effects of GDT:
  - Improved nausea and vomiting[3]
  - Reduced pain scores[3]
  - Better outcomes in abdominal surgery with restrictive fluid administration[4]
  - Shorter length of stay[5]
- Pitfalls in perioperative fluid management algorithms
  - Indices generally accepted in the past like urine output (UO), blood pressure (BP), heart rate (HR), central venous pressure (CVP), pulmonary artery occlusion pressure (PAOP) have been deemed as inadequate markers for optimization of cardiac output (CO) and mixed venous saturation S_vO_2 in the recent years.[6]
  - CVP does not correlate with preload responsiveness. Swan–Ganz catheter has fallen out of favor.[7]
  - Numerous effecting factors including: static (BP, CO, PAOP, HR, LVDEP) vs. dynamic (CO, SV, SVV) parameters, and upstream (DO_2, CVP, PAP) vs. downstream (SvO_2, SV, stroke volume variation, pulse contour analysis, near-infrared spectroscopy-based tissue oxygenation, lactate) indices.[8–10]

Normal Saline vs. Lactated Ringer's vs. Plasma-Lyte

- Type of crystalloid best for resuscitation has not been established.
- Most commonly utilized crystalloids are 0.9% normal saline, lactated Ringer's solution, Plasma-Lyte, and dextrose 5% in water.
- Normal saline (NS) has been associated with decreased renal artery flow and reduced renal cortical tissue perfusion in subjects who received 2 l of NS over 1 hour as compared to Plasma-Lyte 148.[11–13] Possible impaired gastrointestinal and hematological pathways, thrombin generation, and platelet activation due to NS.[14]
- Increased incidence of renal insufficiency but not mortality or length of stay with NS[15]; however, a recent study did not show difference on acute kidney injury (AKI), renal replacement therapy, mortality, or length of stay.[16]

References

1. Myburgh J. A., Mythen M. G. Resuscitation fluids. *The New England Journal of Medicine.* 2013;369(13):1243–51.
2. Grocott M. P., Mythen M. G., Gan T. J. Perioperative fluid management and clinical outcomes in adults. *Anesthesia and Analgesia.* 2005;100(4):1093–106.
3. Chappell D., Jacob M., Hofmann-Kiefer K., Conzen P., Rehm M. A

rational approach to perioperative fluid management. *Anesthesiology.* 2008;109(4):723–40.
4. Nisanevich V., Felsenstein I., Almogy G., et al. Effect of intraoperative fluid management on outcome after intraabdominal surgery. *Anesthesiology.* 2005;103(1):25–32.
5. Thacker J. K., Mountford W. K., Ernst F. R., Krukas M. R., Mythen

M. M. Perioperative fluid utilization variability and association with outcomes: considerations for enhanced recovery efforts in sample US surgical populations. *Annals of Surgery.* 2016;263(3):502–10.
6. Tseng G. S., Wall M. H. Endpoints of resuscitation: what are they anyway? *Seminars in Cardiothoracic and Vascular Anesthesia.* 2014;18(4):352–62.

7. Marik P. E. Obituary: pulmonary artery catheter 1970 to 2013. *Annals of Intensive Care*. 2013;3(1):38.

8. Grocott M. P., Dushianthan A., Hamilton M. A., et al. Perioperative increase in global blood flow to explicit defined goals and outcomes following surgery. *The Cochrane Database of Systematic Reviews*. 2012;11:CD004082.

9. Reddy S., Weinberg L., Young P. Crystalloid fluid therapy. *Critical Care*. 2016;20:59.

10. Finfer S., Bellomo R., Boyce N., et al. A comparison of albumin and saline for fluid resuscitation in the intensive care unit. *The New England Journal of Medicine*. 2004;350(22):2247–56.

11. Shoemaker W. C., Appel P. L., Kram H. B., Waxman K., Lee T. S. Prospective trial of supranormal values of survivors as therapeutic goals in high-risk surgical patients. *Chest*. 1988;94(6):1176–86.

12. Velmahos G. C., Demetriades D., Shoemaker W. C., et al. Endpoints of resuscitation of critically injured patients: normal or supranormal? A prospective randomized trial. *Annals of Surgery*. 2000;232(3):409–18.

13. Chowdhury A. H., Cox E. F., Francis S. T., Lobo D. N. A randomized, controlled, double-blind crossover study on the effects of 2-L infusions of 0.9% saline and plasma-lyte(R) 148 on renal blood flow velocity and renal cortical tissue perfusion in healthy volunteers. *Annals of Surgery*. 2012;256(1):18–24.

14. Brummel-Ziedins K., Whelihan M. F., Ziedins E. G., Mann K. G. The resuscitative fluid you choose may potentiate bleeding. *The Journal of Trauma*. 2006;61(6):1350–8.

15. Yunos N. M., Bellomo R., Glassford N., et al. Chloride-liberal vs. chloride-restrictive intravenous fluid administration and acute kidney injury: an extended analysis. *Intensive Care Medicine*. 2015;41(2):257–64.

16. Young P., Bailey M., Beasley R., et al. Effect of a buffered crystalloid solution vs saline on acute kidney injury among patients in the intensive care unit: the SPLIT Randomized Clinical Trial. *JAMA*. 2015;314(16):1701–10.

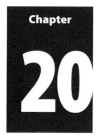

Complications of Anesthesia

Etiology, Prevention, Treatment

Andrew Glasgow

- Most common sources of anesthesia litigation for *brain damage/death*
  1. **Cardiovascular complications** – multifactorial (arrhythmia, hypotension, etc.), pulmonary embolism, inadequate fluid therapy, stroke, hemorrhage, myocardial infarction
  2. **Respiratory complications** – difficult intubation, inadequate ventilation/oxygenation, esophageal intubation, premature extubation, aspiration, airway obstruction
  3. **Medication-related damage** – wrong drug/dose, allergic or adverse reaction, malignant hyperthermia
  4. **Equipment-related damage** – equipment *misuse* more common than *malfunction*. Gas delivery problems most often associated with death
  5. **Block-related damage** – neuraxial cardiac arrest, high spinal/epidural, intravascular injection, absorption
- Most common litigation during MAC anesthesia is a *respiratory event*, due to *over-sedation* (most often in cardiac cath lab and endoscopy suite)[1]
- Most common source of anesthesia litigation → dental injury

Airway-Related Injury

Upper airway facial nerve and mental nerve paresis

- Risk: pressure from rim of mask, rigorous jaw thrust

Nasal epistaxis; nasal septum necrosis; retropharyngeal abscess, sinusitis

- Risk: nasotracheal intubation, nasogastric tube (NGT), nasal temperature, mask
- Important: avoid nasal passage in patients with *basilar skull fractures* or severe facial trauma, due to potential for inadvertent cranial intubation

Laryngeal vocal cord paresis; arytenoid disarticulation; granuloma formation

- Risk: routine and emergent intubations

Tracheal – *Early complications*: tracheal lacerations; hemorrhage; recurrent laryngeal nerve injury; discomfort from tracheostomy. *Late complications*: tracheal stenosis; tracheo-esophageal fistulas; trachea-innominate fistula; tracheomalacia

- Risk: emergent tracheostomy, endotracheal tube (ETT) movement, stylette, ETT cuff > 25 mmHg

Pharyngeal/esophageal tears: abscess, esophageal perforation, mediastinitis

- Risk: age >60, female, difficult intubation, esophageal intubation, NGT, transesophageal echocardiogram (TEE)
- Important: mortality rate up to 50%, monitor esophageal intubations closely

Temporomandibular joint (TMJ) injuries: TMJ disarticulation; pain

- Risk: female, age <60 years old, ASA1/2

Dental injuries: fracture; tooth avulsion

- Risk: laryngoscopy/intubation, airway manipulation, poor dentition, and patient characteristics associated with difficult laryngoscopy, 5th–7th decade occurs in 0.04–0.05% of patients

Respiratory Events

Bronchospasm

Etiology: ETT, desflurane/pungent airway irritant, cold air

Risk factors: reactive airway disease, recent URI

- Prevention: pretreat with inhaled beta-2 agonist
- Treatment: inhaled beta-2 agonist, deepening anesthetic, +/− steroids, +/− epinephrine

Laryngospasm

Involuntary closure of true and false cords, or true cords alone

Risk factors: pediatric patients three times more than adults, recent Upper respiratory infection (URI), gastroesophageal reflux disease (GERD)

- Prevention: vigilance, maintain adequate level of anesthesia
- Treatment: positive pressure ventilation, deepening anesthetic, muscle relaxant

Negative pressure pulmonary edema (NPPE): inspiration against closed airway occurs in 4% of cases of laryngospasm, 0.05–0.1% of general anesthetics

Table 20.1 Ocular injuries, symptoms, risk factors, and rates

	Corneal abrasion	Anterior ischemic optic neuropathy	Posterior ischemic optic neuropathy	Acute angle closure glaucoma
Pain	Yes	No	No	Yes
Vision	Photophobia	Blindness	Blindness	Blurred
Patient risks	Ex-ophthalmos Proptosis Dry eye	HTN, DM, CAD, PVD, CVA, smoker, degenerative eye	Male, HTN, DM, CAD, PVD, obesity Smoker, degenerative eye	Female, elderly, glaucoma
Surgical and anesthesia risks	Prone, lateral	Cardiopulmonary bypass	Prone spine surgery (prolonged, fusion, anemia, hypovolemia, hypotension)	HTN, bucking, coughing, anti-muscarinic pressors – ephedrine
Rate	0.034–0.17%	0.06%	0.013–0.2%	Rare

Central retinal artery occlusion: Common cause of postoperative visual loss, seen most often after prone spine surgeries, caused by extrinsic compression on eye.[3,4]

Risk factors: male, young, OSA, acromegaly, difficult intubation, HEENT surgery[2]

- Pathophysiology: laryngospasm, or compression of airway (ETT/LMA)

1. Negative pressure, -100 to -140 cm H_2O generated → ↑ preload and afterload and ↓ CO) → ↑ pulmonary pressure → ↑ pulmonary capillary hydrostatic pressures → transudate
2. Negative intrapleural pressure → ↑ in interstitial fluid
3. Hypoxia further ↑ pulmonary vascular resistance (PVR) via hypoxic pulmonary vasoconstriction
4. Hyperadrenergic state additionally, ↑ pulmonary blood volume, ↑ PVR, and ↑ hydrostatic pressure
   - Signs and symptoms: acute respiratory distress in an otherwise healthy patient, pink frothy pulmonary secretions, CXR with bilateral interstitial alveolar infiltrates
   - Prevention: use of bite block/spacer, LMA if high risk
   - Treatment: Positive end expiratory pressure (PEEP) via mechanical ventilation or continuous positive airway pressure (CPAP)

Potential role with beta-2 agonists, low tidal volume ventilation strategies, and diuresis, however, further study indicated. Important to determine etiology of pulmonary edema, NPPE vs. cardiogenic, hypervolemic and neurogenic, as treatments can differ

- Resolution: usually occurs in 3–12 hours, however complete resolution may take 12–48 hours. If patient remains intubated after 48 hours, their morbidity and mortality increase significantly.

Aspiration

Aspiration of gastric contents: pain, diabetes, obesity, pregnancy, smoking, alcohol, drug abuse, opioids, and gastrointestinal pathology affect the emptying of solids. Healthy adults who fasted from clear liquids >4 hours have a higher gastric pH and volume than those who fasted between 2 and 4 hours.

Aspiration Management: LMA

If a patient with an LMA regurgitates stomach contents:

1. Place patient in Trendelenberg position
2. Give 100% oxygen
3. Determine risk and benefits of leaving LMA in place vs. placing an ETT tube
4. Evaluation of regurgitation with fiberoptic visualization of trachea and bronchi may be beneficial

Other LMA complications: LMA overinflation, use with nitrous causing LMA distension, use of lidocaine gel → hypoglossal, lingual, and recurrent laryngeal nerve damage (usually temporary)

Aspiration Pneumonitis

- If no symptoms after 2 hours, aspiration unlikely to become serious
- Patients with particulate aspiration may require bronchopulmonary lavage
- Do not use neutralizing solutions
- Do not give prophylactic steroids → may increase mortality
- Do not give prophylactic antibiotics → may increase risk of pneumonia
- Controversial → cricoid pressure has been shown to decrease LES tone without influencing gastric pressure, which potentially can increase the risk of aspiration

Ten Factors That Increase the Risk of Aspiration

1. Emergency surgery
2. Light anesthesia/unexpected motor response
3. Acute or chronic GI pathology
4. Obesity
5. Opioid medication
6. Neurologic disease
7. Lithotomy position
8. Difficult intubation
9. GERD
10. Hiatal hernia

Ocular Injuries

See Table 20.1.

Vascular Complications

Arterial/venous thrombosis, guidewire or catheter embolism, cardiac tamponade pneumothorax, hemothorax, pulmonary artery rupture, carotid artery puncture, central line-associated bloodstream infection (CLABSI), ectopy, hematoma

Central Lines

Acute Complications

- #1 Hematoma or arterial injury
- #2 Cardiac tamponade
- Most common nonserious complication is *ventricular ectopy*

Late Complications

- #1 Infection CLABSI 5% of patients with central lines, overall mortality is unknown. Nosocomial bacteremia associated with mortality rate of 35%
- #2 Thrombosis

Safety Steps

- Where possible use single lumen, heparin-bonded catheters (less risk of infection and thrombus), with bactericidal impregnated patches (less risk of infection) and remove ASAP
- Use multiple confirmation methods: visualization of wire under ultrasound, manometry, pressure waveform monitoring, blood gas measurement, color, and determining nonpulsatile flow

Left-Sided versus Right-Sided Central Line

- Cupola of the pleura is higher on the left (↑ risk of pneumothorax)
- Thoracic duct may be injured on the left
- Left internal jugular (IJ) is usually smaller than the right IJ, and often demonstrates a greater degree of overlap of the adjacent carotid artery
- Left-sided central lines enter the SVC at a more *oblique angle,* → poses a greater risk of vascular perforation and cardiac tamponade
- Left IJ is associated with greater complication rate than right IJ

Location of catheter tip with CXR → decrease risk of cardiac tamponade

- **Right-sided catheters** – CXR location ABOVE the level of the carina
- **Left-sided catheters** – CXR location BELOW the level of the carina
- **Long-term catheters** – PICC, hemodialysis, chemo-specific catheters, should be placed at *cavo-atrial junction,* with radiological supervision (below carina)

Pulmonary Arterial Catheter (PAC)

Minor complications common 50%. Major complications rare 0.1–0.5%

- **Complications related to catheter placement:** Arrhythmias (pretreatment with lidocaine does not prevent arrhythmia), ventricular fibrillation, RBBB, complete heart block, hematoma, scar, pain
- **Catheter residence:** Catheter knots, thromboembolism, pulmonary infarction, infection/endocarditis, endocardial damage, cardiac valve injury, pulmonary artery rupture, pulmonary artery pseudoaneurysm, misinterpretation of data
- **Misuse of equipment:** Three times more likely cause of equipment-related adverse outcomes compared to equipment malfunction

Arterial Lines Complications

Vascular insufficiency thrombosis, vasospasm

- Risk factors: Vasospastic arterial disease, previous arterial injury, thrombocytosis, protracted shock, high-dose vasopressor administration, prolonged cannulation, and infection
- Femoral artery > Radial artery complications
- Brachial lines are associated with potential damage to the median nerve. Bloodstream infections with arterial lines are 1:1,000 catheter days

Intra-osseous (IO) Line Complications

- Extravasation of fluid and meds → compartment syndrome or muscle necrosis, due to improper placement/supervision
- Hematoma, pain, fracture, growth plate injury, fat micro-emboli
- Infection: osteomyelitis and cellulitis (limit use to <72 hours)
- Tibial IO lines have *higher flow* rates than humeral IO lines
- Humeral IO lines reach central circulation faster

Avoid growth plate in pediatric patients; avoid placement in fractured bone. IO lines are a relative contraindication in patients with osteogenesis imperfecta/osteoporosis

Position-Related Peripheral Nerve Complications

Peripheral Neurologic Complications

Etiology: Compression, stretch, ischemia, trauma, and intrinsic patient risk factors – diabetes mellitus, multiple sclerosis, chemotherapy, prolonged immobility, smoking, body habitus, patient position

- Not every nerve injury is due to improper positioning
- Some related to events occurring out of the OR

Ulnar injury: Most common, occurring in 1:2,700 patients

- Risk factors: male, both thin and obese patients, prolonged hospital stay
- More common under GA, although 15% of ulnar injuries occur under MAC or lower extremity regional technique. Supinate arm. May not be related to position

Brachial Plexus

- Avoid stretching or direct compression at axilla (lateral decubitus position – use axillary roll)

Table 20.2 OSHA: anesthetic gases: guidelines for workplace exposure

	OSHA N_2O max	OSHA volatile max
N_2O alone	25 ppm	–
Volatile alone	–	2 ppm
N_2O and volatile	25 ppm	0.5 ppm
Level attainable without scavenging	3,000 ppm	50 ppm

Table 20.3 OSHA maximum limit of radiation for occupational exposure

Prospective annual limit	5 rems/year
Retrospective annual limit	10–15 rems in 1 year
Pregnant women	0.5 rems/gestation

Average exposure in the United States is 0.080–0.2 rem/year.

Peroneal Injury

- Risk factors: prolonged lithotomy (over 2 hours), pressure on lateral aspect of upper fibula (candy cane stirrups), extreme angle, hypotension, thin body habitus, older age, vascular disease, diabetes mellitus, cigarette smoking

Management of postoperative neuropathy: If patient develops minimal to moderate neurologic symptoms that persist longer than 24 hours, consult a neurologist or physiatrist, as physiologic testing can determine if the condition is acute or chronic. If severe, more urgent neurologic consultation warranted.

Fire Hazard

Burn Triad

1. **Ignition source**: cautery, light, fluoroscopic equipment, laser, drills
2. **Oxidizer**: oxygen, nitrous oxide
3. **Flammable material**: drapes, tracheal tube, sponges, gauze

Prevention: Minimize FiO_2 during surgeries involving airway, prevent trapping/pooling of oxygen or flammable antiseptic solution, turn-off fluoroscopic lights when not in use, use lasers and electrocautery with caution

Steps for airway fire: While calling for HELP

1. Remove ETT tube, disconnect from oxygen source, flood field
2. Mask ventilate, → reintubate
3. Examine airway

Predominant mechanism: use of supplemental oxygen during MAC[5]

Chronic Environmental Exposure, Fertility, Carcinogenicity, Teratogenicity, Scavenging

- Nitrous oxide exposure has deleterious reproductive and teratogenic effects in animal studies (Table 20.2)
- Female dentists: ↑ risk of spontaneous abortion when nitrous used in facilities without proper scavenging
- Healthcare providers (HCP) have increased risk of miscarriage, however, may be unrelated to operating room (work hours, stress, etc.)
- Rate of miscarriage, teratogenicity, and infertility is similar for anesthesiologists as it is for non-anesthesiologist physicians

- Trace concentrations of anesthetic vapors do not present a health hazard
- Efforts should be made to keep anesthetic vapors to a minimum

Sources of contamination: inhalation induction, uncuffed ETT, LMAs, circuit disconnects, inadequate scavenging

PACU → unsafe levels of anesthetic gas if air not circulated properly[6]

Radiation Exposure

Ionizing radiation (i.e. X-ray, fluoroscopy, mammogram, CT scan) is associated with cardiovascular disease, thyroid cancer, leukemia, cataracts, glaucoma, dermatitis, and potential effects on fertility (Table 20.3).[7,8]

- 6 ft of air = 9 in. of concrete = 2.5 mm of lead

That is, dosage of radiation varies inversely with the $(Distance)^2$

HCP should wear protective eyewear, utilize lead glass partitions, lead aprons with thyroid shields, and wear detection badges

Lasers

- Eye injury is the greatest risk with lasers, causing burns to cornea or retina, destruction of macula and cataract formation
- Wear protective goggles/lenses
- Lasers may be a source of airway fire, and a cause of HPV transmission from laser plume

Infectious Diseases

Herpetic Whitlow

Etiology: Direct contact with HSV-1, 2 sore. Avoid visible sores, wear gloves

Treatment: Topical 5% acyclovir ointment

HPV Recurrent Respiratory Papillomatosis (RRP) or Laryngeal Papillomatosis

Risk of acquiring RRP is low, however use of N-95 masks and local exhaust ventilation, such as a smoke evacuator, in well-ventilated operating rooms recommended

Needle Stick Injury[9]:

- *Seroconversion rate* depends on infectivity of organism, degree of viremia, size of inoculum, and the immune status of health-care provider (Table 20.4)

Table 20.4 Risk of transmission and PEP after needlestick, HIV, HBV, HCV

	HIV	HBV	HCV
Risk	0.3% (0.09% for mucous membrane)	$\approx$ 22–30% HBeAg-positive source $\approx$ 1–6% HBeAg-negative source	1.8% (negligible for mucous membrane)
PEP/Test	Four-week course (two anti-retroviral medications; three if deemed high risk) HCP should have HIV status checked at time of needlestick and at follow-up	If HBsAg + source or unknown: Unvaccinated: HBIg and HBV vaccine within 24 hours Vaccinated: Check anti-HBsAb level if >10 mIU/ml → done if <10 mIU/ml → give HBIg and HBV vaccine boost If HBsAg − source Unvaccinated: give HBV vaccine Vaccinated: no treatment	PEP not recommended HCP should have HCV status checked within 24 hours and then again >3 weeks

Abbreviated table: See CDC MMWR Recommendations and Reports for detail.

Thermodysregulation

Four Types of Heat Loss

1. Radiation
2. Convection
3. Conduction
4. Evaporation
   - **Redistribution** of heat from the core to periphery is the principal mechanism of heat loss during the first hour/stage of anesthesia

Hypothermia

- **Etiology**
  - Impaired thermoregulation, normally tonic thermoregulatory vasoconstriction keeps core 2°–4° warmer than the peripheral tissue
  - Low ambient temperature of the operating room
- **Prevention**: Forced air warming 30 minutes prevents Phase I cooling. Once in the OR, consider warming the operating room, warming IV fluids, heated humidification of inhaled gases, and forced air warming (most cost effective).

Complications of Hypothermia

- Cardiac arrhythmias and ischemia
- Increase in SVR
- Left shift of Hgb–O_2 saturation curve
- Platelet dysfunction
- Altered mental status, delayed emergence
- Impaired renal function
- Delayed drug metabolism
- Impaired wound healing and increased risk of infection
- Increase stress response
- Increased postoperative protein catabolism
- Postoperative shivering can increase oxygen consumption as much as five times, → decrease oxygen saturation, which can increase the risk of myocardial ischemia

Treatment: warming; meperidine 12.5–25 mg IV can reduce shivering via kappa agonist activity

Active Cooling of Febrile Patient

- May fail to reduce core temperature
- Worsen the situation by triggering thermoregulatory defense responses
- Induce autonomic nervous system activation
- Lead to shivering and potentially patient discomfort

Nonmalignant Hyperthermia/Passive Hyperthermia

Most common in pediatric patients in whom temperature monitoring is either not performed or improperly monitored. Treatment is to stop active warming and remove insulating layers.

Malignant Hyperthermia[10]

1:15,000 pediatric patients, 1:40,000–50,000 adult patients

Risk Factors

Central-core disease, multi-minicore myopathy, King–Denborough syndrome, mostly autosomal dominant, involving ch19q3.1 Ryanodine Receptor type 1 (RYR1), male predominance

- Mortality rate 5% with early detection
- Halothane–caffeine contracture test, false positive rate 10–20%
- False negative rate approximately zero

Mechanism

- Uncontrolled release of intracellular calcium from sarcoplasmic reticulum of skeletal muscle. Calcium removes inhibition of troponin → sustained muscle contraction
- Increase ATPase activity → increase aerobic and anaerobic metabolism

Signs of MH

- Increase CO_2 production → respiratory acidosis
- Increase O_2 consumption
- Decreased O_2 supply, decreasing delivery → cyanosis/lactic acidosis
- Skin mottling
- Tachycardia
- Hypertension

- Arrhythmias
- Hyperthermia
- Rigidity
- Note: Fever is a late sign

Treatment
- Call for help. *MHAUS Hotline*. Stop volatile agent/succinylcholine
- Terminate surgery if possible or continue with nontriggering agent
- Give 100% FiO_2 at 10 L flows and hyperventilate
- Give dantrolene 2.5 mg/kg → up to 10 mg/kg, prn: ↓ rigidity ↓ $EtCO_2$
- Check VBG/ABG and temp
- Treat hyperkalemia, acidosis, and hyperthermia
- Monitor urine output and consider arterial line/central line, +/− diuresis
- Avoid calcium channel blockers

Allergic Reactions

- **Type I Immediate**: atopy, urticarial, anaphylaxis
- **Type II Cytotoxic**: hemolytic transfusion reactions, autoimmune hemolytic anemia, heparin-induced thrombocytopenia
- **Type III Immune complex**: Arthus reaction, serum sickness, acute hypersensitivity pneumonitis
- **Type IV Delayed, cell-mediated**: contact dermatitis, tuberculin-type hypersensitivity, chronic hypersensitivity pneumonitis

Hypersensitivity – exaggerated immunological responses to antigenic stimulation in previously sensitized persons. The allergen may be a protein, polypeptide, or smaller molecule, and even a metabolite/breakdown product

Anaphylaxis – basophils and mast cells release inflammatory agents as a result of antigen interacting with IgE. Most common cause of anaphylaxis during anesthesia are muscle relaxants. 1:3,500–1:20,000 anesthetics

Anaphylactoid – similar, but not IgE-mediated; activation of complement directly or via IgG → inflammatory response; more common than true anaphylaxis

Bottom line: Discontinue drug/agent, administer 100% FiO_2, epinephrine dose 0.01–0.5 mg, consider intubation, IV fluids, diphenhydramine 50–75 mg IV, ranitidine 150 mg, hydrocortisone 200 mg, or methylprednisolone 1–2 mg/kg

Latex allergy – The second most common cause of anaphylaxis during anesthesia 1–5% of the general population has latex allergy, 2–17% of health-care workers. Up to 15% of anesthesiologists, 10% of rubber industry workers, and 70% of patients with *spina bifida, spinal cord injury, and congenital abnormalities of GU tract*

Other risk factors for latex allergy: Patients with certain food allergies, such as avocados, bananas, chestnuts, kiwi fruit, peaches, papayas, potatoes, and tomatoes, may be at higher risk.

References

1. J. Metzner, K. L. Posner, M. S. Lam, et al. Closed claims analysis. *Best Pract Res Clin Anaesthesiol*. 2011; 25(2): 263–76.
2. L. B. Ware, M. A. Matthay. Acute pulmonary edema. *N Engl J Med*. 2005; 353: 2788–96.
3. G. A. Nuttall, J. A. Garrity, J. A. Dearani, et al. Risk factors for ischemic optic neuropathy after cardiopulmonary bypass: a matched case/control study. *Anesth Analg*. 2001; 93(6): 1410–16.
4. L. M. Buono, R. Foroozan. Perioperative posterior ischemic optic neuropathy: review of the literature *Surv Ophthalm*. 2005; 50(1):15–26.
5. S. P. Mehta, S. M. Bhananker, K. L. Posner, et al. Operating room fires: a closed claims analysis. *Anesthesia*. 2013; 118(5):1133–39.
6. US Department of Labor: Occupational Safety and Health Administration. Anesthetic Gases: Guidelines for Workplace Exposures. 2017. www.osha.gov/dts/osta/anestheticgases/ (Accessed February 7, 2017).
7. N. Hamada, Y. Fujimichi. Classification of radiation effects for dose limitation purposes: history, current situation and future prospects. *J Radiat Res*. 2014; 55(4): 629–40.
8. US Department of Labor: Occupational Safety and Health Administration. Maximum permissible dose equivalent for occupational exposure. www.osha.gov/SLTC/radiationionizing/introtoionizing/ionizingattachmentsix.html (Accessed February 7, 2017).
9. Centers for Disease Control. Morbidity and Mortality Weekly Report. Recommendations and Reports Updated US Public Health Service Guidelines for the Management of Occupational Exposures to HBV, HCV, and HIV and Recommendations for Postexposure prophylaxis. June 29, 2001/50 (RR11); 1–42. www.cdc.gov/mmwr/PDF/RR/RR5011.pdf (Accessed February 7, 2017).
10. Malignant Hyperthermia Association of the United States. Managing an MH Crisis. 2017. www.mhaus.org/healthcare-professionals/managing-a-crisis (Accessed February 7, 2017).

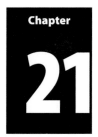

Postanesthesia Recovery Period: Analgesics

Gabriel C. Baltazar, Anuj Malhotra, and Rebecca E. Lee

- **Postoperative analgesic routes**[1,2]
  - **Intravenous**
    - Fastest, most common route of medication delivery
    - Medication doses can quickly be titrated to effect
    - Can be administered by healthcare providers as IV push or infusion, or by the patient through patient-controlled analgesia
      - **Patient-controlled analgesia (PCA)**
        - Device is programmed with specific medication, rate of constant (background) infusion, bolus (demand) dose, and lockout interval
        - Commonly used drugs: fentanyl, morphine, hydromorphone
        - Improved *patient satisfaction* due to control over delivery of pain medications
        - May reduce total opioid consumption and improve pain scores
  - **Oral**
    - Second most common route of medication delivery postoperatively
    - Useful in ambulatory setting and for patients without IV access
    - Bioavailability of oral medications varies widely
    - Generally longer duration of action than IV, but limited utility for managing severe pain due to delayed onset and peak effect
    - Not feasible in NPO patients or those with significant postoperative nausea and vomiting (PONV)
  - **Subcutaneous**
    - Drug injected into subcutaneous fat and absorbed into systemic circulation
    - Generally less painful than IM injection
    - Option for patients without IV access and unable to tolerate PO
    - Absorption of drug varies greatly
    - Larger doses required to reach desired effect
  - **Transcutaneous**
    - Drug absorbed across skin into systemic circulation
    - An option for patients without IV access
    - Transcutaneous patches can slowly release drug into circulation over prolonged periods, providing long-acting pain relief
    - Slow and often unpredictable absorption – drug must be lipophilic for adequate absorption to occur (e.g., fentanyl patch)
  - **Transmucosal**
    - Drug absorbed across mucous membranes into systemic circulation
      - E.g., rectal, sublingual, buccal
    - An option for patients without IV access
    - While generally faster than transcutaneous, absorption is similarly unpredictable
  - **Intramuscular**
    - Drug injected directly into muscle
    - An option for patients without IV access and unable to tolerate PO
    - May not be tolerated due to pain at injection site
  - **Epidural**
    - Excellent modality of analgesia for a wide range of procedures
    - Ability to use local anesthetics and opioids separately or in combination
    - Epidural opioids diffuse into CSF and act on μ receptors in the spinal cord located in the substantia gelatinosa of the posterior horn (Rexed lamina II)
      - Some systemic absorption also occurs
    - Can be placed at many levels of the spinal cord (caudal to cervical), depending on the procedure and desired application:
      - **Caudal** – Groin, pelvic, lower extremity surgery (commonly used in pediatrics)
      - **Lumbar** – Abdominal, pelvic, lower extremity surgery
      - **Thoracic** – Thoracic, upper and lower abdominal, rib fractures
    - Placement of epidural may be difficult or impossible due to patient unwillingness, anatomy, or recent anticoagulation
  - **Spinal**[3]
    - Intrathecal injection has benefit of rapid onset when using local anesthetics or opioids
      - Both act directly on target receptors in the central nervous system (CNS) without systemic effects

- Intrathecal opioids can provide prolonged analgesia from a single injection, particularly if hydrophilic (e.g., intrathecal long-acting morphine)
  - Delayed respiratory depression up to 24 h possible due to eventual rostral spread of cerebrospinal fluid
- Duration and level of block from local anesthetics depend on specific drug properties, total dose, level of injection, patient positioning, and baricity
- **Intrapleural**
  - Local anesthetics and/or analgesics injected in the intrapleural space
  - Produces a multilevel intercostal block for thoracotomies and other thoracic procedure
  - Less reliable technique as the effects vary and depend on patient positioning and volume of injected drug
  - High rate of systemic absorption
- **Opioids**[1,2]
  - **Mechanism of action**
    - Binds to four major opioid receptors located within the CNS: μ, κ, δ, and σ
    - Binding causes activation of G proteins and membrane hyperpolarization
    - Inhibits nociceptive neuronal pathways by preventing release and response to acetylcholine and substance P
  - Can increase the apneic threshold and decrease hypoxic respiratory drive, a significant concern in the postanesthesia setting
  - Tables 21.1 and 21.2 describe commonly used postoperative opioid–agonists and agonist–antagonists
- **Local anesthetics (LA)**[1,4,5] – All bind to intracellular voltage-dependent sodium channels
  - **Lidocaine** – Short-acting amide LA
    - Common uses – Intravenous, topical, infiltration, epidural, peripheral nerve block, and transdermal
      - Intravenous infusions[2] – Useful as part of multimodal pain management strategy. Data supports use during and after major abdominal surgery – reducing postoperative pain and opioid requirements. Postoperative infusion doses range from 1 to 2 mg/kg/h
      - Transdermal patch – 5 percent lidocaine patch applied directly to skin overlying painful area. When applied for the recommended maximum duration of 12 h/day, systemic absorption is minimal
      - IV regional anesthesia (Bier block) – Lidocaine is the drug of choice when performing IV regional anesthesia for the management of intra- and postoperative pain
  - **Chloroprocaine** – Short-acting ester LA

- Common uses: Infiltration, epidural, peripheral nerve block
- Quickest-acting LA
- Low systemic toxicity permits use of high concentrations
- Development of tachyphylaxis with repeated use
  - **Mepivacaine** – Medium-acting amide LA
    - Common uses: Infiltration, epidural, peripheral nerve block
  - **Bupivacaine, Ropivicaine** – Long-acting amide LA
    - Common uses: Infiltration (bupivacaine), peripheral nerve or plexus block, epidural, intrathecal
    - Contraindicated in IV regional anesthesia due to risk of systemic toxicity
    - Ropivicaine – Less lipophilic → less motor block, decreased potential of cardiotoxicity and CNS toxicity
- **Alpha-2 agonists**[1,5]
  - **Clonidine** – Specific, central-acting alpha-2 agonist with hypnotic, sedative, anxiolytic, sympatholytic, analgesic properties
    - Intra- and postoperative use associated with improved pain control and decreased opioid requirements
    - Most efficacious when administered via neuraxial route (epidural, intrathecal) either alone or in combination with local anesthetics
    - Side effects include sedation and hypotension
  - **Dexmedetomidine** – Specific, central-acting alpha-2 agonist with similar effects as clonidine but with higher specificity for alpha-2 receptors
    - Intraoperative use as part of multimodal pain management strategy decreases intra- and postoperative opioid requirements
    - Postoperatively can be used as a low dose intravenous infusion (0.2–0.7 mcg/kg/h) or added to neuraxial or peripheral local anesthetics to potentiate their effect
- **Nonsteroidal anti-inflammatory drugs (NSAIDs)**[2,5,6]
  - Analgesic, anti-inflammatory, anti-pyretic compounds
  - Mechanism: Inhibition of cyclooxygenase → decreased synthesis of prostaglandins
  - When given alone they provide analgesia for mild and moderate pain
  - When given as adjuncts and part of a multimodal analgesic regimen, they can provide significant pain relief and decrease opioid consumption
  - Common side effects: GI upset/ulceration, platelet dysfunction, renal dysfunction
  - Selective COX-2 inhibitors theoretically have fewer GI and platelet effects but show increased risk of stroke and myocardial infarction

Table 21.1 Commonly used postoperative opioid agonists

Drug	Route	Dose (adult)	Onset	Duration of action	Comments
Morphine	IV	2–15 mg	5–10 min	4–5 h	– Risk of respiratory depression and excess sedation in renal failure (from morphine-6-glucoronide metabolite)
	IM	5–20 mg	10–30 min	4–5 h	
	Oral (immediate release)	10–30 mg	30 min	3–5 h	
	Oral (extended release)	15–60 mg (or greater)	Variable	8–12 h	
	Epidural (bolus)	1–5 mg	30–60 min	12–24 h	
	Epidural (continuous)	0.1–1 mg/h	30–60 min	Continuous	
	Intrathecal	0.1–0.3 mg	30–60 min	18–24 h	
Fentanyl	IV	25–100 µg	Immediate	30–60 min	– Can rarely cause chest wall rigidity (especially in children)
	IM	25–100 µg	7–8 min	1–2 h	
	Transdermal	12.5–100 µg/h	6 h	72–96 h	
	Transmucosal	100–200 µg	5–15 min	Variable	
	Epidural (bolus)	50–100 µg	5–10 min	60 min	
	Epidural (continuous)	25–100 µg/h	5–10 min	Continuous	
	Intrathecal	5–25 µg	Immediate	60 min	
Meperidine	IV	50–75 mg	5 min	2–3 h	– Smaller doses used for postoperative shivering (12.5–25 mg IV)
	IM	50–75 mg	10–15 min	24 h	– Metabolite normeperidine lowers seizure threshold
	SubQ	50–75 mg	10–15 min	2–4 h	– Mild anticholinergic effect
	Oral	50–150 mg	10–15 min	2–4 h	
Hydromorphone	IV	0.2–1 mg	5–10 min	3–4 h	– Safer in renal failure vs. morphine (no renally excreted active metabolites)
	SubQ	0.8–1 mg	5–10 min	3–4 h	
	Oral	2–4 mg	15–60 min	3–4 h	
	Epidural (bolus)	0.5–1 mg	15 min	8–12 h	
	Epidural (continuous)	0.1–0.2 mg/h	15 min	Continuous	
	Intrathecal	0.04–0.1 mg	5 min	10–20 h	
Methadone	IV	2.5–10 mg	10–20 min	6–8 h	– Watch for QTc prolongation
	Oral	5–10 mg	30–60 min	Variable	– Exhibits NMDA antagonism, MAOI activity
Codeine	Oral	15–60 mg	30–60 min	4–6 h	– Metabolized by CYP2D6 to morphine – "Slow" metabolizers show increased drug sensitivity – "Fast" metabolizers show drug resistance – Avoid in pediatric tonsillectomy patients
Oxycodone	Oral (immediate release)	5–15 mg	10–30 min	3–6 h	– Commonly combined with acetaminophen
	Oral (extended release)	10–80 mg	60 min	12 h	
Hydrocodone	Oral	5–10 mg	10–30 min	4–6 h	– Commonly combined with acetaminophen
Tramadol	Oral	50–100 mg	30–60 min	4–6 h	– Also exhibits SNRI activity – Generally not recommended in children <17 years old

Table 21.2 Opioid agonist–antagonists

Drug	Route	Dose (adult)	Onset	Duration of action
Buprenorphine (partial µ agonist, κ antagonist)	IV	0.3–0.6 mg	5–15 min	6–13 h
	IM	0.3–0.6 mg	15–30 min	6–13 h
Butorphanol (κ agonist, partial µ antagonist)	IV	0.5–2 mg q3–4 h	30–60 min	8–24 h (dose-dependent)
	IM	2 mg q3–4 h		
Nalbuphine (κ agonist, partial µ antagonist)	IV	10 mg/70 kg q3–6 h	2–3 min	3–6 h
	IM		5–15 min	3–6 h
	Subq		5–15 min	3–6 h
Pentazocine (κ agonist, partial µ antagonist)	IV	5–30 mg q3–4 h	15 min	1 h
	IM			2 h
	Subq			2 h

Table 21.3 Common postoperative NSAIDs

Drug	Route	Dose (adult)	Onset	Duration of action
Ibuprofen (COX-1 and COX-2)	Oral	200–400 mg q4–6 h	30–60 min	4–8 h
	IV	400–800 mg q6 h		4–8 h
Naproxen (COX-1 and COX-2)	Oral	250–500 mg q6–8 h	30–60 min	6–10 h
Ketorolac (COX-1 and COX-2)	IV or IM	15–30 mg q6 h	30–60 min	3–6 h
Celecoxib (COX-2)	Oral	400 mg once or 200 mg q12 h	30–60 min	8–12 h
Diclofenac	Oral	50 mg 2–3 times daily	30–60 min	8–12 h
	Topical	Apply twice daily	Variable	Variable
Meloxicam	Oral	7.5–15 mg daily	30–60 min	Up to 24 h
Indomethacin	Oral	20–40 mg q12 h	30–60 min	4–6 h

- ○ Table 21.3 describes commonly used postoperative NSAIDs
- **N-methyl-aspartate (NMDA) receptor blockers**[5,6]
  - ○ **Ketamine**
    - Sedative-hypnotic NMDA receptor antagonist with activity at opioid, cholinergic, monoaminergic receptors
    - Also acts as Na^+ channel blocker
    - Results in dissociative state producing anesthesia and analgesia
    - Side effects – Salivation, hallucinations (attenuated by benzodiazepine administration), bronchodilation, sympathomimetic activity
  - ○ **Magnesium**
    - In the CNS acts as a non-competitive NMDA receptor antagonist
    - When infused as adjunct intraoperatively in doses of 8 mg/kg/h, some studies demonstrate decreased perioperative pain
    - Potentiates the effects of neuraxial opioids when given intrathecally
    - Side effects include hypotonia
  - ○ **Amantadine**
    - Non-competitive NMDA antagonist
    - Most often used for chronic neuropathic, musculoskeletal, postoperative pain
- **Tricyclic antidepressants (TCAs)**[5,6]
  - ○ Examples – Amitriptyline, nortriptyline, imipramine, clomipramine
  - ○ Primarily act in the CNS as serotonin–norepinephrine reuptake inhibitors
  - ○ Demonstrate efficacy in treating neuropathic pain and fibromyalgia, but also as adjuncts in the postoperative period
  - ○ Mechanism of analgesia likely related to neuromodulation of descending pain pathways
- **Selective serotonin/norepinephrine inhibitors (SNRIs)**[5,6]
  - ○ Examples – Venlafaxine, duloxetine
  - ○ Mechanism thought to be similar to TCAs
- **Gabapentinoids**[5–7]
  - ○ Examples – Gabapentin, pregabalin
  - ○ Inhibit α-2-σ voltage-gated calcium channels in the CNS → modulate nociceptive pathways
  - ○ Effective in treating neuropathic, chronic, and postoperative pain
  - ○ Synergistic effects when given in conjunction with NSAIDs and opioids
  - ○ Can be given preoperatively for multi-modal postoperative pain control
- **Other regional techniques**[5,6]
  - ○ **Peripheral nerve and plexus blocks**
    - Local anesthetics are injected and/or infused around a peripheral nerve or plexus, resulting in anesthesia in those nerve distributions
    - Provide excellent intra- and postoperative analgesia for surgery involving the upper and lower extremities
  - ○ **Transverse abdominal pain (TAP) blocks**
    - Controls incisional pain after large abdominal surgeries
    - Local anesthetic delivered in fascial plane between transversus abdominis and internal oblique, blocking somatic afferents from T8–L1
    - No effect on visceral pain
  - ○ **Rectus sheath block**
    - Useful for postoperative analgesia for midline abdominal surgeries, especially umbilical hernia repairs
    - Local anesthetic is injected between rectus abdominis and posterior rectus sheath
      - Acts on T9–T11 dermatomes

- o **Paravertebral blocks**
  - Used to manage pain from thoracic, breast, upper abdominal surgeries, and rib fractures
  - Local anesthetic is injected into paravertebral space along the spinal column, targeting the spinal nerves as they exit the intervertebral foramina
  - Results in ipsilateral somatic and sympathetic block in a dermatomal distribution
  - Complications – Pneumothorax, intravascular injection, epidural or intrathecal injection
- **Postoperative analgesia – Other techniques**[6,7]
  - o **Transcutaneous electrical nerve stimulation (TENS)**
    - Involves placement of transcutaneous electrodes to deliver current resulting in nerve excitation
    - Continuous stimulation of nerve pathways results in downregulation of nociceptive impulse transmission (gate-theory)
    - Useful as adjunct in postoperative period
    - Associated with reduced postoperative analgesic use, however efficacy varies by study and many patients cannot tolerate the sensation of electrical stimulation
  - o **Cryotherapy (cryoanalgesia)**
    - Temporary but prolonged neurolysis (weeks to months) by freezing and thawing peripheral nerves using cold cryo probe
    - Mostly used for post-thoracotomy pain
    - Analgesia may not reach full effect for 48 h
  - o **Acupuncture**
    - Involves insertion of needles into discrete, anatomically defined points (meridians)
    - Needles may be twisted or have electrical current applied
    - Mechanism of action has been debated, but possibly related to release of endogenous opioids

- Naloxone administration can reverse effects of acupuncture
  - In some studies acupuncture appears to reduce postoperative pain, decrease opioid-requirements, and decrease opioid-related side effects
  - Relatively safe, devoid of systemic effects
- o **Hypnosis**
  - Relaxation technique meant to alter arousal and decrease sympathetic tone associated with pain
  - Pain perception altered by having patient focus on other sensations, localize pain to another site, and dissociate from a painful experience
  - Benefit greatest for patients with pre-existing musculoskeletal disorders

Postoperative analgesia in patients on opioid maintenance [2,6]

- **Methadone**
  - o Continue peri-operatively
  - o Full opioid agonist; can aid in analgesia
  - o Half-life of 12–72 h, analgesic duration of 6–8 h, consider split dosing to BID or TID
- **Buprenorphine**
  - o Discontinue 3 days prior to elective procedures
  - o Partial opioid agonist/antagonist with ceiling effect and very high-affinity binding for mu-opioid receptor, difficult to displace with perioperative opioids
  - o Half-life of 20–37 h, analgesic duration of 6–13 h, highly variable based on route of administration
- **Oral naltrexone**
  - o Discontinue 3 days prior to elective procedures
  - o Full opioid antagonist
  - o Half-life of 4 h, active metabolite 9 h
- **Depot naltrexone**
  - o Stop 1 month prior to elective procedures
  - o Monthly high-dose subcutaneous injection, effect wanes by end of 4 weeks

References

1. Nicholau T. K. The postanesthesia care unit. *Miller's Anesthesia*, 8th edn, R. D. Miller, et al. (eds.), 2014; Chapter 96, 2924–46. Philadelphia, PA: Elsevier Inc.
2. Sinatra R. S., Jahr J. S., Watkins-Pitchford J. M. *The Essence of Analgesia and Analgesics*. 2010. New York, NY: Cambridge University Press.
3. Hindle A. Intrathecal opioids in the management of acute postoperative pain. *Contin Educ Anaesth Crit Care Pain* 2008; 8(3): 81–5.
4. Weibel S., Jokinen J., Pace N. L., et al. Efficacy and safety of intravenous lidocaine for postoperative analgesia and recovery after surgery: a systematic review with trial sequential analysis. *Br J Anaesth* 2016; 116(6): 770–83.
5. Butterworth J. F., Mackey D. C., Wasnick J. D., Morgan G. E., Mikhail M. S. *Morgan and Mikhail's Clinical Anesthesiology*, 5th edn, 2013. New York, NY: The McGraw-Hill Companies.
6. Chou R., Gordon D. B., de Leon-Casasola O. A., et al. Management of Postoperative Pain: A Clinical Practice Guideline from the American Pain Society, the American Society of Regional Anesthesia and Pain Medicine, and the American Society of Anesthesiologists' Committee on Regional Anesthesia, Executive Committee, and Administrative Council. *The Journal of Pain* 2016; 17(2): 131–57.
7. Malhotra A., Malhotra V., Rawal N. *Perioperative Pain Management. Yao & Artusio's Anesthesiology: Problem-Oriented Patient Management*, 8th edn, Fun-Sun F., Yao, M. D., Manuel L., Fontes, M. D., Vinod Malhotra M. D. (eds.). 2016. Philadelphia, PA: Lippincott Williams & Wilkins.

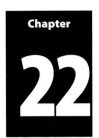

Chapter 22

Postanesthesia Recovery Period: Common Scenarios

Gabriel C. Baltazar and Rebecca E. Lee

Respiratory Consequences of Anesthesia and of Surgical Incisions

- **Loss of pharyngeal tone**[1-3]
  - Most common cause of postoperative airway obstruction – increased risk in sedated, obtunded patients → loss of tone leads to soft tissue/airway collapse and subsequent airway obstruction
  - Due to combined effects of residual anesthetics, inadequate reversal of neuromuscular blockade, and opioid overdose
  - Treatment:
    - Jaw thrust, continuous positive airway pressure (CPAP), oral or nasal airway, laryngeal mask airway, and possible intubation with endotracheal tube
    - Reversal of pharmacologic agents with naloxone, flumazenil, neostigmine/sugammadex
- **Residual neuromuscular blockade**[1]
  - Residual neuromuscular blockade may affect diaphragm, pharyngeal muscles, and accessory muscles of respiration → risk of respiratory failure
- **Atelectasis**
  - Occurs in dependent lung fields (West Zone 3) in nearly all patients receiving anesthesia
    - Multifactorial etiology – Prolonged patient immobility, change in respiratory physiology, decreased lung volumes, impaired gas exchange, obesity, postoperative pain
  - Intraoperatively – Prevention with positive end-expiratory pressure (PEEP) and recruitment maneuvers
  - Postoperatively – Can be managed with CPAP, incentive spirometry, pain control, and patient upright repositioning
- **Laryngospasm**[1]
  - Sudden spasm of vocal cords leading to partial or complete occlusion of larynx
  - Patients are most susceptible on emergence from general anesthesia and immediately post-extubation (children > adults)
  - Increased risk with use of volatile anesthetics compared with propofol
  - Treatment: CPAP, propofol, or succinylcholine to break laryngospasm

- **Bronchospasm**[1]
  - Can occur in any patient, but more likely in those with preexisting reactive airway disease
  - Risk increases with pharyngeal or tracheal stimulation, suctioning, or aspiration
  - Treatment: Inhaled beta agonists or anticholinergics, IV anticholinergics, IV epinephrine
- **Airway edema**[1]
  - Swelling of tissue in and around airway
  - More likely in:
    - Prolonged procedures in prone or Trendelenburg position
    - Surgeries requiring large volume of fluid administration
    - Surgeries of the head and neck in close proximity to airway
  - External signs – e.g., facial swelling – may be absent and do not necessarily predict a lack of oropharyngeal or laryngeal edema
- **Airway hematoma**[1]
  - A possibly devastating consequence of head and neck procedures causing direct compression of airway
  - Treatment options: Urgent evacuation of hematoma, swift return to OR for awake fiberoptic intubation, emergent tracheostomy
- **Obstructive sleep apnea (OSA)**[1,2]
  - Redundant oropharyngeal tissue or other anatomic abnormalities → airway obstruction when patient is asleep, sedated, or anesthetized
  - Universally underdiagnosed – STOP-BANG assessment can be utilized to assess risk
  - Majority of OSA patients are NOT obese
  - CPAP and judicious use of sedating medications can diminish risk of obstruction
  - Patients on CPAP are more likely to be placed in a monitored unit in the immediate postoperative setting
- **CO_2 narcosis**[1]
  - Volatile anesthetics and opioids decrease the brain's sensitivity to increased levels of CO_2
  - Respiratory drive is depressed, leading to decreased minute ventilation

- Without prompt diagnosis, the result may be patient confusion, obtundation, even coma
- Can be treated with naloxone 0.04 mg every 5 min as needed

- **Diffusion hypoxia**[1]
  - Nitrous oxide (N_2O) administration during anesthesia results in rapid diffusion of N_2O into alveoli when the gas is discontinued
    - Results in dilution of alveolar oxygen → decreasing PAO_2 → arterial hypoxemia
  - Supplemental oxygen should be given to all patients after receiving nitrous oxide, as the effect of diffusion hypoxia may persist up to 10 min

- **Post-obstructive (negative pressure) pulmonary edema**[1]
  - Transudative edema due to exaggerated negative intrathoracic pressure
    - Caused by attempts at inspiration against a closed glottis, most commonly with obstructed endotracheal tube or laryngospasm
  - Radiographic evidence of bilateral fluffy pulmonary infiltrates
  - Treatment is supportive: Supplemental oxygen, diuresis, positive pressure ventilation if warranted

- **Transfusion-related acute lung injury (TRALI)**[1]
  - Non-cardiogenic pulmonary edema occurring within 6 h of transfusion
  - Must be considered in any patient receiving blood products, especially plasma-derived components
  - Mechanism thought to be secondary to leukocyte antibodies in the transfused product causing inflammation, vascular leakage, and pulmonary edema

- **Pulmonary embolism**[1]
  - Considered in postop patients with sudden onset of hypoxemia, dyspnea, tachycardia, hypotension, and chest pain
    - In unconscious or sedated patients, the classic findings may be attenuated or absent
  - May be a result of embolization from deep vein thrombosis, fat (long bone trauma/surgery), or amniotic fluid (following delivery)

- **Pneumonia**[1]
  - Occurs in up to 9 percent of high risk surgery patients
  - General anesthesia itself can predispose to pneumonia due to alterations in:
    - Mucociliary clearance, forced vital capacity, and alveolar macrophage activity
  - Patients needing extended ventilator support postoperatively are at higher risk

- **Pneumothorax**[1]
  - Entrainment of air into pleural cavity leads to lung collapse
  - Common causes:
    - Surgical trauma
    - Rupture of surface blebs
    - Central line placement

- Aggressive positive pressure ventilation
- Bronchoscopy
- Presents as hypoxia, tachycardia, decreased breath sounds, hypotension
  - Circulatory collapse is possible with tension pneumothorax
- Management:
  - One hundred percent FiO_2, needle decompression, chest tube placement

Cardiovascular Consequences of General and Regional Anesthesia

- **Postoperative hypertension**[1,2]
  - Patients with preexisting hypertension prior to undergoing anesthesia are at greatest risk of hypertension in the postoperative period
    - Carotid endarterectomies and intracranial surgeries in particular are most commonly associated with postoperative hypertension
  - Other causes of hypertension and their treatments include:
    - Pain leading to increased sympathetic tone
      - Treatment: Pain medication, regional anesthetic/analgesic techniques
    - Hypercarbia
      - Treatment: Invasive and noninvasive ventilatory support
    - Urinary retention/bladder distention
      - Treatment: Bladder catheterization
    - Intubated patients with inadequate sedation
      - Treatment: Sedation, pain control
    - Nausea and vomiting
      - Treatment: Pharmacologic and antiemetics

- **Postoperative hypotension**[1,2]
  - Etiologies of postoperative hypotension can be characterized as:
    - Hypovolemic
      - Decreased intravascular volume due to insufficient fluid resuscitation, surgical bleeding, third-space translocation
      - Treat with IV crystalloid, colloid, blood products, vasopressors, cardiac inotropes
    - Cardiogenic
      - Pump failure secondary to myocardial ischemia or infarction, cardiac tamponade, dysrhythmias, cardiomyopathy
      - Diagnose with ECG monitoring, echocardiography, central venous pressure monitoring, pulmonary artery catheter monitoring (situation-dependent)
      - Treatment depends on etiology and may include a combination of vasopressors, inotropes, volume resuscitation, anti-arrhythmics, cardioversion, or defibrillation

- Distributive
  - Most commonly a result of sympathectomy, allergic reactions, and systemic inflammatory response syndrome (SIRS)/sepsis
  - Sympathectomy: Due to neuraxial/regional anesthetic techniques or surgical complication. Treatment may include volume resuscitation and direct/indirect acting vasopressors such as phenylephrine, vasopressin, ephedrine, norepinephrine, and epinephrine
  - Allergic reactions: Include anaphylactic and anaphylactoid reactions. Most commonly implicated triggers are in order of most common: neuromuscular blockers, antibiotics, and latex
  - SIRS/sepsis: Systemic inflammatory response resulting in decreased systemic vascular resistance and hypotension. Management consists of cardiovascular support and treatment of inciting cause or infectious agent
- Arrhythmias (be familiar with ACLS algorithms)[1,2]
  - **Sinus bradycardia**
    - Medication-related:
      - Anticholinesterases, opioids, beta-blockers
    - Procedure-related:
      - Increased intracranial pressure, high spinal anesthesia, increased intraocular pressure, bowel distention
  - **Sinus tachycardia**
    - Most often a consequence of pain, hypovolemia, agitation, fever/hyperthermia, sepsis, or medications (anticholinergics)
  - **Atrial dysrhythmias**
    - Atrial fibrillation (AFib), atrial flutter (AFL), premature atrial complexes (PACs)
    - New onset of atrial dysrhythmias may occur in up to 10 percent of patients postoperatively, with higher rates after cardiothoracic procedures
    - For acute-onset AFib, treatment is aimed at controlling the ventricular response rate
      - Beta-blockers and calcium channel blockers are first-line agents
  - **Ventricular dysrhythmias**
    - Immediately postoperative, premature ventricular contractions (PVCs), and ventricular bigeminy are most commonly encountered
      - Can be secondary to underlying cardiac pathology, electrolyte abnormalities, hypercapnia, and increased sympathetic tone
      - PVCs are frequently benign and are usually managed by treating the above causes
    - Ventricular tachydysrhythmias (e.g., ventricular tachycardia, ventricular fibrillation) are rare but can occur, especially, in patients with underlying cardiac pathology

Nausea and Vomiting

- Postoperative nausea and vomiting (PONV) occur in up to 30 percent of patients, and together are the second most common complaint after pain in the postoperative period
- **Physiology**[4,5]
  - Nausea refers to the subjective feeling of the need to vomit, while vomiting (emesis) is the actual oral expulsion of gastrointestinal contents
  - Input from the cerebral cortex, GI tract vagal afferents, the vestibular system, and the central chemoreceptor trigger zone (CRTZ) act on the area postrema in the medulla oblongata
  - Efferent signals are then sent to visceral and somatic nuclei, resulting in the physical act of emesis as well as the accompanying sympathetic and vagal symptoms (e.g., sweating, tachycardia, salivation)
  - Neurotransmitters implicated in nausea and vomiting pathways include:
    - Serotonin (5-HT), acetylcholine (ACh), substance P, dopamine (DA), and histamine
- **Etiology**[3–5]
  - **Toxins inside the gastrointestinal lumen**
    - Examples include hypertonic saline, copper sulfate, syrup of ipecac
    - Cause release of 5-HT from enterochromaffin cells, stimulating vagal afferents to the brainstem and eventual activation of the area postrema
  - **Circulating toxins and drugs**
    - Can cause nausea and vomiting by direct stimulation of the CRTZ
    - The CRTZ is unique in that it lacks a blood–brain barrier, allowing it to detect emetogenic substances in the bloodstream
    - Intravenous and volatile anesthetics, opioids, and a myriad of other substances can trigger nausea and vomiting in this manner
  - **Activation of the vestibular system**
    - Classically implicated in motion sickness, Meniere's disease, procedures involving the inner ear
    - Drugs such as opioids have also been implicated in increasing the sensitivity of the vestibular system
- **Risk factors**[4,5]
  - **Patient-related factors**
    - Female sex (the strongest predictor)
    - Non-smokers
    - History of PONV or motion sickness
    - Older age, anxiety, and history of migraines have also been implicated, but data is less convincing
- **Anesthesia-related factors**
  - Perioperative opioids
  - Volatile anesthetics – Specific agent has no effect
  - Nitrous oxide – No more emetogenic than volatiles, however risk is additive with simultaneous nitrous oxide and volatile administration

Table 22.1 Simplified risk score for PONV in adults

Number of risk factors	Risk of PONV (%)
0	10
1	20
2	40
3	60
4	80

Table 22.2 Simplified risk score for postoperative vomiting (POV) in children

Number of risk factors	Incidence of POV (%)
0	9
1	10
2	30
3	55
4	70

- o Duration of anesthesia – Longer and more invasive procedures increase risk
- **Surgical-related factors**
  - o Strabismus surgery in children (but not adults) – Most well-established independent surgical risk factor for PONV
    - Most commonly implicated procedures include middle- and inner-ear surgeries, adenoidectomy and tonsillectomy, gynecologic surgery, laparoscopic abdominal surgery
- **Risk assessment**[6,7]
  - o In adults, an additive scoring system can be used to predict the risk of PONV
    - 1 point is given for each of the following: female gender, nonsmoking status, history of PONV or motion sickness, postoperative opioid use
    - Table 22.1 describes the relationship between number of risk factors and risk of PONV
  - o In the pediatric population, a similar additive scoring system is utilized
    - 1 point is given for each of the following independent variables: surgical duration ≥30 min, age ≥ 3, strabismus surgery, history of POV in patient or immediate relative.
    - Table 22.2 describes the relationship between number of risk factors and incidence of POV.
- **Preventive strategies**[1,4,5]
  - o Avoid exposure to opioids, volatile anesthetics, and nitrous oxide when feasible
  - o Administer propofol for induction and maintenance of general anesthesia, as this decreases early PONV (defined as initial 6 h postoperatively)
  - o Opt for regional over general anesthesia
  - o Utilize a multimodal pain management strategy to reduce the need for opioids in the intra- and postoperative period

- o Administer PONV prophylactic medications
  - For low risk patients with no risk factors (see above), prophylaxis is generally not warranted
  - For patients with one risk factor, a single prophylactic agent (ondansetron) should be used, with the option of adding a second agent (dexamethasone)
  - For higher risk patients with two or more risk factors, at least two agents should be used
- o Aggressively hydrate patients in the perioperative period with crystalloid
  - In some studies, liberal crystalloid supplementation was shown to be as effective as an antiemetic
  - Mechanism is possibly related to decreasing the release of arginine vasopressin (known to have emetic properties) during episodes of hypovolemia
- **Failed or absent prophylaxis**[8]
  - o If pharmacologic prophylaxis fails, an antiemetic should be administered from a class of drug different from those given for prevention
    - The benefit of re-dosing the same agent postop is minimal
  - o Propofol in small doses (20 mg IV) can be considered as a rescue antiemetic, however the effects are generally short-lived
  - o The dose of ondansetron as a rescue agent (1 mg) is less than that given for prophylaxis (4 mg)
- **Antiemetic agents**[3–5]
  - o Table 22.3 describes the commonly used agents for PONV prophylaxis and treatment
- **Multimodal therapy**[4,5,8]
  - o Greatest quantifiable decrease in PONV is observed when adding a single prophylactic agent
  - o Utilization of more agents will further reduce risk, however the benefits become less pronounced as more are added
    - Especially true once two agents have been given
  - o Combining multiple pharmacologic agents with other preventive strategies (e.g., hydration, oxygen, total intravenous anesthetic) significantly decreases the overall PONV incidence
- **Acupressure and acupuncture**[4,5,8]
  - o Stimulation of the P6 meridian pressure point of the wrist reduces risk of nausea and vomiting to a similar degree as traditional antiemetics
  - o Acupuncture, acupressure, and transcutaneous nerve stimulation are hence effective means to prevent PONV
- **Antacids, histamine-2 (H2) blockers, and proton pump inhibitors (PPIs)**[4,5]
  - o Effective for pre- and postoperative neutralization of gastric acids
  - o Examples:
    - Antacids – Calcium carbonate tablets, citric acid/sodium citrate
    - H2 blockers – Cimetidine, famotidine, ranitidine
    - PPIs – Omeprazole, esomeprazole, lansoprazole, pantoprazole

Table 22.3 Commonly used agents for PONV

Drug	Mechanism	Dose (adult)	Comments
Ondansetron	5-HT$_3$ (serotonin) antagonist	4 mg IV (ppx) 1 mg IV (rescue)	– More effective when given near end of surgery – QTc prolonging – Caution in patients taking other serotonergic agents due to risk of serotonin syndrome
Dolasetron	5-HT$_3$ antagonist	12.5–50 mg IV	
Granisetron	5-HT$_3$ antagonist	1 mg IV	
Metoclopramide	D$_2$ (dopamine) antagonist Minor 5-HT$_3$ antagonist	10–50 mg IV	– Minimal antiemetic benefit from 10 mg dose, greater efficacy at 25 or 50 mg – Promotes gastric motility – QTc prolonging
Droperidol	D$_2$ antagonist	1 mg IV 0.5 mg IM	– FDA black box warning for QTc prolongation has made its use more controversial, although at doses used for PONV the risk is likely minimal
Haloperidol	D$_{2,3,4}$ antagonist 5-HT$_2$ antagonist	0.5–1 mg IV 0.5 mg IM	– QTc prolonging – IV use is off-label
Prochlorperazine	D$_2$ antagonist	6.25–12.5 mg IV/IM 3–6 mg buccal	
Diphenhydramine	H$_1$ (histamine) antagonist	12.5–50 mg IV	– Anticholinergic side effects – Caution in elderly and others at risk of delirium
Promethazine	H$_1$ antagonist	12.5–25 IV/IM	
Aprepitant	NK1 (neurokinin) antagonist	40 mg PO	– Blocks substance P binding to NK receptor – Better at preventing vomiting than nausea – Expensive – Must be administered hours before surgery
Dexamethasone	Unknown	4–8 mg	– Effective only as prophylaxis – Administer shortly after induction – Similar PONV benefit with either 4 or 8 mg
Scopolamine	Muscarinic ACh antagonist	1.5 mg transdermal patch × 24 h	– Can be applied the night before surgery or immediately preop as onset is > 4 h

- No direct antiemetic effects
- Possibly useful as adjuncts for preventing and treating gastroesophageal reflux disease (GERD), indigestion, and dyspepsia, which may contribute to PONV

Neuromuscular Consequences of Anesthesia

- **Residual paralysis**[1,2]
  - Persistent residual neuromuscular blockade in the PACU due to incomplete antagonism of non-depolarizing neuromuscular blocking drugs
  - Associated with:
    - Generalized muscle weakness
    - Difficulty in phonation – Laryngeal muscle weakness
    - Diplopia – Extraocular muscle weakness
    - Difficulty swallowing and increased aspiration risk – Impaired coordination of pharyngeal constriction and relaxation of upper esophageal sphincter
    - Upper airway obstruction – Pharyngeal muscle weakness
    - Atelectasis
  - Ultimate consequence may be hypoxia, hypercarbia, respiratory failure, and prolonged ventilator time

- **Muscle soreness**[9]
  - Myalgias may occur after administration of succinylcholine for muscle relaxation
  - Incidence is difficult to quantify, with reported rates as high as 89 percent
    - Less common in children and patients over age 50
    - Possibly less common in those with greater muscle fitness
  - Mechanism not entirely understood, but likely due in part to uncoordinated nature of muscle contractions leading to muscle fiber rupture or damage
  - Prevention:
    - NSAIDs, lidocaine, and small doses of non-depolarizing muscle relaxants may lessen the risk of myalgias
- **Recovery of airway reflexes**[1]
  - Examples of airway reflexes include:
    - Pharyngeal (gag) reflex – Prevents unintended objects from entering the pharynx
      - Stimulation of posterior tongue, posterior pharyngeal wall, or soft palate results in bilateral pharyngeal muscle contraction

113

- Cough reflex – Enhances clearance of secretions/airway particulates and protects from aspiration of foreign objects
  - Stimulation of sensory nerves in ciliated epithelium of upper airways results in coordinated activity of diaphragm, thoracic muscles, and abdominal muscles
  - The protective airway reflexes are blunted during general anesthesia and neuromuscular blockade

Neurologic Consequences of Anesthesia

- **Confusion**[1]
  - Anesthesia results in a depressed level of consciousness – Impairs memory, attention, and reaction time
  - May last for hours postoperatively, despite outward appearance of wakefulness and alertness
  - Commonly manifests as unawareness of surroundings, repetitive questioning, emotional lability
- **Delirium**[10]
  - Acute and fluctuating disturbance in cognition, awareness, and/or level of consciousness unexplained by a preexisting neuro-cognitive disorder
  - Occurs in 10 percent of patients ≥50 years old undergoing elective surgery
  - Incidence highest in surgical repair of hip fractures and bilateral knee replacements
  - **Patient risk factors**
    - Advanced age (≥70 years old)
    - Preoperative cognitive impairment
    - Decreased functional status
    - Alcohol abuse
    - Severe illness
    - Vision impairment
    - History of delirium
  - **Intra- and postoperative risk factors**
    - Bleeding (Hct < 30 percent)
    - Blood transfusions
    - Use of anticholinergics, antihistamines, narcotics, and sedative-hypnotics
  - **Management:**
    - Exclude and treat iatrogenic causes – Electrolyte abnormalities, hypoxia, dehydration, endocrine dysfunction, pain, infection, anemia, and others

- Repeatedly reorient to surroundings
- Promote sleep hygiene, remove excessive stimulation
- Remove restraints and tethers if possible such as monitors, catheters, and physical restraints
- Judiciously utilize typical and atypical antipsychotics

- **Postoperative cognitive dysfunction (POCD)**[11]
  - Defined as a deterioration in cognitive function lasting days, weeks, months, or longer after undergoing anesthesia
  - **Risk factors**
    - Cardiac surgery (although the disorder has been well described after non-cardiac surgery as well)
      - Incidence as high as 70 percent at 1 week, up to 40 percent at 1 year
    - Lengthier surgery/time under general anesthesia
    - Intraoperative organ ischemia and damages
    - Age > 60
    - Preexisting cerebral, cardiac, or vascular disease
    - History of alcohol abuse
  - **Mechanism**
    - Unclear, but likely a complex interplay of genetics, drug toxicity, inflammatory mediators, hormones, and tissue hypoxia
- **Delayed emergence from anesthesia**[1,2]
  - **Pharmacologic**
    - Residual effects of administered anesthetics – IV and volatile anesthetics, opioids
    - Excessive sedation
    - Inadequate reversal of neuromuscular blockade
    - Central anticholinergic syndrome
      - Treatment: Physostigmine – crosses blood–brain barrier
    - Patient intoxication with illicit substances
  - **Metabolic:**
    - Electrolyte, glucose, or acid/base abnormalities, hypo/hyperthermia
    - Other systemic disorders – e.g., hepatic or uremic encephalopathy
      - **Neurologic:** Ischemic or embolic stroke, TIA, intracerebral hemorrhage, seizure increased intracranial pressure

References

1. Nicholau T. K. The postanesthesia care unit. *Miller's Anesthesia*, 8th edn. R. D. Miller, et al. (eds.), 2014; Chapter 96, 2924–46. Philadelphia, PA: Elsevier Inc.
2. Butterworth J. F., Mackey D. C., Wasnick J. D., Morgan G. E., Mikhail M. S. *Morgan and Mikhail's Clinical Anesthesiology*, 5th edn., 2013.
3. Sinatra R. S., Jahr J. S., Watkins-Pitchford J. M. *The Essence of Analgesia and Analgesics*. 2010. New York, NY: Cambridge University Press.
4. Apfel C. Postoperative nausea and vomiting. *Miller's Anesthesia*, 8th edn.

New York, NY: The McGraw-Hill Companies.

R. D. Miller, et al. (eds.), 2014; Chapter 97, 2947–73. Philadelphia, PA: Elsevier Inc.
5. Prashant S., Yoon S. S., Kuo B. Nausea: a review of pathophysiology and therapeutics. *Therap Adv Gastroenterol*, 2016; 9(1): 98–112.

6. Apfel C., Laara E., Koivuranta M., et al. A simplified risk score for predicting postoperative nausea and vomiting: conclusions from cross-validations between two centers. *Anesthesiology*, 1999; 91: 693–700.

7. Eberhart L. H., Geldner G., Kranke P., et al. The development and validation of a risk score to predict the probability of postoperative vomiting in pediatric patients. *Anesth Analg*, 2004; 99: 1630–7.

8. Gan T. J., et al. Consensus guidelines for the management of postoperative nausea and vomiting. *Anesth Analg*, 2014; 118(1): 85–113.

9. Wong S. F., Chung F. Succinylcholine-associated postoperative myalgia. *Anaesthesia,* 2000; 55(2): 144–52.

10. Miller M. O. Evaluation and management of delirium in hospitalized older patients. *Am Fam Physician*, 2008, Dec 1; 78(11): 1265–70.

11. Rasmussen L. S., Stygall J. S., Newman S. P. Cognitive dysfunction and other long-term complications of surgery and anesthesia. *Miller's Anesthesia*, 8th edn. R. D. Miller, et al. (eds.), 2014; Chapter 99, 2999–3010. Philadelphia, PA: Elsevier Inc.

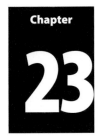

Chapter 23

Central and Peripheral Nervous System

Connie Yue and Jung Kim

Brain

Cerebral Blood Supply

- Anterior cerebral circulation: Provided by anterior cerebral arteries (ACA) and middle cerebral artery (MCA) from internal branch of carotid artery.

    ACA stroke: Contralateral lower limb motor and sensory defect.

    MCA stroke: Contralateral facial and upper limb motor and sensory defect.

- Posterior cerebral circulation: Provided by vertebral arteries
- Circle of Willis provides collateral circulation (Figure 23.1 and Table 23.1)

Cerebral Blood Flow and Cerebral Metabolism

- CPP = MAP − ICP or CVP whichever is higher
- CBF receives 15 percent of cardiac output.

Physiological factors that affect CBF (Graphs 1 and 2)

- $CMRO_2$
    - Coupled with CBF under normal conditions
    - Increase $CMRO_2$ increases CBF
- Autoregulation
    - Between MAP 60 and 160
    - This range is "right-shifted" in chronic hypertension.
    - Can be impaired by brain tumor, injury or stroke. Under these conditions CBF becomes pressure-dependent. Small change in MAP can lead to profound changes in CBF.
- $PaCO_2$: 1 mmHg $PaCO_2$ decrease leads to 1–2 ml/100 g/min decrease in CBF.

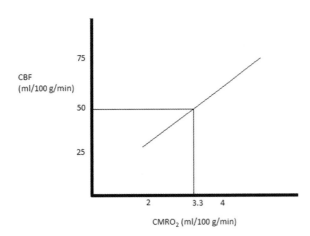

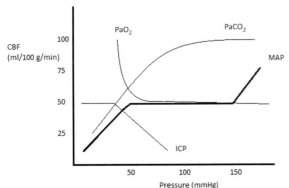

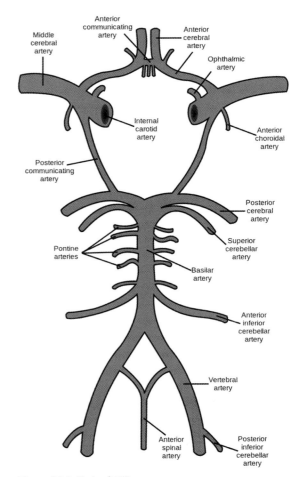

Figure 23.1 Circle of Willis

Table 23.1 Normal values

Cerebral perfusion pressure (CPP)	80–100 mmHg
Intracranial pressure (ICP)	5–12 mmHg
Cerebral blood flow (CBF)	50 ml/100 g/min
Cerebral metabolic rate of oxygen ($CMRO_2$)	3 ml/100 g/min 50 ml/min

Table 23.2 Drug effects on cerebral parameters

	CBF	$CMRO_2$	ICP
Volatiles	↑	↓	↑ (MAC >1)
Nitrous oxide Ketamine	↑	↑	↑
Propofol Etomidate	↓	↓	↓

CBF: Cerebral Blood Flow
$CMRO_2$: Cerebral Metabolic Rate
ICP: Intracranial Pressure

- PaO_2: Only affects CBF in severe hypoxemia usually when $PaO_2 < 50$ mmHg.
- Energy substrates for cerebral metabolism:
  - Glucose in normal conditions
  - Ketone bodies during starvation

Anesthetic Effect on Cerebral Blood Flow

- Desflurane, isoflurane, and sevoflurane cause:
  - Dose-dependent vasodilation and increase in CBF:
    Desflurane > Isoflurane > Sevoflurane
  - Dose-dependent decrease in $CMRO_2$ and impaired autoregulation
  - Uncoupled $CMRO_2$ and CBF (Table 23.2).
- Nitrous oxide causes increase in $CMRO_2$ and CBF from vasodilation.
- Hypocarbia can blunt the effect of volatile anesthetic-induced increase in CBF.
- *Circulatory steal phenomenon*: Volatiles increase blood flow in the normal area of the brain, but not in the ischemic areas, results in redistribution of blood away from the ischemic area.
- *Reverse steal phenomenon (Robin Hood)*: Barbiturates cause cerebral vasoconstriction in normal area and allow blood to redistribute to ischemic area.
- IV induction agents lower CBF and $CMRO_2$ (Table 23.2).

Cerebrospinal Fluid and Cerebral Protection

- Normal CSF pressure = 8–15 mmHg
- Normal CSF volume = 150 ml
- At higher altitude CSF becomes more alkaline to offset the hypoxic ventilatory drive.
- Pathophysiology of cerebral ischemia: Decreased perfusion or glucose cause ATP depletion and ATP pump failure. Raised intracellular calcium level leads to lipase and proteases activation, and neuron damage.

Table 23.3 Anesthetics effects on evoked potential amplitude and latency

Visual (VEP)	Via CN III
Motor (MEP)	Via lateral corticospinal tract
Somatosensory (SSEP)	Via dorsal column to medial lemniscus pathway
Brainstem auditory (BAEP)	Via CN VIII Useful for posterior fossa surgery

- Hypothermia:
  - The most effective method of cerebral protection
    - For every 1°C decrease, $CMRO_2$ decreases by 6–7 percent.
  - Mild hypothermia (33°C–35°C) improves neurological function in patient with return of spontaneous circulation (ROSC).[1]

Spinal Cord

- Spinal cord (conus medullaris) ends at L1 in adult and L3 in infant.
- Anterior spinal artery provides 75 percent of spinal cord circulation.
  - Artery of Adamkiewicz from aorta arises from T9 to T12 and joins with anterior spinal artery to supply lower spinal cord. Injury to this artery can cause spinal cord ischemia.
- Anterior spinal syndrome
  - Lower extremity motor temperature and pain sensation defect
  - Intact proprioception and vibration
- Posterior spinal cord is supplied by two posterior spinal arteries.
- *Autonomic hyperreflexia*: Seen in patient with T7 and above spinal cord injury. Stimulation below the lesion causes vasoconstriction in lower extremities and reflex vasodilation in upper extremities, which results in severe hypertension and bradycardia. Prevented by spinal anesthesia.
- Three major sensory tracts:
  - Spinothalamic (pain, temperature, touch)
  - Spinocerebellar (proprioception)
  - Posterior column (touch, pressure, vibration)
- Abnormal if amplitude decrease more than 50 percent or latency increase.
- In order of sensitivity to inhaled anesthetics: VEP >MEP > SSEP >BAEP (Table 23.3)[2]

	Amplitude	Latency
Isoflurane Sevoflurane Desflurane Propofol	↓	↑
Ketamine Etomidate	↑	↑
Opioid Benzodiazepine	No effect	No effect

Neuromuscular and Synaptic Transmission

- At the neuromuscular junction (NMJ), acetylcholine (ACh) released from the presynaptic neuron binds to nicotinic ACh receptors (NAChR) on the postsynaptic muscle membrane. This leads to Na^+ influx and membrane depolarization (from -90 mV to $+50$ mV).[5]
- Presynaptic ACh release is triggered by Ca^{2+} voltage-gated channel. Lambert–Eaton syndrome has antibody to this Ca channel.
- Postsynaptic AChR requires two ACh binding at its alpha sites to be activated. Myasthenia gravis has antibody to the postsynaptic AChR.
- Action potential:
  - Occurs in an "all-or-none" fashion
  - Results from Na influx from voltage-gated Na^+ channel
- Local anesthetics inhibit Na^+ channel by binding to intracellular portion of Na^+ channel.
- *Upregulation of postsynaptic receptors*: from decreased stimulation over time. Increases risk of hyperkalemia with succinylcholine (Box 23.1).

Box 23.1 Conditions causing NAChR upregulation

Stroke, spinal cord injury
Burn injury (24 h after injury up to 2 years)
Prolonged immobility
Prolonged exposure to neuromuscular blockade
Multiple sclerosis, Guillain–Barré syndrome, amyotrophic lateral sclerosis
Duchenne muscular dystrophy[3]

Skeletal Muscle Contraction

- Muscle contraction occurs by a sliding filament mechanism between actin and myosin.
- At rest, the attraction of myosin and actin filaments is blocked by troponin–tropomyosin complex.
- Action potential depolarizes muscle membrane and triggers calcium release from sarcoplasmic reticulum.
- Calcium removes the inhibitory effect of troponin–tropomyosin complex on actin and myosin and initiates contractile process.
- Energy is produced from splitting ATP by myosin head, which is also an ATPase.
- Reattachment of ATP to myosin causes myosin and actin release, after which a new cycle can start.[4]

References

1. Butterworth J. F., Mackey D. C., Wasnick J. D. Eds. Chapter 26 Neurophysiology & Anesthesia, *Morgan & Mikhail's Clinical Anesthesiology*, 5th edn. New York, NY: The McGraw-Hill Education LLC, 2013, 575–92.
2. Barash P. G., Cullen B. F., Stoelting R. K., et al. Eds. Chapter 36 Anesthesia for Neurosurgery, *Clinical Anesthesia*, 7th edn. Philadelphia, PA: Lippincott Williams & Wilkins, a Wolters Kluwer Business, 2013, 996–1029.
3. Murray M. J., Harrison B. A., Mueller J. T., et al. Eds. Chapter 44 Physiology of Neuromuscular Transmission, *Faust's Anesthesiology Review*, 4th edn. Philadelphia, PA: Saunders, 2014, 98–100.
4. Hall J. E. Chapter 6 Contraction of Skeletal Muscle, *Guyton and Hall Textbook of Medical Physiology*, 13th edn. Philadelphia, PA: Elsevier, 2016, 75–88.
5. Murray M. J., Harrison B. A., Mueller J. T., et al. Eds. Chapter 39–41, Autonomic Nervous System, The Sympathetic Nervous System: Anatomy and Receptor Pharmacology, The Parasympathetic Nervous System: anatomy and receptor Pharmacology, *Faust's Anesthesiology Review*, 4th edn. Philadelphia, PA: Saunders, 2014, 85–93.

Pain Mechanisms and Pathways

Chapter 24

James Yeh and Yury Khelemsky

Introduction

Pain is "an unpleasant sensory and emotional experience associated with actual or potential tissue damage," as defined by the International Association for the Study of Pain.[1] Other important pain-related definitions are listed in Box 24.1.

In the neurophysiologic classification, pain is divided into three categories based on mechanism[2]:

1. Inflammatory
   - Caused by tissue damage and the resultant inflammatory response
2. Pathological
   - The result of a dysfunctional nervous system. This includes:
     - Neuropathic pain, which is a result of damage to the nervous system (e.g., diabetic neuropathy)
     - Dysfunctional pain, which occurs in the absence of nerve damage or inflammation (e.g., fibromyalgia)
3. Nociceptive
   - Caused by the activation of specific neural pathways by potentially harmful stimuli

Box 24.1 Definitions for commonly encountered vocabulary in pain medicine[1,2]

Allodynia	Perception of a non-noxious stimulus as painful
Analgesia	Absence of pain in response to a normally painful stimulus
Anesthesia dolorosa	Pain in an area without sensation
Dysesthesia	An unpleasant abnormal sensation, with or without stimulus
Hyperalgesia	Increased pain in response to a noxious stimulus
Hyperesthesia	Increased sensitivity to sensory stimuli (includes allodynia and hyperalgesia)
Hyperpathia	An abnormally painful response to a stimulus, especially a repetitive one, and an increased threshold
Hypoalgesia	Decreased pain in response to a noxious stimulus
Hypoesthesia	Decreased sensitivity to sensory stimuli
Paresthesia	An abnormal sensation, with or without stimulus

   - Serves as a warning for impending or current tissue damage

Pain can also be classified temporally[2]:

- Categorized as chronic or acute based on the duration of symptoms.
- The cutoff is arbitrary, however 3 months and 6 months are the most commonly used values to define chronic pain.

Nociceptors and Nociceptive Afferent Neurons

Nociception involves four complex processes:

1. **Transduction** is the conversion of the noxious stimuli to an electrical impulse.
2. **Transmission** involves the conduction of this signal from its origin into the central nervous system (CNS).
3. **Modulation** of the pain signal can occur in the spinal cord via various inhibitory pathways.
4. **Perception** is the end result of this pathway and involves the subjective experience of noxious stimuli.

Nociceptors

- They are the specialized receptors located at the terminals of afferent neurons.
- They convert mechanical, thermal, and chemical stimuli into action potentials that are carried into the CNS.[3] These receptors include:
  - Mechanonociceptors – Respond to pinch and pinprick
  - Silent nociceptors – Respond to inflammation
  - Polymodal mechanoheat nociceptors – The most common; stimulated by extreme pressure or temperature and certain noxious compounds, including bradykinin, histamine, prostaglandins, and capsaicin.[4]

Transmission of the pain signal from the site of stimulation to the cortex involves:

- **First-order neurons**, with cell bodies in the dorsal root ganglia
- **Second-order neurons**, with cell bodies in the dorsal horn of the spinal cord
- **Third-order neurons**, with cell bodies in the thalamus

Dorsal Horn Transmission and Modulation, Wind-Up Phenomenon

1. Signals from nociceptors are transmitted by first-order neurons into the dorsal horn of the spinal cord.

- First-order neurons are comprised of myelinated A delta and unmyelinated C fibers.

2. They synapse selectively with *second-order neurons* in the *ipsilateral dorsal horn*, which is comprised of Rexed laminae I–VI.
   - *Rexed lamina II*, also known as the *substantia gelatinosa*, is notable for having large numbers of interneurons and opioid receptors and likely plays a significant role in the modulation of pain.[5]
   - Second-order neurons are composed of:
     - Wide dynamic range (WDR) neurons, which respond to the full range of noxious and non-noxious stimuli
     - Nociceptive specific neurons, which respond only to painful stimuli
3. These fibers then cross midline and ascend in the *contralateral spinothalamic tract* to the *thalamus.*
4. They then synapse with third-order neurons which project to the *postcentral gyrus* and *superior wall of the sylvian fissure.*[4,6]
5. The *spinoreticular tract* is responsible for the transmission of signals from the spinal cord to the *reticular formation* and may play a role in the motivational and emotional components of pain.[7]

"Wind-up" phenomenon

- Occurs in spinal cord neurons and is implicated in the *development of chronic pain.*
- When exposed to the same stimulus repeatedly, WDR neurons have a progressive increase in their response per stimulus.
- The neurotransmitters *glutamate and aspartate*, as well as *NMDA receptors*, are believed to be involved in this process.[4]

Spinal and Supraspinal Neurotransmission and Modulation

Pain may be modulated by inhibitory mechanisms at multiple different levels throughout its pathway from the periphery to the cortex.

- In the periphery, tissue damage results in the release of endogenous opioid peptides by leukocytes, which interact with peripheral opioid receptors, resulting in attenuation of the pain response.[3]
- In the spinal cord, non-noxious sensation transmitted by afferent fibers can disrupt the transmission of the pain signal by WDR neurons and the spinothalamic tract.
  - This contributes to the "gate theory" of pain processing and is mediated by *glycine and GABA.*[4]

Supraspinal pathways are involved in the inhibition of pain transmission in the spinal cord.

- Inhibitory pathways interact with primary afferent neurons and interneurons.
  - Utilizes alpha-2 adrenergic, serotonergic, and opioid-mediated mechanisms

- This inhibitory signal originates in the *periaqueductal gray area* and *reticular formation*, is conducted to the *nucleus raphe magnus* and *medullary reticular formation*, and is then transmitted to the *dorsal horn neurons.*[4]

Autonomic Contributions to Pain

Areas of the nervous system involved in the processing of pain can overlap with areas dedicated to the regulation of the autonomic nervous system (ANS).

- Altered ANS function can contribute to pain syndromes, such as complex regional pain syndrome (CRPS).[8]
- The sympathetic nervous system has been shown to play roles in neuropathic, vascular, and visceral pain.
- Many interventional pain procedures specifically target the sympathetic nervous system. Commonly performed procedures include[9]
  - Stellate ganglion blocks for upper extremity pain
  - Celiac plexus blocks for abdominal pain
  - Hypogastric plexus blocks for pelvic pain
  - Ganglion impar blocks for perineal pain
  - Lumbar sympathetic blocks for lower extremity pain.

Psychological Influences on Pain Perception

The experience of pain is not solely limited to the physiological processes of nerves and neurotransmitters. Psychological and cognitive factors can greatly influence a patient's perception of pain and impact treatment outcomes.[10]

- Fear: The threat of pain or re-injury may prevent patients from pursuing beneficial physical therapy.
- Loss of control: The feeling that pain is uncontrollable can lead to decreased motivation in seeking out new management strategies.
- Depression: Common in chronic pain, with an estimated prevalence of at least 50 percent of patients in specialized pain centers.
  - While depression is generally thought to be a result of chronic pain, it has also been identified as a risk factor for developing chronic pain.

Gender and Age Differences in Pain Perception

Gender and Pain

Gender can influence the perception of pain and there is some evidence of differential responses to pain depending on gender, but results have been inconsistent.

- Women have been shown to have greater pain sensitivity, greater use of pain-relieving medication, and are at increased risk for chronic pain.
  - The reason for this is thought to be multifactorial, involving psychological, social, and physiologic elements.[11]

Aging and Pain

- Aging is associated with the development of chronic painful conditions.
  - Arthritis, back pain, neuropathies, previous fractures

- There are numerous age-related changes in pathways involved in the processing of pain.
  - ○ *Damage* or degeneration of *sensory fibers*
  - ○ Lower levels of neurotransmitters of primary sensory nerves

- There is an increase in pain thresholds in the elderly, which has been shown to be a result of decreased sensitivity to low-intensity pain.
  - ○ Subsequently, the elderly may be at increased risk for tissue damage.[12,13]

References

1. IASP Taxonomy 2012. Available from: www.iasp-pain.org/Taxonomy.

2. Nagda J. V., Bajwa Z. H. Definitions and Classification of Pain. In: Z. H. Bajwa, R. J. Wootton, C. A. Warfield (eds.), *Principles and Practice of Pain Medicine*, 3rd edn. New York, NY: McGraw-Hill Education; 2016.

3. Stein C., Kopf A. Anesthesia and Treatment of Chronic Pain. In: R. D. Miller (ed.), *Miller's Anesthesia*, 8th edn. Philadelphia, PA: Elsevier/ Saunders; 2015, 1898–918.

4. Rosenquist R. W., Vrooman B. M. Chronic Pain Management. In: J. F. Butterworth, D. C. Mackey, J. D. Wasnick (eds.), *Morgan & Mikhail's Clinical Anesthesiology*, 5th edn. New York, NY: The McGraw-Hill Companies; 2013.

5. Kleiner J. S. Substantia Gelatinosa. In: J. S. Kreutzer, J. DeLuca, B. Caplan (eds.), *Encyclopedia of Clinical Neuropsychology*. New York, NY: Springer New York; 2011, 2432–3.

6. D'Mello R., Dickenson A. H. Spinal Cord Mechanisms of Pain. *BJA: British Journal of Anaesthesia* 2008; 101(1): 8–16.

7. Cohen R. I. Anatomy and Physiology of Pain. In: Z. H. Bajwa, R. J. Wootton, C. A. Warfield (eds.), *Principles and Practice of Pain Medicine*, 3rd edn. New York, NY: McGraw-Hill Education; 2016.

8. Gill J. S. Sympathetic Blocks. In: Z. H. Bajwa, R. J. Wootton, C. A. Warfield (eds.), *Principles and Practice of Pain Medicine*, 3rd edn. New York, NY: McGraw-Hill Education; 2016.

9. Menon R., Swanepoel A. Sympathetic Blocks. *Continuing Education in Anaesthesia Critical Care & Pain* 2010; 10(3): 88–92.

10. Turk D. C., Okifuji A. Psychological Aspects of Chronic Pain. In: Z. H. Bajwa, R. J. Wootton, C. A. Warfield (eds.), *Principles and Practice of Pain Medicine*, 3rd edn. New York, NY: McGraw-Hill Education; 2016.

11. Bartley E. J., Fillingim R. B. Sex Differences in Pain: A Brief Review of Clinical and Experimental Findings. *BJA: British Journal of Anaesthesia* 2013; 111(1): 52–8.

12. McCarberg W. Pain in the Elderly. In: Z. H. Bajwa, R. J. Wootton, C. A. Warfield (eds.), *Principles and Practice of Pain Medicine*, 3rd edn. New York, NY: McGraw-Hill Education; 2016.

13. Lautenbacher S., Peters J. H., Heesen M., Scheel J., Kunz M. Age Changes in Pain Perception: A Systematic-Review and Meta-Analysis of Age Effects on Pain and Tolerance Thresholds. *Neuroscience & Biobehavioral Reviews* 2017; 75: 104–13.

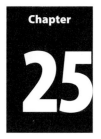

Autonomic Nervous System

Thomas Palaia, Joseph Park, Nakiyah Knibbs, and Jeffrey Ciccone

Sympathetic System

- **Receptors:** Sympathetic receptors are G protein-coupled with two main groups: α and β. Dopamine receptors also play a role in sympathetic stimulation.
  - There are two types of α receptors, α1 (Gq-coupled receptor) and α2 (Gi-coupled receptor).
  - There are three types of β receptors, β1, β2, and β3, all of which are Gs-coupled. β2 receptors are mainly stimulated by epinephrine. All of these increase the level of cAMP, which is the second messenger.
  - Dopamine receptors are sympathetic receptors found on blood vessels and are also G protein-coupled.[1]
- **Transmitters:** Sympathetic preganglionic neurons originating from T1 to L2–L3 of the spinal cord travel to ganglia and release acetylcholine (ACh). Upon being stimulated by the ACh in the ganglia (usually paravertebral or prevertebral ganglia), the nicotinic postganglionic receptor causes the release of:
  - Norepinephrine (NE)
  - Dopamine (from the kidneys)
  - Acetylcholine (from sweat glands)
  - Epinephrine (from chromaffin cells in the adrenal medulla with which preganglionic neurons synapse directly)

  These neurotransmitters activate target tissues that lead to the effects seen with the sympathetic nervous system (see Table 25.1).[2]
- **Synthesis:** Sympathetic neurotransmitters are synthesized from tyrosine as follows: tyrosine → DOPA → dopamine → NE → epinephrine. The first step is the rate limiting step, catalyzed by tyrosine hydroxylase.
  - All of these steps, except for the transformation from NE to epinephrine, occur in the *postganglionic sympathetic nerve ending.*
  - NE transforms to epinephrine in the adrenal medulla. They are stored in vesicles until postganglionic nerve is stimulated.[1,2]
- **Release:** Once the nicotinic postganglionic nerve or adrenal medulla is stimulated, storage vesicles containing NE, ACh, dopamine, or epinephrine merge with cell membrane and release contents into synapse and the receptors located on target organs are activated.[1]
- **Responses:** See Table 25.1.

- **Termination of action:** Most NE and epinephrine are removed from synaptic cleft *via reuptake* into storage vesicles. The small amount not taken up by vesicles enters circulation where it is *metabolized by monoamine oxidase (MAO), catechol-o-methyl transferase (COMT),* or both in blood, liver, and kidney. About 25 percent of *NE is removed by the lungs,* whereas dopamine and epinephrine are not affected.[3]

Parasympathetic System

- **Receptors:** There are five types of muscarinic receptors: M1, M2, M3, M4, and M5. Of these, M2 and M3 receptors affect the patients' hemodynamics.
  - M2 receptors are Gi-coupled receptors found in the heart.
  - M3 receptors are Gq-coupled receptors located in various parts of the body that lead to increased intracellular calcium.[4]

  The location and action of these receptors are detailed in Table 25.1.
- **Transmitters:** The main neurotransmitter used in the parasympathetic system is ACh. Parasympathetic preganglionic neurons originating from brainstem nuclei CN III, VII, IX, and X as well as sacral levels S2–S4 travel to ganglia (usually located on target organ) where it releases ACh. This ACh acts on nicotinic postganglionic receptors which also release ACh, activating target tissues and leading to effects seen with the parasympathetic nervous system (see Table 25.1).
- **Synthesis:** ACh is synthesized in the preganglionic and postganglionic neurons from the compounds choline and acetyl coenzyme A (acetyl-CoA) by the enzyme choline acetyltransferase (ChAT).[4]
- **Release:** ACh is located within vesicles of preganglionic and postganglionic neurons until its release into the synapse. The influx of calcium stimulates the docking, fusion, and ultimately the release of ACh-containing vesicles.[4,5]
- **Responses:** See Table 25.1
- **Termination of action:** ACh is inactivated within the synapse by the enzyme acetylcholinesterase (AChE) that hydrolyzes the ACh into its component choline and acetic acid.[4]
- **Pharmacologic agents:** Two classes of medications that manipulate the PNS with anesthetic relevance are *muscarinic antagonists and cholinesterase inhibitors.*

Table 25.1 Autonomic responses of target organs

Organ		Sympathetic response		Parasympathetic response		Dominant response
		Response	Receptor	Response	Receptor	
Heart	Force of contraction	Increase	β1	Decrease	M2	P
	Rate of contraction	Increase	β1	Decrease	M2	P
Blood vessels	Arteries	Vasoconstriction	α1 (α2)			S
	Veins	Vasoconstriction	α2 (α1)			S
	Skeletal muscle	Vasodilation	β2			S
Bronchial tree		Bronchodilation	β2	Bronchoconstriction	M3	P
Splenic capsule		Contraction	α1			S
Uterus		Contraction	α1	Variable		S
Vas deferens		Contraction	α1			S
Gastrointestinal tract		Relaxation	α2	Contraction	M3	P
Eye	Radial muscle (iris)	Contraction (mydriasis)	α1			S
	Circular muscle (iris)			Contraction (miosis)		P
	Ciliary muscle	Relaxation	β2	Contraction (accommodation)	M3	P
Kidney		Renin secretion	β1			S
Bladder	Detrusor	Relaxation	β2	Contraction	M3	P
	Trigone and sphincter	Contraction	α1	Relaxation	M3	Neither
	Ureter	Contraction	α1			S
Pancreas – insulin release		Decrease	α2			S
Fat cells – lipolysis		Increase	β1/β3			S
Liver glycogenolysis		Increase	α1/β2			S
Hair follicles, smooth muscle		Contraction (piloerection)	α1			S
Nasal secretion		Decrease	α1/α2	Increase		P
Salivary glands		Increase secretion	α1	Increase secretion		P
Sweat glands		Increase secretion	α1	Increase secretion		P

S = sympathetic, P = parasympathetic.

Source: Adapted from *Brody's Human Pharmacology: Molecular to Clinical (Table 9.2)*, by L. Wecker, L. M. Crespo, T. M. Brody, G. Dunaway, C. Faingold. Philadelphia, PA: Mosby/Elsevier; 2010. Copy Year 2010 by Mosby/Elsevier.

o *Muscarinic antagonists:* Competes with ACh specifically at muscarinic receptors. Used for their chronotropic, sedative, and anti-sialogogue effects. For example, glycopyrrolate is usually paired with an anticholinesterase to mitigate bradycardia during neuromuscular blockade reversal.

- These anti-muscarinics exhibit similar efficacy in receptor blockade with some notable differences in the robustness of response (Table 25.2). For example, atropine causes a greater heart rate response, whereas scopolamine has increased sedative effects. As an exception, glycopyrrolate (a quaternary ammonium compound) does not cross the blood–brain barrier and therefore has no CNS or ophthalmic effects.

Table 25.2 Comparative pharmacologic characteristics of muscarinic antagonists

	Atropine	Scopolamine	Glycopyrrolate
Antisialogogue effect	++	+++	+++
Bronchodilation	++	+	++
Sedation	+	+++	0
CNS toxicity	+	+++	0
Cycloplegia/mydriasis	+	+++	0
Increased heart rate	+++	+	++

0, None; +, mild effect; ++, moderate effect; +++, marked effect.

- Due to their tertiary amine structure, atropine and scopolamine both cross the blood–brain barrier and their use could potentially lead to CNS toxicity, evidenced by altered mental status. This can be treated with the anticholinesterase, physostigmine, that can also cross the blood–brain barrier.
  - *Cholinesterase inhibitors:* Used for the reversal of neuromuscular blockade and for the diagnosis and treatment of myasthenia gravis. These medications reversibly bind the cholinesterase enzyme, rendering it inactive and increasing the amount of ACh available to bind at both nicotinic and muscarinic receptors.[6]
    - The use of these drugs (neostigmine, physostigmine, pyridostigmine, edrophonium) leads to bradycardia, bronchospasm, salivation, increased GI motility, and miosis.

Ganglionic Transmission

- **Sympathetic**: Sympathetic preganglionic neurons, which are *relatively shorter,* arise from T1 to L2 of spinal cord and travel to paravertebral ganglion (or prevertebral ganglion for the celiac, superior mesenteric, and inferior mesenteric ganglia).
  - Here they synapse with postganglionic neurons, which are relatively longer. At the synapse, ACh is released by the preganglionic neurons that activate the nicotinic ACh receptors on the postganglionic neurons.
  - The postganglionic neurons will then release their neurotransmitters, primarily NE but also epinephrine, dopamine, or ACh, which then affects the target organ.
- **Parasympathetic**: Parasympathetic preganglionic fibers, which are *relatively longer,* arise from cranial nuclei or the sacral plexus (S2–S4 of spinal cord) and travel to small ganglia located near the target organ.
  - Here they synapse with postganglionic neurons, which are relatively shorter. At the synapse, ACh is released by preganglionic neurons which activate the nicotinic ACh receptors (much like the sympathetic system).
  - The postganglionic neurons will then release ACh which then affects the target organ.[7]

Reflexes

- **Afferent limbs:** Sensory neurons that receive input from viscera have cell bodies located in the sensory ganglia of either a cranial nerve for parasympathetic fibers or a paravertebral ganglion versus a prevertebral ganglion for sympathetic fibers. These project to the central nervous system and initiate the efferent portion of the reflex.
- **Efferent limbs:** Starts with the preganglionic neuron cell body, which for the sympathetic system is located in the T1–L2 region of the spinal cord and for the parasympathetic system is located in the cranial nuclei or sacral plexus. This axon extends to ganglia where it synapses with the postganglionic neuron which projects to the smooth muscles of the target organ or cardiac muscle. The effect on the organ will depend on which system sympathetic or parasympathetic is predominating at the time.[8]

Temperature Regulation

Temperature Sensing, Central, and Peripheral

The process of thermoregulation is controlled by multiple distinct tissue types and thermally sensitive cells throughout the body in three distinct phases:

- **Afferent thermal sensing**
  - Cold signals travel typically along A delta fibers and increase action potential and firing with decreased temperatures while warm signaling is transmitted via unmyelinated C fibers.
    - C fibers also transmit pain which is why it is not possible to distinguish high temperature from sharp pain.
  - Thermal input transmitted diffusely across spinothalamic tract of anterior spinal cord.[9]
- **Central regulation**
  - The hypothalamus receives afferent thermal input from skin surfaces, deep tissues, and the central nervous system.
    - It appears that thermal information is processed within the spinal cord and central nervous system to a certain degree prior to reaching the hypothalamus which is why patients with high spinal cord transections are still able to regulate core body temperature.[10]
- **Efferent response**
  - Changes in both peripheral and core temperature begin an autonomic response that alters both metabolic heat production and environmental heat loss.
    - Typically the body attempts to conserve both heat and energy maximally by employing energy-efficient techniques such as vascular tone modulation (vasoconstriction or vasodilation) prior to metabolically taxing activities such as shivering/sweating.
  - Even in response to inhibition of thermoregulatory techniques (shivering inhibited by muscle relaxant administration), core body temperature remains normal unless temperature-regulating techniques are unable to compensate.
  - Illness, medications, and advanced age all diminish the efficacy of the thermoregulatory response.[9]

Temperature Regulating Centers: Concept of Set Point

- **Hypothalamus** is responsible for maintaining core body temperature within narrow range known as the *interthreshold range* (range that does NOT induce an autonomic response).
  - Core body temperature that rises above *interthreshold range* will induce peripheral vasodilation and sweating.

- Core body temperature that falls below this *inter-threshold* range will induce vasoconstriction and shivering.[11]
- Exact mechanism that maintains the temperature threshold remains unknown, although it is believed to be mediated by a complex interaction of various neurotransmitters (NE, Dopamine, 5-hydroxytryptamine, ACh, PGE-1, various other neuropeptides).
  - Response controlled primarily by thermal input from core structures and tissues (up to 80 percent)
- Circadian rhythm (times of day), sex, age (marginally impaired in older adults), menstrual phase, exercise, nutritional intake, endocrine conditions such as hyper/hypothyroidism, and drugs (anesthetics, alcohol, CNS stimulants/depressants) all constantly modify the *interthreshold range*.[9]

Heat Production and Conservation

- Decrease in central core temperature below the *interthreshold range* will first induce energy-efficient temperature conservation by inducing **vasoconstriction** prior to shivering thermogenesis.
  - Vasoconstriction mediated by α-adrenergic sympathetic nerves decreases the metabolic heat loss by mitigating convection and radiation (primary source of heat loss) from surface of the skin.
  - Capillaries (up to 10 μm in diameter) supply the nutritional component of blood flow to the skin that are not affected by thermoregulation and provide blood flow independent of thermoregulatory response.
    - Arteriovenous (AV) shunts (up to 100 μm) are the predominant thermoregulatory vasculature component. It can hold up to 10,000 times as much blood in comparison to an equal length of capillary.
    - Sympathetic activation induces vasoconstriction of AV shunts thereby returning more warm blood to core tissues and organs.
- **Non-shivering thermogenesis:** Mechanism whereby skeletal muscle and brown fat increase metabolic heat production without mechanical work
  - More pronounced in infants (can nearly double heat production) versus a minimal increase in heat production in adults
  - Controlled primarily by NE release from adrenergic nerve terminals
- **Shivering thermogenesis:** Centrally mediated rapid tremor and unsynchronized muscular activity that can increase metabolic heat production by 50–100 percent in adults
  - Does not occur in infants, and mechanism not entirely developed until 7 years of age.[9]

Heat Loss: Mechanisms

- **Radiation:** Heat loss to the environment that occurs anytime the temperature of the patient is above absolute zero (always).
  - Most significant portion of total heat loss (up to 67 percent) in certain studies.[12]
  - Proportional to the temperature difference between any two sources raised to the fourth power.
- **Convection:** Heat loss secondary to air movement
  - Mechanism by which forced air warming devices and blankets protect from intraoperative convection heat loss.
- **Conduction:** Heat loss that occurs through direct contact
  - Use of table padding with foam or rubber on the operating room table will insulate the patient and minimize heat loss via conduction.
- **Evaporation:** Sweating is suppressed under general anesthesia and therefore a minor contributor to heat loss.

Body Temperature Measurement, Sites, Gradients

- Temperature monitoring is indicated for all general and neuraxial anesthetics extending beyond 30 minutes. It detects intraoperative hypothermia, hyperthermia, and possible incidence of malignant hyperthermia.
  - Temperatures vary greatly throughout body and each reading has its own distinct physiologic and practical significance.
- Core temperatures are typically more uniform and higher when compared to peripheral skin temperatures, and are most useful when used to detect malignant hyperthermia or quantify hypothermia.
  - Core body temperature should be maintained >36°C whenever possible, unless hypothermia (cerebral/cardiovascular protection during cardiopulmonary bypass) is indicated.
  - True core body temperature sites: tympanic membrane, pulmonary artery catheter, distal esophagus, and nasopharynx should be used whenever possible.
    - Oral, axillary, bladder, rectal temperatures all provide reasonable estimations of core temperature.
  - Skin temperature will be lower in comparison to central core temperature and may be used as an estimate of core temperature, but the values must be interpreted with caution.
    - Especially during cases with large, rapid swings in temperature (i.e., cardiopulmonary bypass), skin temperature readings are of minimal utility when used to guide intraoperative thermal management.[9]

Effect of Drugs/Anesthesia on Temperature Regulation

- **Redistribution:** Occurs during both general anesthesia (secondary to pharmacological effects of anesthetic agents) and during neuraxial anesthesia (secondary to loss of sympathetic tone)
  - Phase 1: Thermal energy (warm blood volume) from "central" compartments such as abdomen and thorax to the extremities and peripheral tissues secondary to anesthetic-induced vasodilation
    - 1–2°C decrease during first hour of general anesthesia
    - Forced air warming devices used preoperatively to pre-warm patient may mitigate this phase of heat loss by neutralizing central–peripheral temperature gradient.[13]
  - Phase 2: Continued heat loss to environment over next 3–4 hours of general anesthesia
    - Much more gradual than Phase 1
    - Also minimized with the use of forced air warming devices, warmed IV fluids and increasing ambient temperature of operating room.
  - Phase 3: Steady state, in which the production of heat is approximately equal to metabolic heat production (>4 hours from anesthesia induction).[13]
- **Central thermoregulation inhibition:** Anesthetic agents inhibit reflexive responses from the hypothalamus that maintain the interthreshold range
  - For each percentage of inhaled isoflurane, there is approximately a 3°C decrease in the temperature threshold that induces vasoconstriction.[3]
    - Primarily occurs under general anesthesia, although occurs to some degree during neuraxial techniques which is thought to be due to altered perception of the hypothalamus to the temperature of the anesthetized dermatomes.[13]
  - Shivering is generally absent while under general anesthesia especially with co-administration of neuromuscular blocking agents.

- **Postoperative shivering**
  - More common with longer surgical duration and greater volatile anesthetic concentrations used during surgery[13]
  - Hypothermia upon reactivation of the interthreshold range by the hypothalamus
  - Increased risk of myocardial ischemia during severe shivering, as this may increase oxygen consumption five times that of a normothermic patient[13]
  - **Frequent** during the post-partum period
    - Thought to be a combination of central heat redistribution secondary to peripheral vasodilation and interruption of sympathetic tone
    - May be attributed to possible hormonal response in the immediate post-partum period as 23–44 percent of patients exhibit shivering even after natural child birth without neuraxial anesthesia[14]
- **Harmful effects of hypothermia in intra-operative and postoperative period**
  - Increased incidence of myocardial ischemia secondary to shivering, increased oxygen consumption, and increased vascular resistance
  - Cardiac arrhythmias
  - Decreased oxygen release by RBCs due to leftward shift of hemoglobin–oxygen saturation curve
  - Coagulopathy and possibly increased transfusion requirements
    - Mild hypothermia (1–2°C below 37°C) can increase the need for allogenic transfusions by 20 percent
  - Potentiation of neuromuscular blockade
  - Delayed wound healing and increased infection risk (up to three times wound infection rate)
  - Decreased drug metabolism and anesthetic requirements[9]
    - Minimum alveolar concentration (MAC) reduced by approximately 5 percent per °C below 35°C[15]

References

1. Brody T. M., Larner J., Minneman K. P., Wecker L. (eds.). Chapter 9: Introduction to the Autonomic System. *Brody's Human Pharmacology: Molecular to Clinical.* Philadephia, PA: Elsevier Mosby; 2005, 93–106.
2. Philipson L. H. β-Agonists and Metabolism. *J Allergy Clin Immunol.* 2002 Dec 31; 110(6): S313–7.
3. Miller R. D., Eriksson L. I., Fleisher L. A., Wiener-Kronish J. P., Young W. L. Chapter 16: The Autonomic Nervous System. *Anesthesia,* 7th edn.

Philadelphia, PA: Elsevier/Saunders; 2009, 346–86.
4. Siegel G. J., Agranoff B. W., Albers R. W., et al. (eds.) Chapter 7: Acetylcholine. *Basic Neurochemistry: Molecular, Cellular and Medical Aspects,* 6th edn. Philadelphia, PA: Lippincott-Raven; 1999, 186–207.
5. Wessler I. Acetylcholine Release at Motor Endplates and Autonomic Neuroeffector Junctions: A Comparison. *Pharmacol Res.* 1996 Feb 29; 33(2): 81–94.

6. Martyn J. A. J. Neuromuscular Physiology and Pharmacology. R. Miller (ed.), *Miller's Anesthesia,* 8th edn. Philadelphia, PA: Elsevier Saunders; 2015, 423–43.
7. David G., Hirst S., Bramich N. J., Edwards F. R., Klemm M. Transmission at Autonomic Neuroeffector Junctions. *Trends Neurosci.* 1992 Feb 29; 15(2): 40–6.
8. Binder M. D., Hirokawa N., Windhorst U. (eds.). Autonomic Reflexes. *Encyclopedia of Neuroscience.* Berlin, Heidelberg: Springer; 2009, 272–81.

9. Miller R. D. *Miller's Anesthesia*, 8th edn. Philadelphia, PA: Churchill Livingstone/Elsevier; 2015.

10. Simon E. Temperature Regulation: The Spinal Cord as a Site of Extrahypothalamic Thermoregulatory Functions. *Rev Physiol Biochem Pharmacol.* 1974; 71: 1–76.

11. Butterworth J. F., Mackey D. C., Wasnick J. D. *Morgan & Mikhail's Clinical Anesthesiology*, 5th edn. New York, NY: The McGraw-Hill Companies, Inc; 2013.

12. Sessler D. I. Mild Perioperative Hypothermia. *N Engl J Med.* 1997; 336(24): 1730–7.

13. Sessler D. I. Perioperative Heat Balance. *Anesthesiology.* 2000; 92(2): 578–96.

14. Harper R. G., Quintin A., Kreynin I., Brooks G. Z., et al. Observations on the Post Partum Shivering Phenomenon. *J Reprod Med.* 1991; 36: 803–7.

15. Eger E. I., Johnson B. H. MAC of I-653 in Rats, Including Test of the Effect of Body Temperature and Anesthetic Duration. *Anesth Analg.* 1987; 66: 974–6.

Central Nervous System Anatomy

Devon Flaherty and Jonathan Gal

Monro-Kellie Doctrine[1]: The intracranial space is a fixed space composed of: (1) brain parenchyma, (2) cerebrospinal fluid, and (3) blood. An increase in the volume of one must result in a decrease in one or both of the remaining two volumes.

The Brain

Cerebral hemispheres have three components: cerebral cortex (gray matter), sub-cortical white matter, and the basal ganglia (also gray matter).

Cerebral cortex is functionally divided into Brodmann areas (47 in total). Anatomically divided by sulci into lobes and specific gyri.

- o **Primary motor cortex** – Located on the precentral gyrus. Critical for voluntary motor movement of contralateral side of the body. Stimulated with transcranial motor evoked potentials. Organized into a motor homunculus. See Figures 26.1 and 26.2.
- o **Premotor cortex** – Also involved in motor function, as well as planning and mediating motor impulses.
- o **Primary somatosensory cortex** – Located on the post-central gyrus. Receives sensory information from the contralateral side of the body. Also arranged as a homunculus.
- o **Wernicke's area** – Located in the dominant temporal Lobe. Critical for language comprehension. Lesion

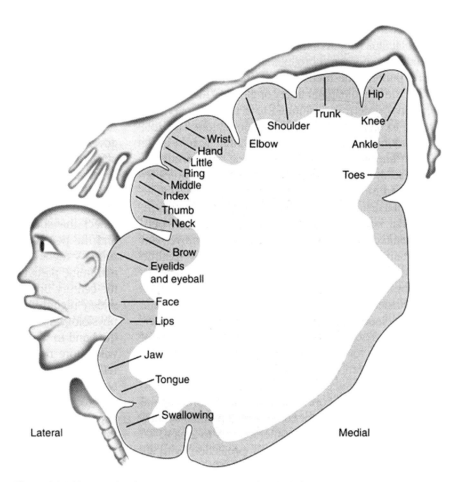

Figure 26.1 Homunculus – lower extremity is represented medially, followed by upper extremity and head as you move more laterally along the gyrus

results in Wernicke's aphasia, which is a fluent aphasia ("word salad"). Connects to Broca's area via the arcuate fasciculus.

- o **Broca's area** – Located in the dominant inferior frontal lobe. Critical for speech production. Damage results in Broca's aphasia, which is an expressive aphasia.
- o **Longitudinal fissure** – Separates the cerebrum into the right and left hemispheres
- o **Transverse fissure** – Divides the cerebrum from cerebellum
- o **Central sulcus** – Separates the precentral gyrus (anterior) from the postcentral gyrus (posterior)
- o **Lateral sulcus** – Separates the frontal and parietal lobes from the temporal lobe[2,3]

Basal Ganglia

- Composed of three nuclei: caudate nucleus, putamen, and globus pallidus interconnected by the internal capsule
- Essential for motor control
- Functionally they work with the *substantia nigra, subthalamic nuclei,* and other midbrain structures to form the *extrapyramidal system*
- *Parkinson's disease:* Loss of dopaminergic neurons in the substantia nigra
- *Huntington's disease*: Neuron loss in the caudate and putamen

Brainstem

The brainstem is comprised of the *midbrain, pons, and medulla.*

The *reticular formation* (also known as the reticular activating system) – constellation of nuclei located in the tegmentum of the brainstem, lateral hypothalamus, and thalamus (medial, intralaminar, and reticular nuclei)

- Functions to control consciousness and arousal
- Communicates with the cerebral cortex, often using serotonin or norepinephrine as neurotransmitters
- Also has descending tracts (*reticulospinal tract*) that regulate spinal reflexes, autonomic function, and respiratory control

Area postrema (medulla) – A chemoreceptor trigger zone for emesis. Lacks blood–brain barrier and is a direct interface between parenchyma, blood, and cerebrospinal fluid (CSF). It is exposed to emetogenic agents in blood and CSF. Not essential for vomiting from motion or vagal stimuli.

Dorsal vagal complex (medulla) – Area postrema + nucleus of the solitary tract + vagal dorsal motor nucleus. Implicated in nausea and vomiting by receiving signals from the chemoreceptor trigger zone and the viscera.

Nausea/vomiting impulses can also come from the vestibular system, midbrain, and cerebral cortex.[4,5]

How Is Respiration Controlled?

1. **Primary respiratory center** (medulla) – Also known as "medullary respiratory center" is comprised of dorsal and ventral respiratory groups
   a. **Dorsal respiratory group** – Initiates inspiration. Down-stream effects activate phrenic and intercostal nerves. Active during quiet breathing. Stimulated either by intrinsic pacemaker function, or possibly by extrinsic pacing by the *Pre-Botzinger complex.*
   b. **Ventral respiratory group** – Both inspiratory and expiratory neurons. Stimulated by intense activity in the dorsal respiratory group. Inactive during quiet breathing, but functions during active exhalation.
2. **Apneustic center** (pons, reticular formation) – Modulates signals from the primary respiratory center. Stimulates inspiratory neurons, inhibits expiratory neurons.
3. **Pneumotaxic center** (pons, nucleus parabrachialis, and Kolliker Fuse nucleus) – Modulates signals from the primary respiratory center. Inhibits inspiratory neurons or apneustic center.
   - o Respiratory centers contain chemoreceptors that detect pH levels and adjust ventilation accordingly. Peripherally, aortic and carotid bodies contain chemoreceptors that increase ventilation in response to decreased pH, increased $PaCO_2$, and decreased PaO_2.
   - o **Aortic body** afferent impulses transmitted along *the vagus nerve.*
   - o **Carotid body** afferent impulses transmitted along *the glossopharyngeal nerve.*
   - o Many drug classes such as opiates and sedative/hypnotic agents inhibit transmission in the dorsal respiratory group of the primary respiratory center causing respiratory depression.[6]

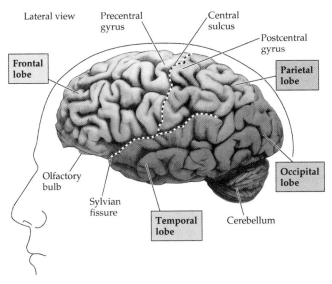

Figure 26.2 Lobes of the cortex – the brain is divided into four lobes (frontal, parietal, occipital, and temporal). The precentral and postcentral gyri are separated by the central sulcus. The frontal and temporal lobes are separated by the lateral sulcus
By Allan Ajifo [CC BY 2.0 (http://creativecommons.org/licenses/by/2.0), via Wikimedia Commons

Cerebral Circulation

Major vessels course through the subarachnoid space before entering the brain parenchyma. A ruptured aneurysm in these vessels will lead to subarachnoid hemorrhage rather than parenchymal hemorrhage.

Arterial System

Circle of Willis – Allows for anastomosis between both sides of the brain and is composed of:

- Anterior communicating artery ×1
- Anterior cerebral arteries ×2, A1 segments (horizontal)
- Internal carotid arteries ×2
- Posterior communicating arteries ×2
- Posterior cerebral arteries ×2, P1 segments (horizontal)
- Basilar artery ×1
    - Highly variable anatomy, only ~25 percent of population has a complete vascular ring.
    - When clamping the internal carotid artery during a carotid endarterectomy, the mean arterial pressure is transiently elevated to increase the perfusion pressure through the contralateral internal carotid artery, perfusing the Circle of Willis and subsequently the contralateral brain tissue.
    - Vertebral artery injection is commonly implicated in local anesthetic systemic toxicity following brachial plexus blocks and cervical blocks.[7]

Venous System

- Internal regions of the brain are drained by the internal cerebral veins, which empty into the great cerebral *vein of Galen.*
- All other regions of the brain are drained by *venous sinuses,* which are enveloped within the layers of dura and ultimately drain into the *internal jugular veins or pterygoid plexus.*
- *Emissary veins* connect venous sinuses to extracranial veins acting as a potential route for intracranial transmission of infection.
- *Bridging veins* traverse the dura and can be torn with applied traction (e.g., trauma or CSF drainage after a spinal tap), which can lead to a subdural hematoma.
- Venous sinuses in the skull are kept patent by connections to the dura and surrounding osseous structures even when intraluminal pressure decreases such as in hypovolemia or head-up position. This allows for the entrainment of air and the possibility of venous air embolism when open sinuses are exposed to atmospheric air (i.e., craniotomy in sitting position).

The Spinal Cord

Spinal cord blood supply:

- One anterior spinal artery
    - Formed from the two vertebral arteries.
    - Narrows around T4 and becomes the *anterior medial spinal artery.* Gets contributions from the *radicular arteries* – branches from intercostal arteries (T1–L1, highly variable).
    - *Artery of Adamkiewicz* is the largest radicular artery, usually arises at T9–T12 (highly variable) and supplies the lower half of the anterior spinal cord.
- Two posterior spinal arteries
    - Formed from either vertebral arteries (25 percent of population) or posterior–inferior cerebellar arteries (75 percent of population)
    - Supply dorsal white columns, and dorsal gray matter

Notable tracts:

- Ascending tracts
    - **Spinothalamic tract** – Carries *pain and temperature input.*
        - First-order neurons with cell bodies in *dorsal root ganglion* (DRG) are stimulated via their peripheral free nerve endings.
        - Axons travel through Lissauer's tract to synapse on to second-order neurons in the dorsal horn *(substantia gelatinosa or nucleus proprius).*
        - Secondary neuron's axons decussate within 1 to 3 vertebral levels via the *ventral white commissure* and travel to the contralateral *ventral posterolateral nucleus of the thalamus.*
        - Third-order neurons send impulses along the internal capsule to the somatosensory cortex.
    - **Dorsal column/medial lemniscus** – Carries tactile discrimination, proprioception, form recognition, and vibratory input.
        - First-order neurons are in the DRG and give rise to either the fasciculus gracilis (lower extremity) or fasciculus cuneatus (upper extremity).
        - Ascend ipsilaterally, until they synapse with second-order neurons in the medulla, at either the *gracile or cuneate nuclei.*
        - Fibers of the second-order neurons decussate, forming the *medial lemniscus* and synapse on to the *contralateral ventral posterolateral nucleus of the thalamus.*
        - Third-order neurons send axons along the posterior limb of the internal capsule to the *somatosensory cortex.*
- Descending tracts
    - **Corticospinal tracts**: Voluntary control of skeletal muscle to the body.
        - Originates from upper motor neurons in the primary motor cortex. Decussate in the medulla. Synapse on to lower motor neuron in ventral horn of spinal cord. Lower motor neuron interacts directly with skeletal muscle.
    - **Corticobulbar tract**: Voluntary control of skeletal muscle to regions of the body controlled by cranial nerves.

- Originates in the primary motor cortex (upper motor neurons), travels down the internal capsule, crosses to contralateral side in the brainstem to innervate motor nuclei of cranial nerves (innervates some cranial nerves bilaterally).[8]

The Spine

It is comprised of cervical (7), thoracic (12), lumbar (5), sacral (5), and coccygeal (4) vertebrae.

Important landmarks:

- Chassaignac's tubercle – C6 transverse process
- Vertebra prominens – C7
- Inferior angle of the scapular – T7
- Lower rib margin – T10
- Tuffier's line – Imaginary line between iliac crests, estimates L4 vertebral body or L4/5 interspace
- Posterior iliac spines – S2
- Sacral cornu – S5

Key locations:

- Spinal cord extends from skull base to conus medullaris ~L1/2 in adults, L3 in infants

Table 26.1 Dermatomal sensory blockade with anatomical landmark correlate, as required for different types of surgery

Sensory level	Landmark	Surgery/site
T4	Nipple	Entire peritoneum, cesarean section, upper abdominal
T6	Xiphoid process	Hernia repair, lower abdominal surgery (gynecologic, urologic)
T10	Umbilicus	Hip surgery, TURP, labor/vaginal delivery
L1	Inguinal ligament	Thigh/knee surgery
L2	Knee	Ankle and foot surgery
S1	N/a	Perineal and anal surgery

- Dural sac extends from foramen magnum to S2 in adults and S3/4 in infants
- Maximum thoracic kyphosis at T4
- Maximal lumbar lordosis at L3[9]
- Dermatomal blockade at certain anatomical sites can be used to assess adequacy of block height (Table 26.1)

Regional differences in vertebral morphology:

- Cervical: Small vertebral bodies, transverse processes come off vertebral body.
- Thoracic: Spinous processes are sharply angled inferiorly. Increasing vertebral body size. Transverse processes attached to pedicle/lamina. Articulations with ribs.
- Lumbar: Spinous processes are perpendicular to neuraxis. Large vertebral bodies, transverse processes attached to pedicles/lamina.

Atlantoaxial instability: Associated with Down syndrome, longstanding rheumatoid arthritis, trauma, and ankylosing spondylitis.

Paravertebral Space

- Borders: Parietal pleura (anterolateral), superior costotransverse ligament (posterior), vertebral body/disk, and intervertebral foramina (medial)
- Contains spinal nerves very loosely invested in fascia, allowing for great exposure to local anesthetics

Facet joints – See Figure 26.3

- Small stabilizing joints between vertebrae. Often implicated as a source of axial back pain.
- Innervated by the *medial branch of the posterior division* of spinal nerves. Can be blocked by a "medial branch block."
- A single facet joint is only sufficiently blocked if both the above and below branches are blocked.

Meninges

Three layers of meninges are dura, arachnoid, and pia mater.

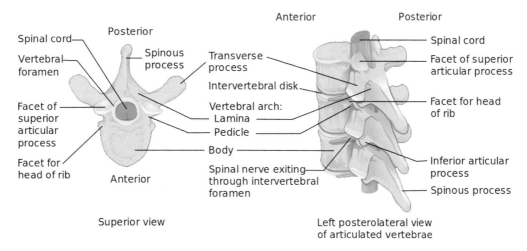

Figure 26.3 Vertebral anatomy – transverse and sagittal views of the vertebral column depicting the vertebral body, transverse processes, lamina, spinous processes, and facet joints

In general, the dura imparts structure while the arachnoid imparts impermeability.

As loosely covered ventral and dorsal roots fuse to form spinal nerves, they are enveloped by a dural sleeve (dura and arachnoid mater).

What layers does a midline spinal needle pass through?
- Skin > subcutaneous fat > supraspinous ligament > interspinous ligament > ligamentum flavum > epidural space > dura > subdural space > arachnoid mater > subarachnoid space

What layers does a paramedian spinal needle pass through?
- Skin > subcutaneous fat/skeletal muscle > ligamentum flavum > epidural space > dura > subdural space > arachnoid mater > subarachnoid space

What are the borders of the epidural space?
- Superiorly – Foramen magnum (a "high epidural" wouldn't block the cranial nerves)
- Inferiorly – Sacrococcygeal ligament
- Anteriorly – Posterior longitudinal ligament
- Posteriorly – Lamina and ligamentum flavum
- Laterally – Pedicles

What is contained in the epidural space?
- Fat, nerves, vessel
- *Internal vertebral plexus* (also known as Batson's plexus) – Venous drainage of the epidural space. The plexus is valveless and communicates with both the basilar plexus and deep pelvic veins.
  - Veins can act as a pathway for spread of infection or malignancy.
  - Veins are more prominent in lateral epidural space, providing an explanation for the higher rate of intravascular catheters with a paramedian epidural approach.

- Patients with IVC compression or elevated intraabdominal or intracranial pressures have more distention of epidural veins leading to a higher likelihood of intravascular injection as well as increased spread of local anesthetic (less non-vascular volume in the epidural space).

Where is the epidural space the largest?
- ~L2 (roughly 6 mm in the midline)
- The mid thoracic region also contains a large epidural space (~5 mm).[9]

Cranial Nerves

Use this mnemonic to remember the function of the 12 cranial nerves (i.e., motor, sensory, or both). **SSMMBMBSBBMM**: "Some say money matters but my brother says big brains matter most" (Table 26.2).[10]

Olfactory
- Function may be lost during tissue swelling with pregnancy, tumors, or basilar skull fractures from trauma.

Optic
- Ischemia can result in *ischemic optic neuropathy*, either anterior (affecting the optic disk) or posterior (retrobulbar optic nerve ischemia) and presents as *painless visual loss.*
  - Anterior ischemic optic neuropathy (AION): Usually after cardiac surgery
  - Posterior ischemic optic neuropathy (PION): After spine surgery

Oculomotor
- Controls the majority of eye motion via extraocular muscles.
- "Down and out." Patients with a palsy of this nerve have an *inferior and lateral diversion* to their pupil, as well as *mydriasis.*
- During herniation, this nerve is stretched by the medial temporal lobe leading to an ipsilateral palsy.

Table 26.2 Cranial nerves listed by number, name, location, and functions

CN #	Name	Location	M/S/B	Function
1	Olfactory	Telencephalon	S	Smell
2	Optic	Diencephalon	S	Vision
3	Oculomotor	Midbrain	M	Extrinsic eye muscles
4	Trochlear	Midbrain	M	Extrinsic eye muscles
5	Trigeminal	Pons	B	General facial sensation; Muscles of mastication
6	Abducens	Midbrain/Pons	M	Abduction of eye
7	Facial	Midbrain/Pons	B	Taste; Facial muscles
8	Vestibulocochlear	Midbrain/Pons	S	Hearing, balance
9	Glossopharyngeal	Medulla	B	Taste; Sensation (see below)
10	Vagus	Medulla	B	Mixed (see below)
11	Accessory	Spinal cord	M	Sternocleidomastoid and trapezius motor
12	Hypoglossal	Medulla	M	Tongue movements

M = Mixed, S = sensory, B = both motor and sensory functions.

Trochlear

- Innervates the superior oblique muscle (crucial for extorting and depressing the eye)
- Lesions of this nerve result in the inability to intort the eye
  - Patients cock their head to the opposite site to allow for compensatory intortion of contralateral eye.
- Who gets trochlear nerve lesions?
  - Blunt head trauma
  - Elevated ICP
  - Compressive lesions (i.e., posterior circulation aneurysm, tumor)
  - Cavernous sinus lesions, because nerve travels through subarachnoid space and cavernous sinus
- CN IV has the longest intracranial course outside of brainstem leaving it susceptible to shearing or compressive forces.

Trigeminal

- Three distributions – Ophthalmic (V1), maxillary (V2), and mandibular (V3)
- Controls the muscles of mastication, such as the masseter (these muscles can be directly stimulated with a peripheral nerve stimulator to give "false twitches").
- Affected in trigeminal neuralgia, most commonly V2 or V3.
- Branches can be blocked for supraorbital (V1), infraorbital (V2), greater palatine (V2), or nasopalatine (V2) nerve blocks.
- Mandibular nerve provides general sensory innervation to anterior two-third of the tongue.
- Oculocardic reflex initiated by V1 due to compression of globe or traction on extraocular muscles.

Abducens

- Controls *abduction* of the eye via the *lateral rectus muscle*.
- A lesion results in the inability to abduct eye.
  - CN VI palsy is the most common ocular motor paralysis.

Facial nerve

- Five branches control facial muscles: (1) temporal, (2) zygomatic, (3) buccal, (4) mandible, and (5) cervical branches.
- Branches pass through but do not innervate the parotid gland. These nerve branches are often monitored intraoperatively during parotidectomies.
- Activity of orbicularis oculi via stimulation of the zygomatic branch of CN VII is often used for neuromuscular blockade monitoring.
- Taste sensation from the anterior two-thirds of the tongue is carried by the chorda tympani.

Vestibulocochlear

- Connects to the dorsal vagal complex, allowing for nausea with motion. Post-operative nausea and vomiting is associated with ear surgeries and a history of motion sickness.
- Aminoglycosides are classic ototoxic agents:
  - Gentamicin total dose is associated with ototoxicity and vestibulopathy.
  - Gentamicin administration rate and peak plasma levels are associated more with nephrotoxicity.
- Transient partial hearing loss is relatively common after spinal anesthesia in the parturient.

Glossopharyngeal

- Sensory innervation of soft palate, posterior one-third of tongue, and posterior oropharynx
  - Vallecula is innervated by glossopharyngeal (via pharyngeal plexus) and the vagus nerve.
  - The underside of the epiglottis is innervated solely by the vagus nerve (via internal branch of the superior laryngeal nerve).
- Blocked by topicalized local anesthetic administration or injection at the base of the anterior tonsillar pillar (anesthetizes the tonsillar, lingual, and pharyngeal branches)
  - Often utilized prior to an awake fiberoptic intubation

Vagus

- Motor innervation to the larynx via the recurrent laryngeal nerve and external branch of the superior laryngeal
- Sensory innervation
  - Internal branch of the superior laryngeal nerve
    - Hypopharynx
    - Vallecula (shared with CN IX)
    - Epiglottis
    - Larynx at and above vocal cords
  - Recurrent laryngeal nerve
    - Below vocal cords, including trachea and lower airways
- A Miller blade is theoretically more likely to induce laryngoscopy-related bradycardia than a Macintosh blade because the underside of the epiglottis is innervated by the vagus nerve. The vallecula is innervated by both the glossopharyngeal and vagus nerves.
- Unilateral palsy of the recurrent laryngeal nerves leads to hoarseness and is not an airway emergency.
  - Hoarseness after interscalene block may be from transient unilateral recurrent laryngeal nerve block.
  - Recurrent laryngeal nerve palsies are often in the context of thyroid and parathyroid surgery.
  - Nerve palsy has been described in cases of prolonged intubation with an over-inflated endotracheal tube cuff.
  - Recurrent laryngeal nerve may be severed or damaged during sternotomy or aortic arch repair because its path loops under the aortic arch.
- Bilateral complete palsy of recurrent laryngeal nerves leaves vocal cords flaccid and rarely results in complete airway obstruction.

Table 26.3 Cranial nerve reflexes

Reflex	Afferent nerve	Efferent nerve
Corneal	V$_1$	VII
Oculocardiac	V$_1$	X
Lacrimation	V$_1$	VII
Pupillary	II	III
Gag	IX	X

- Bilateral incomplete palsy of the recurrent laryngeal nerves leaves the vocal cords with unopposed adduction forces resulting in complete airway obstruction. This is an airway emergency.
  - Posterior cricothyroid muscle is the only muscle that can abduct the vocal cords.
- CNX provides parasympathetic innervation diffusely including the respiratory tract (bronchoconstriction and secretions).

  - Opposing sympathetic innervation is provided from T1 to T4 (cardioaccelerator fibers).

Spinal Accessory

- Motor innervation of sternocleidomastoid and trapezius
- When sacrificed during neck dissection leads to shoulder discomfort and weakness
- May be injured during posterior cervical triangle lymph node biopsies, central line placement, and facial nerve blocks

Hypoglossal

- Innervates intrinsic and extrinsic muscles of the tongue except for palatoglossus (CN X)
- Very rare unilateral lesions have been described after oral airway, LMA, and orotracheal tube placement.
  - Patient may have dysphagia, dysphonia, and ipsilateral tongue deviation (Table 26.3).

References

1. Mokri B. The Monro-Kellie Hypothesis Applications in CSF Volume Depletion. *Neurology*. 2001; 56: 1746–9.
2. Waxman S. G. Cerebral Hemispheres/ Telencephalon. In: Waxman S. G. (ed.), *Clinical Neuroanatomy*, 27th edn. New York, NY: McGraw-Hill; 2013. http://eresources.library.mssm .edu:2751/content.aspx?bookid=673& sectionid=45395972.
3. Jacobson S., Marcus E. M. Motor System II: Basal Ganglia. In: *Neuroanatomy for the Neuroscientist*, 2nd edn. New York, NY: Spinger Science + Business Media, LLC; 2011: 207–24.
4. Waxman S. G. The Brain Stem and Cerebellum. In: Waxman S. G. (ed.), *Clinical Neuroanatomy*, 27th edn. New York, NY: McGraw-Hill; 2013.
5. Hornby P. J. Central Neurocircuitry Associated with Emesis. *Am J Med*. 2001; 111(8): 106–12.
6. Balofsky A., George J., Papadakos P. Neuropulmonology. *Handb Clin Neurol*. 2017; 140(2006): 33–48. Doi: 10.1016/B978-0-444-63600-3.00003-9.
7. Waxman S. G. Vascular Supply of the Brain. In: Waxman S. G. (ed.), *Clinical Neuroanatomy*, 27th edn. New York, NY: McGraw-Hill; 2017.
8. Waxman S. G. The Spinal Cord. In: Waxman S. G. (ed.), *Clinical Neuroanatomy*, 27th edn. New York, NY: McGraw-Hill; 2013.
9. Cousins M., Bridenbaugh P. Anatomy of the Neuraxis. In: Brown B., Dernoski N., (eds.), *Cousins & Bridenbaugh's Neural Blockade in Clinical Anesthesia and Pain Medicine*, 4th edn. Philadelphia, PA: Lippincott Williams & Wilkins; 2009.
10. Monkhouse S. General Considerations. In: Monkhouse S. (ed.), *Cranial Nerves: Functional Anatomy*, 1st edn. Cambridge: Cambridge University Press; 2009.

Respiratory Physiology

Chapter 27

Maria Castillo

Lung Volumes and Capacities

Tidal volume (TV): Volume inspired and expired during quiet breathing cycle (~500 mL)

Residual volume (RV): Volume left in lungs after maximum expiratory effort (~2 L)

Expiratory reserve volume (ERV): Maximal volume that can be forcibly exhaled from end-expiratory position of a tidal volume

Inspiratory reserve volume (IRV): Volume that can be inspired with maximal effort above the normal resting end-inspiratory position of a tidal volume[2,3]

Total lung capacity (TLC): Volume in lung after maximum inspiration (6–8 L). TLC is increased in COPD and decreased in restrictive lung disease

$$TLC = IRV + ERV + TV + RV = VC + RV$$

Vital capacity (VC): Maximum volume that can be exhaled after maximal inspiration (4–6 L). VC is decreased in both restrictive and obstructive lung disease

$$VC = TLC - RV = IRV + ERV + TV$$

Functional reserve capacity (FRC): Volume in lungs after an ordinary expiration (3–4 L). FRC is increased with increased height and age and decreased in pregnant women, obese patients, supine position, and general anesthesia

$$FRC = ERV + RV$$

Inspiratory vital capacity (IVC): Maximal volume inhaled from the point of maximum expiration[2–4]

Time constants (Tau) τ: Describes the rapidity of change in an exponential curve

τ = Time required to inflate lung (τ = 63%; 2τ = 87%; 3τ = 95%; 4τ = 99%)

τ = Total compliance × airway resistance[4]

Spirometry: Measures lung function, volume, flow, and breathing pattern

FEV_1 (Forced expiratory volume in 1 second) – volume exhaled by the end of the first second of forced expiration

FVC (Forced vital capacity) – vital capacity determined from a maximally forced expiratory effort

Dead space (physiological): The volume of gas ventilating the conducting airways and unperfused alveoli (anatomic dead space ~2 mL/kg)

Closing capacity: Volume at which small airways lacking cartilaginous support begin to close in dependent parts of the lung. Highly dependent on lung volume and the radial traction of the surrounding lung tissue to keep open. Increases with age, meaning respiratory bronchioles will collapse at higher volume than in younger people.[2,4,5]

Methods of Measurement of Lung Volumes

Nitrogen washout: Patient breathes O_2 for several minutes to eliminate N_2; then, the quantity of N_2 eliminated is measured. Thus, if 2 L of N_2 is eliminated, and initial alveolar concentration was 80 percent, then the initial volume of the lung was 2.5 L.[3]

Helium: Use as a tracer gas. If 50 mL of helium is introduced to lungs and concentration is measured to be 1 percent, then the lung volume is 5 L.

Plethysmograph: Gas-tight box in which changes in the volume of the body can be determined as a change in pressure within the box.

O_2 uptake: Oxygen diffuses into erythrocytes down the pressure gradient, O_2 partial pressure of atmosphere = 160 mmHg; in alveolus = 150 mmHg; in pulmonary arterial blood in capillaries ~20–40 mmHg. Increasing FIO_2 to 100 percent increases alveolar partial pressure, increasing gradient, aiding O_2 diffusion.[3]

Increased O_2 uptake: Caused by left shift, transfusion, increased alveolar ventilation, and increased FIO_2

Decreased O_2 uptake: Caused by anemia, blood dyscrasias, dead space, V/Q mismatch, COPD, and diffusion limitations

CO_2 production: Parallels O_2 consumption according to respiratory quotient. Only 80 percent as much CO_2 is produced as O_2 is consumed.

Respiratory quotient (RQ): CO_2 produced/O_2 consumed which is under normal conditions is 0.8. It indirectly indicates whether proteins, carbohydrates, or fats are primarily being used for energy consumption. When RQ is >0.8, carbohydrates are being metabolized. When <0.8, lipids are being metabolized. At 0.8, a combination of proteins, lipids, and carbohydrates are metabolized.[2]

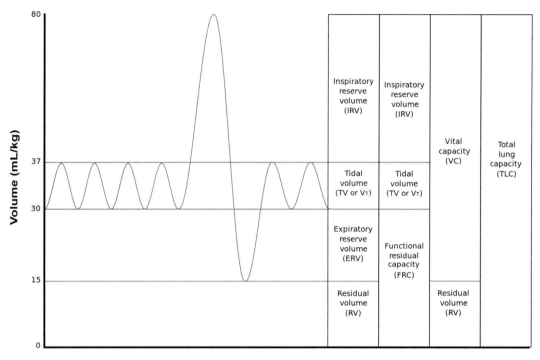

Figure 27.1 Lung volumes[1]

Exercise testing: Heart rate and ventilation plotted against O_2 consumption

Excessive increase in heart rate – primarily cardiac causes of exercise limitation

Excessive increase in ventilation – primarily respiratory causes of limitation

Both are increased – likely pulmonary vascular disease (Figure 27.1)[1]

Lung Mechanics

$$\text{Compliance} = \Delta V/\Delta P$$

Dynamic compliance: Volume change divided by the peak inspiratory trans-thoracic pressure

Static compliance: Volume change divided by the plateau inspiratory trans-thoracic pressure[2,6,7]

Total compliance is calculated using lung compliance and chest wall compliance, defined as:

$$1/C_{total} = 1/C_W + 1/C_L$$

Pleural pressure gradient: Due to lung density, gravity, and conformation of the lung within the thorax, which predominates in the basal lung tissue, pleural pressure is less negative at the base than at higher portions of the lung.

Flow-volume loops: Plot of Y-axis = rate of airflow; X-axis = total volume inspired or expired during maximally forced inspiratory and expiratory maneuvers (Figure 27.2)

Hysteresis: Pressure–volume curves of the lung compliance during inflation and deflation, which are different due to additional energy required during inspiration to recruit alveoli[7]

Surfactant: Secreted by type II alveolar epithelial cells; profoundly lowers surface tension of the alveolar lining fluid, increasing compliance of the lung, decreasing work of expanding the lung, inhibiting transudation of fluid, increasing stability of alveoli, decreasing atelectasis[7]

LaPlace's law: The pressure in an alveolus (P) is greater than ambient pressure by an amount dependent on the surface tension in the liquid lining (T) and the radius of the alveolus (R): **P = 2T/R**

Resistance: Airway resistance $R = \Delta P/\Delta V$

For air to flow into lungs, ΔP must be developed to overcome airway resistance. ΔP depends on caliber of airway and rate and pattern of airflow.[2-4]

Principles of Gas Flow Measurement

Laminar flow occurs when the gas passes down parallel-sided tubes at less than a critical velocity; the pressure drop is proportional to the flow rate as per **Poiseuille's equation:**

$\Delta P = 8QL\mu/\pi r^4$ otherwise written as $Q = \Delta P\pi r^4/8\mu L$

ΔP: Pressure difference between two ends

Q: Gas flow rate

L: Length of the tube

μ: Viscosity

r: Radius of the tube[2,7]

Turbulent flow: Pressure proportional to the volume of gas flow squared times a gas density constant. There is more resistance with turbulent flow, which occurs at airway branch points and airway wall irregularities.[3]

Orific flow occurs at severe constriction such as stenosis or obstruction of the upper airway; the pressure drop is

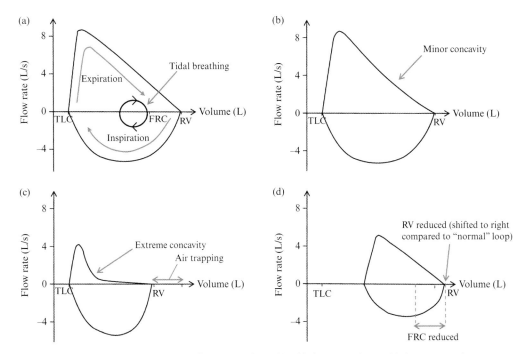

Figure 27.2 Flow-volume loop (a) normal flow-volume loop, (b) mild obstructive disease, (c) obstructive pulmonary disease, (d) restrictive pulmonary disease[1]

dependent on density of the gas rather than viscosity, which is why using helium decreases resistance to flow.

Note: At *low flow rates*, there is *laminar flow* which depends on the *viscosity* of the gas. At *high flow rates*, there is *turbulent flow* which depends on the *density* of the gas.[3]

Work of breathing: Potential energy is stored by the lung during inspiration and expended during expiration, thus expiration is passive.

Work against elastic resistance is increased when breathing is slow and deep; work against air flow resistance is increased when breathing is rapid and shallow.

Increased elastic resistance (pulmonary fibrosis, pulmonary edema) – Rapid and shallow is favored

Increased airway resistance (asthma, obstructive lung disease) – Deep and slow is favored[3]

Regulation of airway caliber: Neural control of airway smooth muscle and there is pharmacological modulation of this input

Acetylcholine (Ach) acts on muscarinic subtypes, especially M_3 receptors for contractile response; epinephrine and norepinephrine act on α- and β-adrenergic receptors; vasoactive intestinal peptide (VIP), nitric oxide (NO), substance P, and neurokinin A act via second messenger cascades.[2,3,6]

Ventilation–Perfusion

Distribution of ventilation: In low flow states, distribution is determined by compliance. In high flow states, distribution is determined by resistance. In upper, more expanded regions of the lung, resistance is lower, so flow rate is increased, equalizing distribution of ventilation.

Distribution of perfusion: Determined by gravity and hydrostatic pressure; decreased blood flow to apex; with positive pressure ventilation, apical alveoli can compress surrounding capillaries, preventing blood flow[2]

Zones

Zone 1 – Alveolar pressure P_A > arterial P_a > venule P_v, creating decreased transmural pressure causing collapse of blood vessels and minimal blood flow. Includes apical area of lungs.

Zone 2 – Transition region below Zone 1 where P_a > P_A > P_v, resulting in resistance to flow during most but not all of the respiratory cycle

Zone 3 – Dependent region where P_a > P_v > P_A, thus blood flow is unimpeded and gas exchange happens continuously; includes most of the lung

Zone 4 – Atelectatic portion of the lung[3]

Hypoxic pulmonary vasoconstriction: Adaptive vasomotor response to alveolar hypoxia, which redistributes blood to optimally ventilated lung segments by an active process of vasoconstriction, thereby improving ventilation–perfusion matching[2]

Alveolar gas equation:
$$PAO_2 = [FiO_2 \times (Patm - PH_2O)] - PaCO_2/RQ$$
$$PAO_2 = \text{Alveolar } O_2 \text{ tension}$$

Diffusion

Pulmonary diffusion capacity: Amount of gas that can diffuse across a membrane in a given period

Diffusing capacity of lung for carbon monoxide (DLCO) is determined by the surface area of gas exchange, the

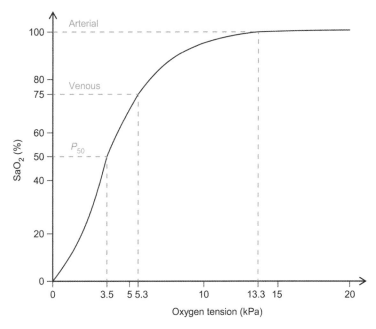

Figure 27.3 Hemoglobin–oxygen dissociation curve[1]

membrane thickness, the pressure gradient between the gas phase in the alveolus and the plasma in the capillary, the molecular weight, and solubility

> CO used as the test gas, inhaled at a small concentration to TLC just after a maximal expiration, held, then deeply exhaled to RV; inhaled CO – exhaled CO = quantity either taken up by the blood or remaining in the lung (RV); RV can be determined if an insoluble gas is administered with CO[2]

Apneic oxygenation: Diffusion of oxygen to alveoli in absence of ventilation

Diffusion hypoxia: When nitrous oxide is discontinued, large quantities cross from the blood into the alveolus down its concentration gradient, diluting the O_2 and CO_2 in the alveolus, causing a decrease in the partial pressure of oxygen resulting in hypoxia; can be avoided by increasing fractional inspired O_2 concentration.[2,3,6]

Blood Gas

O_2 transport: As RBC passes alveolus, O_2 diffuses into the plasma, increasing PaO_2. As PaO_2 increases, O_2 diffuses into the RBC and combines with hemoglobin (Hb).

O_2 physical solubility: Oxygen exists in dissolved form or combined with Hb.

Oxyhemoglobin (Hb–O_2) saturation: Each Hb consists of four heme molecules attached to a globulin molecule; each heme consists of glycine, α-ketogluteric acid, and iron in the ferrous form. Each ferrous ion can bind loosely to one oxygen molecule; as they bind, the Hb becomes saturated.[2,3,6,7]

Hb–O_2 dissociation curve: Relates the saturation of Hb to the PaO_2

> Hb is fully saturated at 700 mmHg; the flat part of the curve signifies 95–98% saturation and $PaO_2 \sim 90$–100 mmHg; when $PaO_2 < 60$, saturation falls steeply. PaO_2 of 60 is roughly a saturation of 90 percent (Figure 27.3)[1]

Rightward shift means increased oxygen unloading at a given PO_2; can be caused by increased temperature, increased H+, increased PCO_2, and increased 2,3-DPG.

2,3-Diphosphoglycerate (2,3-DPG): An end-product of red cell metabolism

> Shifts O_2 dissociation curve to the right; increased in chronic hypoxia and chronic lung disease

P_{50}: PO_2 at which Hb is 50 percent saturated; ~**26.7** mmHg

Blood O_2 content: In arterial blood, 98 percent is oxyhemoglobin, <2 percent is dissolved in plasma

$$CaO_2 = (Hgb \times 1.39 \times SaO_2\%) + (PaO_2 \times 0.003)$$
1.39 mL = amount of O_2 bound per gram Hb at 1 atm
0.003 mL = amount of dissolved O_2 in blood[4]

Respiratory enzymes: Oxidases catalyze the transfer of electrons from its substrate to molecular oxygen

CO_2 transport: CO_2 and O_2 move between the systemic capillary blood and tissue cells, and between the capillary blood and alveolar gas in the lungs by *passive diffusion*

> CO_2 diffuses 20 times faster than O_2
> In plasma, CO_2 exists in physical solution and hydrated to *carbonic acid (H_2CO_3)* and as *bicarbonate (HCO_3^-)*; in erythrocytes, CO_2 combines with Hb as *carbaminohemoglobin (Hb-CO_2)*

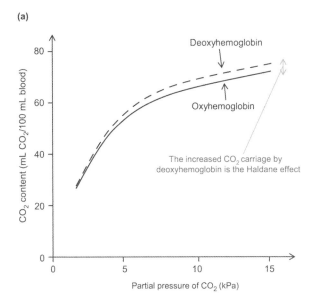

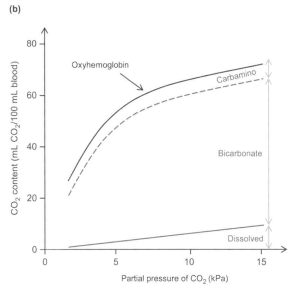

Figure 27.4 CO_2 dissociation curve[1]

Carbonic anhydrase: Speeds up first part of reaction inside RBCs

HCO_3 – Diffuses out of the cell more easily than H^+, so Cl^- ions diffuse into the cell (chloride shift); some of the H^+ ions bind to Hb due to the fact that reduced Hb is less acidic than the oxygenated form[4]

Reduced Hb in peripheral blood helps with loading of CO_2, while oxygenation in pulmonary capillaries assists with unloading

$$CO_2 + H_2O \Longleftrightarrow H_2CO_3 \Longleftrightarrow H^+ + HCO_3$$

Hemoglobin (Hb) as a buffer: H^+ is then buffered by Hb

$$H^+ + Hb \Longleftrightarrow HHb$$

CO_2 dissociation curve: Total CO_2 is plotted against the PCO_2, illustrating the amount of each form of CO_2 in the blood (Figure 27.4)[2,4,5]

Bohr effect: Shift of the Hb–O_2 dissociation curve caused by changes in CO_2 or pH

Shift is to the right in systemic capillaries where PCO_2 is higher and pH is lower, increasing offloading of O_2 to tissues

Shift is to the left in pulmonary capillaries where CO_2 is lower, increasing O_2 binding to Hb[2,4]

Haldane effect: Deoxygenation of blood increases its ability to carry CO_2; the lower the saturation of Hb with O_2, the larger the CO_2 concentration for a given PCO_2[4]

Systemic Effects of Hypercarbia and Hypocarbia

Hypercarbia: Restlessness, tremor, slurred speech, mood changes, increased cerebral blood flow (CBF) leading to headache, increased CSF pressure, papilledema, increased catecholamine release, ↑ HR, ↑ BP

Hypocarbia: Decreased CBF, decreased cerebral blood volume, decreased cerebral oxygen delivery, decreased

ICP, decreased myocardial oxygen supply, increased coronary vascular resistance, increased risk of coronary artery spasm, increased coronary microvascular leakage, increased myocardial oxygen demand, increased intracellular calcium concentration, increased platelet count and aggregation[2,4]

Systemic Effects of Hyperoxia and Hypoxemia/Hypoxia

Hyperoxia: Increased production of cytotoxic oxygen free radicals that can cause damage to the alveolar-capillary membrane, increased mucous plugging and atelectasis, increased risk of ARDS, retrolental fibroplasia, nausea, vomiting, numbness, twitching, dizziness, possibly seizures

Hypoxia: Increased catecholamine release, ↑ HR, decreased CBF, headache, somnolence, mental status changes, heart failure, renal function impairment, sodium retention, proteinuria, shock, ventricular fibrillation asystole[2,4]

Basic interpretation of arterial blood gas: Normal room air $PO_2 = \sim100$, $PCO_2 = \sim40$

Respiratory acidosis: ↑PCO_2 → ↓HCO_3^-/PCO_2 ratio; ↓pH

Respiratory alkalosis: ↓PCO_2 → ↑HCO_3^-/PCO_2 ratio; ↑pH

Metabolic acidosis: ↓HCO_3^-/PCO_2 → ↓pH

Metabolic alkalosis: ↑HCO_3^-/PCO_2 → ↑pH

If PCO_2 cannot account for value of pH, compensatory changes may be creating a mixed picture.[2–4,6,7]

Control of Ventilation

Respiratory Center

Dorsal medullary respiratory group – Receives afferent visceral input from CN IX and X; regulates timing of the respiratory cycle; inspiration-intrinsic periodic firing generates repetitive bursts of action potentials

Ventral medullary respiratory group – Expiration-quiescent during normal breathing but become active during exercise and then begin firing expiratory cells; control over musculature of pharynx, larynx, and tongue

The cortex, the apneustic center in lower pons, the pneumotaxic center in upper pons, the limbic system, and the hypothalamus can also affect breathing pattern.[4]

Central chemoreceptors: Located near ventral surface of medulla, surrounded by brain extracellular fluid (ECF); increased H^+ or dissolved CO_2 stimulates breathing, decreases inhibition

Peripheral chemoreceptors: Carotid bodies – located at the bifurcation of the common carotids; aortic bodies – located above and below aortic arch; respond to decreased arterial PO_2 and pH as well as increased arterial PCO_2[4,7]

Proprioceptive receptors: Pulmonary stretch receptors inhibit further inspiration and slow respiratory frequency; juxtacapillary "J" receptors respond to engorgement of capillaries via vagus nerve[4]

Respiratory Muscles, Reflexes, Innervation

Diaphragm: Thin, dome-shaped sheet of muscle attached to lower ribs and spine; innervated by the phrenic nerves (C3–C5)

External intercostal muscles: Connect adjacent ribs; slope downward and forward causing increased lateral and anteroposterior diameters of the thorax when they contract; innervated by intercostal nerves of the same level

Internal intercostal muscles: Pull ribs downward and inward, decreasing thoracic volume

Abdominal wall (rectus abdominis, internal and external obliques, transversus abdominis): Raise intra-abdominal pressure by contracting, pushing diaphragm upward

Accessory muscles of inspiration: Scalene muscles elevate first two ribs; sternomastoids raise the sternum[7]

CO_2 and O_2 response curves: Central and peripheral chemoreceptors sensing an increase in H^+ activate a negative feedback loop to change rate of ventilation

Opioids cause a right-shift in the response curve, while hypoxemia causes a left-shift. Benzodiazepines and propofol decrease the slope of the curve, while volatile anesthetics decrease the slope and cause a right shift.[2,3,6]

Non-respiratory Functions of the Lungs

Metabolic: Pulmonary endothelial cells metabolize endogenous substances and can affect pharmacokinetics.[4]

"First-pass" uptake – Amount of substance removed from blood on first cycle through the lungs

Lungs have substantial concentrations of P_{450} isoenzymes as well as a high concentration of angiotensin-converting enzyme (**ACE**)

Mast cells and neuroendocrine cells can produce serotonin (**5-HT**), and the lungs can extract from blood and metabolize 5-HT to 5-HIAA.

Lungs also metabolize leukotrienes, cyclo-oxygenase, prostaglandins, thromboxane, and prostacyclin.[6]

Immune: Cytoplasmic vesicles and caveolae are involved in endocytosis.

Airway surface film has antimicrobial properties. Respiratory epithelium contains *ciliated columnar cells* that help move out mucus and particles and goblet cells that secret mucus.

Other cells include submucosal secretory cells, Clara cells which produce detoxifying proteins, mast cells, macrophages, monocytes, and alveolar epithelial cells which also produce surfactant.

Lungs are also a vascular reservoir due to the capacity of the pulmonary vessels and a physical filter for particles and pathogens, and they humidify inhaled air.[6]

Perioperative Smoking

Physiologic Effects

Nicotine affects the sympathetic nervous system, causing hypertension and tachycardia.

Carbon monoxide takes the place of oxygen on the Hb molecule, shifting the Hb–O_2 dissociation curve to the left and decreasing oxygen availability in the tissues.

Smoking increases mucus production, damages cilia, which impairs clearing of secretions, irritates bronchial tree, and inhibits immune function.[8]

Cessation of Smoking

48–72 hours – May have more reactive airways and increased secretions, less hypertension and tachycardia, less carbon monoxide, thus less carboxyhemoglobin, less tissue hypoxia, increased ciliary function

2–4 weeks – Decreased mucus production, less reactive airways

4–6 weeks – Immune functions normalize

<8 weeks – Possibly an increase in complications

>8 weeks – Decreased postoperative morbidity and mortality[8]

References

1. Miller R. D., Cohen N. H., Eriksson L. I., et al. *Miller's Anesthesia*, eighth edition. Philadelphia, PA: Elsevier, 2015; pp. 442–72.

2. Barash P. G., Cullen B. F., Stoelting R. K., et al. *Clinical Anesthesia*, seventh edition. Philadelphia, PA: Lippincott Williams & Wilkins, 2013; pp. 263–86.

3. Benumof J. L. *Anesthesia for Thoracic Surgery*, second edition. Philadelphia, PA: W.B. Saunders, 1995; pp. 43–122.

4. Slinger P. *Principles and Practice of Anesthesia for Thoracic Surgery*. New York: Springer, 2011; pp. 51–69, 103–19.

5. West J. B. *Pulmonary Physiology and Pathophysiology: An Integrated, Case-Based Approach*. Baltimore, MD: Lippincott Williams & Wilkins, 2001; pp. 16–30.

6. Butterworth J. F., Mackey D. C., Wasnick J. D. *Morgan & Mikhail's Clinical Anesthesiology*, fifth edition. New York: McGraw-Hill, 2013; pp. 487–526.

7. Katznelson R., Beattie W. S. Perioperative smoking risk. *Anesthesiology* 2011; 114: 734–6.

8. Chambers D., Huang C. L., Matthews G. *Basic Physiology for Anaesthetists*. Cambridge, UK: Cambridge University Press, 2015.

Respiratory System Anatomy

28

Samuel Hunter and Daniel Katz

Nose[1]

- Structure – Cartilage and bone; divided by septum into similar halves
  - External nares → nasal conchae → nasopharynx
- Blood supply – Dual supply from internal carotid and external carotid
  - Majority of epistaxis from anterior nose, Kiesselbach's plexus
  - Posterior bleeds are less common, harder to control
- Innervation – Cranial nerves (CN) V_1 (ophthalmic branch) and V_2 (maxillary branch)
- Clinical relevance: Most airway resistance in nasal passages
  - Nasal approach to fiberoptic intubation
    - Topical anesthesia to V_1 and V_2
    - Topical vasoconstrictor for decreased bleeding
  - Sinus surgery

- Controlled hypotension to optimize surgical field
- Regional nerve blocks – Infraorbital nerve block for V_2, sphenopalatine block for nasal mucosal anesthesia and vasoconstriction

Pharynx[1]

- Anatomy – Nasopharynx, oropharynx, laryngopharynx
- Innervation
  - Nasopharynx – Maxillary branch of trigeminal (V_2)
  - Oropharynx – Glossopharyngeal (CN IX): posterior one-third of tongue, superior epiglottis, gag reflex (Figure 28.1)

Larynx[1]

- Sensory innervation
  - Internal branch of superior laryngeal nerve (X): Inferior epiglottis to cords

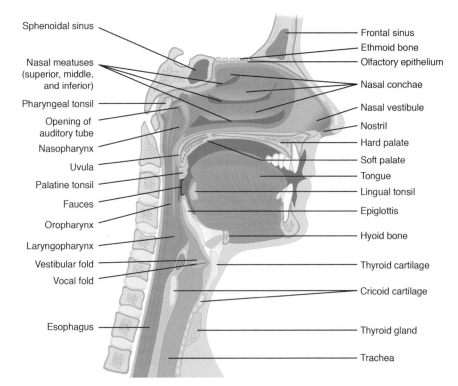

Sphenoidal sinus
Nasal meatuses (superior, middle, and inferior)
Pharyngeal tonsil
Opening of auditory tube
Nasopharynx
Uvula
Palatine tonsil
Fauces
Oropharynx
Laryngopharynx
Vestibular fold
Vocal fold
Esophagus

Frontal sinus
Ethmoid bone
Olfactory epithelium
Nasal conchae
Nasal vestibule
Nostril
Hard palate
Soft palate
Tongue
Lingual tonsil
Epiglottis
Hyoid bone
Thyroid cartilage
Cricoid cartilage
Thyroid gland
Trachea

Figure 28.1 Pharynx

- ▪ Block inferior to the greater cornu of the hyoid bone within the thyrohyoid membrane for awake intubation
  - ○ Recurrent laryngeal nerve (CN X): Mucosa below cords
    - ▪ Transtracheal block through cricothyroid membrane for awake intubation
- Motor innervation
  - ○ External branch of superior laryngeal nerve (SLN; CN X): Cricothyroid muscle
  - ○ Recurrent laryngeal nerve (CN X): All other laryngeal muscles
- Notable muscles
  - ○ Cricothyroid – Vocal cord tensor and adductor; only muscle innervated by SLN
  - ○ Posterior cricoarytenoid – Only pure abductor of cords (Figure 28.2)
- Bones and cartilages
  - ○ Hyoid bone – Most superior
  - ○ Thyroid cartilage – Most prominent, "Adam's apple"
  - ○ Cricoid cartilage – Most inferior, only complete ring of cartilage
    - ▪ Margin of safety with percutaneous access, as posterior cartilage protects other neck structures
- Nerve injury patterns

  - ○ Superior laryngeal nerve injury – Fixed partially abducted cords leading to hoarseness and vocal fatigability, aspiration risk
  - ○ Partial recurrent laryngeal nerve injury – Complete adduction of cords due to unopposed cricothyroid action, loss of abductor function
    - ▪ Bilateral partial injury may lead to stridor and complete airway obstruction
  - ○ Complete recurrent laryngeal nerve injury – Partial adduction of cords into a fixed position, hoarseness (Figure 28.3)

Trachea[1]

- Connects larynx to lungs; anterior to esophagus in the neck
- Approximately 20 cartilaginous partial rings with posterior muscle and connective tissue
  - ○ 2nd through 4th rings covered by thyroid isthmus
- Jugular veins run anterolateral; common carotid arteries run posterolateral
- Posterior to aorta and superior vena cava in mediastinum
  - ○ Innominate artery adjacent to trachea, can predispose to tracheoinnominate fistulas in context of tracheostomies
- Left main bronchus crosses directly under aortic arch
  - ○ Left bronchus can be compressed by aortic aneurysms

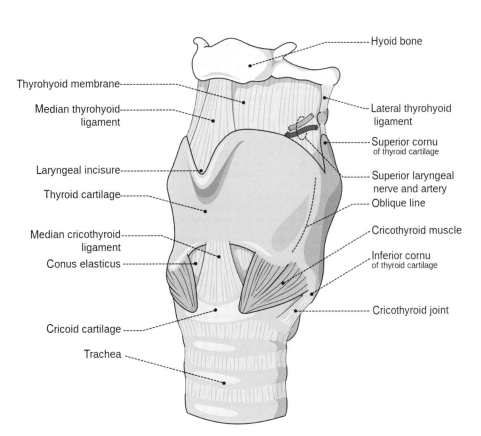

Thyrohyoid membrane
Median thyrohyoid ligament
Laryngeal incisure
Thyroid cartilage
Median cricothyroid ligament
Conus elasticus
Cricoid cartilage
Trachea

Hyoid bone
Lateral thyrohyoid ligament
Superior cornu of thyroid cartilage
Superior laryngeal nerve and artery
Oblique line
Cricothyroid muscle
Inferior cornu of thyroid cartilage
Cricothyroid joint

Figure 28.2 Larynx

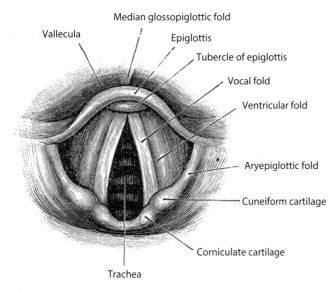

Figure 28.3 Vocal cord

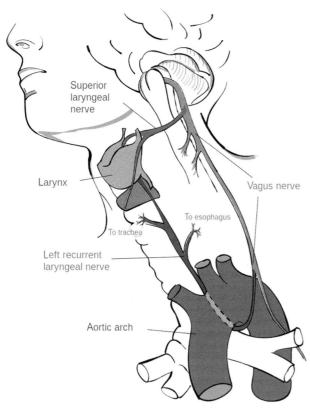

Figure 28.4 Recurrent laryngeal nerve

- Left recurrent laryngeal can be compromised by aortic dissection or aneurysm (Figure 28.4)
- Neck: highly vascular area with intricate muscle and nerve anatomy
  - Location of major anatomy in neck from medial → lateral: recurrent laryngeal nerve → carotid artery → vagus nerve → internal jugular vein → phrenic nerve
  - Important to be aware of neck anatomy for procedures including central line placement, stellate ganglion blocks, and cervical plexus blocks

- Thoracic duct: Lymphatic vessel containing chyle that runs from T12 to root of neck and drains into systemic circulation at junction of left subclavian and internal jugular veins. Left-sided thoracic duct is bigger in diameter than right
  - Concern for damage to left thoracic during left-sided central venous line placement resulting in chylothorax
- Subclavian artery and vein: Travel alongside each other above the first right rib but below the clavicle, putting them at risk for compression in pathologies resulting in thoracic outlet syndrome
  - Subclavian artery: Located between the two heads of the anterior scalene muscle
  - Subclavian vein: Located anterior to the anterior scalene muscle
- Brachial plexus: Located between the anterior and middle scalene muscle

Lung[2]

- Nerve innervation: Parasympathetic innervation to lung provided by the vagus nerve, and sympathetic by T1–T4 nerves through the stellate ganglion
- Blood supply:
  - Pulmonary circulation: Pulmonary artery → pulmonary capillaries → pulmonary veins
  - Bronchial circulation: Left heart → bronchial artery supplying airway → pulmonary circulation (as above)
  - "Onion effect": Blood flow greater in hilum (inner) than in periphery (outer)
- Structure: Right bronchus take-off is 2 cm below carina with a steep angulation which is the reason for more foreign body obstructions on right rather than left
  - Right lung: Three lobes (upper, middle, lower) with approximately 53 percent of the ventilation
  - Left lung: Two lobes (upper, lower) with approximately 47 percent of the ventilation
- West's zones of the lung: Conceptual organization of pulmonary hemodynamics based on gravity
- Zone 1: Airway pressures (P_a) > pulmonary artery (P_A) pressure > pulmonary venous pressure (P_v)
  - With this pressure gradient there is no blood perfusion despite ventilation which normally does not exist. However, with high PEEP or low P_a pressure such as with general anesthesia zone 1 may occur.
- Zone 2: $P_A > P_a > P_v$
  - Blood flow is proportional to difference between P_a and P_A
- Zone 3: $P_A > P_v > P_a$
  - Blood flow is proportional to the difference between P_A and P_v.
  - Body positioning can also be used to decrease blood flow to abnormal areas of the lung such as in unilateral pneumonia encouraging patient to lie on non-diseased side.

- In an upright position, Zone 3 falls in the most dependent portion of the lung and thus there is *both* increased ventilation and perfusion with increased gravity.
- Pneumocytes (alveolar cells): Line the alveoli in the lungs
  - Type I cell: Thin cells that line 97 percent of the alveolar surface, ideal for gas diffusion
  - Type II cell: Line 3 percent of the alveolar surface, secrete pulmonary surfactant to decrease the alveolar tension
- Muscles of respiration
  - Diaphragm
  - Innervated by phrenic nerve – "C3, 4, 5 keeps the diaphragm alive"
  - Contraction moves diaphragm down, decreasing intrathoracic pressure and causing inspiration
  - Mostly type 1, slow-twitch muscle – Prevents fatigue. Neonatal diaphragms proportionally more type 2 fast-twitch, predisposing to respiratory fatigue
  - Openings in the diaphragm allow passage to the abdominal cavity:
    - Vena cava at T8
    - Esophagus at T10
    - Aorta at T12
  - Intercostals
  - External intercostals aid inspiration
  - Internal intercostals aid exhalation
  - Accessory muscles of respiration – More prominently utilized in respiratory fatigue
  - Sternocleidomastoid
  - Scalene muscles
  - Minor – Pectorals, trapezius, latissimus dorsi, serratus muscles
  - Exhalation– Passive during normal breathing
  - Forceful exhalation aided by abdominal wall and internal intercostals
- Pediatric airway
  - Funnel-shaped larynx and trachea
  - Anteriorly slanted vocal cords
  - More cephalad larynx – C4 in infants versus C6 in adults
  - Narrowest portion at cricoid cartilage in infants versus at vocal cords in adults
  - Infants have a long, floppy, omega-shaped epiglottis which is more difficult to lift indirectly with a Macintosh blade
  - Relatively larger tongue and occiput predispose to obstruction

References

1. Pawha P., Jiang J., Shpilberg K., Luttrull M., Govindaraj S. Gross and radiographic anatomy. In: DeMaria S., Jr. (ed.), *Anesthesiology and Otolaryngology*. New York, NY: Springer; 2013, 3–33.
2. Hansen J., Koeppen B., Netter F. *Netter's Atlas of Human Physiology*. Tererboro, NJ: Icon Learning Systems; 2002.

Respiratory System: Pharmacology

Kyle James Riley and Daniel Katz

Bronchodilators

Overview

Bronchodilators relax smooth muscle and expand the airways.[1,2] Beta-2 agonists and anticholinergics are the two bronchodilators most commonly used for this purpose.[3,4]

Typical route of administration: inhaler or nebulizer, but for some medications, oral and injection choices are available.[4]

- Basic inhalation options:
  - Metered-dose inhaler (MDI)[5]
  - Dry-powder inhaler (DPI)[5]
  - Soft-mist inhaler (SMI)[6]
  - Nebulizer[5]

Beta-2 Agonists

Beta-2 agonists stimulate the beta-2 receptors in the airway muscles, relaxing the muscles, thereby widening constricted airways.[7]

Bronchoconstriction Mechanism

Increased rhythmic Ca^{2+} concentration oscillations activate myosin light-chain kinase (MLCK) phosphorylation. This increases the contractile interaction of actin and myosin,[8] resulting in increased bronchoconstriction.[9–11]

Beta-2 Agonists Effects

Beta-2 agonists reduce Ca^{2+} concentration through beta-2 receptor stimulation of the cAMP-PKA (protein kinase A) pathway resulting in increased bronchodilation.[9–11]

Some beta-2 agonists can indirectly decrease bronchospasm by other mechanisms that include:

- Inhibiting the release of acetylcholine by action at cholinergic nerve presynaptic beta-2 receptors[12]
- Preventing the release of inflammatory mediator from human lung mast cells[13]

Although many of these medications are receptor-specific, at high doses their specificity may decrease, resulting in crossover reactions. For example, high doses of albuterol may cross-react with beta-1 receptors to cause tachycardia.

Beta-2 Agonists Drug Examples

Short-acting beta agonists (SABAs): albuterol and fenoterol[4]

Long-acting beta agonists (LABAs): salmeterol and formoterol[3,4]

Anticholinergics

Anticholinergics act on cholinergic nerve signal transmission, including the parasympathetic nervous system, by blocking the binding of the neurotransmitter acetylcholine to its receptors.[14]

Bronchoconstriction Mechanism

In the smooth muscle cells of the bronchi and bronchioles, increases in cytoplasmic Ca^{2+} results in contraction of the muscle cells leading to bronchoconstriction.[14]

Postganglionic parasympathetic neurons release acetylcholine → activate smooth muscle cell muscarinic M_3 receptors → activate a Gq class protein → upregulate the phospholipase C pathway → release inositol triphosphate (IP3) into cellular cytoplasm[14,15] → IP3 molecules bind to sarcoplasmic reticulum Ins3P receptors on a Ca^{2+} channel → sarcoplasmic reticulum release of Ca^{2+} → increase concentration of cytoplasmic Ca^{2+} → increase in contractile interaction of actin and myosin → bronchoconstriction.[15,16]

Anticholinergic Effects

Muscarinic anticholinergics will bind to the muscarinic M3 receptors, which reduces the binding of acetylcholine to the same M3 receptors. The reduced binding allows natural cellular pathways to reduce the concentration of cytoplasmic Ca^{2+}, resulting in bronchodilation.[14]

These medications can act systemically, especially if given via the IV or IM route, and may produce other anticholinergic side effects such as tachycardia, dry mouth, and confusion if the medication crosses the blood–brain barrier (e.g., atropine).

Anticholinergics Drug Examples

Short-acting anticholinergic medications: ipratropium and oxitropium[7]

Long-acting anticholinergic drugs also known as long-acting muscarinic agents (LAMAs): tiotropium[4]

Anti-Inflammatory Medications

The following classes of anti-inflammatory medications have been shown to be effective treatments in controlling asthma symptoms and attacks:[17,18]

- Corticosteroids
- Leukotriene modifiers
- Mast cell stabilizers
- Immunoglobulin E (IgE) blockers

Corticosteroids

Corticosteroids, specifically glucocorticosteroids, work in responsive cells by activating glucocorticoid receptors to directly and indirectly regulate the transcription of target genes.[19]

Glucocorticosteroids can increase the levels of anti-inflammatory proteins.

- Glucocorticoid receptor dimers bind to DNA at sites in the promoter region of steroid-responsive anti-inflammatory genes, usually increasing transcription with resulting increase in anti-inflammatory protein synthesis.

Glucocorticosteroids inhibit gene transcription of inflammatory mediator proteins. Many of the genes for inflammatory mediator proteins are upregulated in asthmatic airways by transcription factors like nuclear-factor-kappaB (NF-kappaB).

Corticosteroids and beta-2 agonists can also have mutually synergistic effects.

- Corticosteroids → increase the transcription of the beta-2 receptor gene → restoring G-protein/beta-2 receptor coupling → inhibiting beta-2 receptor downregulation.[20]
- Beta-2 agonists → increase in the nuclear translocation of glucocorticoid receptors → enhancing the suppression of the transcription of inflammatory genes.[21]

Corticosteroid Drug Examples

Inhaled glucocorticosteroids: budesonide and fluticasone[4]

Oral systemic corticosteroids: prednisone and methylprednisolone[3,4]

Leukotriene Modifiers

Leukotrienes, a family of eicosanoid inflammatory mediators, are synthesized in a number of different immune system cells, including eosinophils, leukocytes, and mast cells.[22]

- Leukotrienes activate G-protein-coupled receptors found in structural cells including glandular epithelium, smooth muscle cells, and in inflammatory cells like basophils, eosinophils, and neutrophils.[23]
- Cysteinyl leukotrienes' primary effect is through their binding to cysteinyl leukotriene receptor 1 (CysLTR1). CysLTR1 activation causes airway bronchoconstriction, edema, influx of eosinophils and neutrophils, smooth muscle proliferation, mucin secretion by goblet cells, and respiratory epithelial cell hypertrophy.

Leukotriene modifier drugs (or antileukotrienes) function either as:

- 5-Lipoxygenase pathway inhibitors – inhibiting the formation of both cysLTs and LTB4
- Cysteinyl leukotriene receptor CysLTR1 antagonists, blocking the actions of cysLTs on target cells like bronchial smooth muscle cells[23]

Leukotriene Drug Examples

Oral leukotriene receptor antagonists (LTRAs): montelukast and zafirlukast[3]

Oral 5-lipoxygenase inhibitor: zileuton[3]

Mast Cell Stabilizer

The degranulation of mast cells and eosinophils release potent inflammatory mediators including histamine and leukotrienes.[24] Mast cell stabilizers work by stabilizing the plasma membranes of eosinophils and mast cells through the blocking of a calcium channel essential for cell degranulation. The blockade prevents the release of inflammatory mediators from the cell granules.[24]

Mast Cell Stabilizer Drug Example

Mass cell stabilizer nebulizer: cromolyn[3]

Immunoglobulin E (IgE) Blocker

IgE antibodies can increase the levels of an individual's proinflammatory mediator proteins by:

1. Production of allergen-specific IgE antibodies, which is triggered by an atopic person's initial exposure to the allergen.[25]
2. These IgE molecules can then become attached to inflammatory cells including basophils, macrophages, and especially mast cells, through its Fc portion linking with the cell Fc receptors.
3. Release of proinflammatory mediators, including histamine, leukotrienes, and cytokines, is triggered by subsequent allergen exposure where cross-bridging between IgE on the inflammatory cells' surface and the allergen provokes cell degranulation.[25,26]

IgE blockers work by blocking the binding of IgE to an inflammatory cell's Fc receptors by binding to the IgE molecules Fc portion themselves. This prevents IgE from attaching to inflammatory cells and being able to cause a cell's degranulation when exposed to allergens.[25]

IgE Blockers Drug Example

Immunomodulators subcutaneous injection: omalizumab[3]

References

1. CDC/National Center for Health Statistics. Asthma. 2017; www.cdc.gov/nchs/fastats/asthma.htm. Accessed February 28, 2017.

2. National Center for Chronic Disease Prevention and Health Promotion, Division of Population Health. Chronic Obstructive Pulmonary Disease (COPD). 2016; www.cdc.gov/copd/index.html. Accessed February 28, 2017.

3. National Heart, Lung, and Blood Institute, National Institutes of Health.

Asthma Care Quick Reference. Guidelines from the National Asthma Education and Prevention Program. Expert Panel Report 2. 2012; www.nhlbi.nih.gov/files/docs/guidelines/asthma_qrg.pdf. Accessed February 27, 2017.

4. Rabe K. F., Hurd S., Anzueto A., et al. Global strategy for the diagnosis, management, and prevention of chronic obstructive pulmonary disease: GOLD executive summary. *Am J Respir Crit Care Med.* 2007; 176(6): 532–55.

5. Ram F. S., Sestini P. Regular inhaled short acting beta2 agonists for the management of stable chronic obstructive pulmonary disease: Cochrane systematic review and meta-analysis. *Thorax.* 2003; 58(7): 580–4.

6. Buhl R., Maltais F., Abrahams R., et al. Tiotropium and olodaterol fixed-dose combination versus mono-components in COPD (GOLD 2–4). *Eur Respir J.* 2015; 45(4): 969–79.

7. Cooper C. B., Tashkin D. P. Recent developments in inhaled therapy in stable chronic obstructive pulmonary disease. *BMJ.* 2005; 330(7492): 640–4.

8. Pfitzer G. Invited review: regulation of myosin phosphorylation in smooth muscle. *J Appl Physiol (1985).* 2001; 91(1): 497–503.

9. Bai Y., Sanderson M. J. Airway smooth muscle relaxation results from a reduction in the frequency of $Ca2+$ oscillations induced by a cAMP-mediated inhibition of the IP3 receptor. *Respir Res.* 2006; 7: 34.

10. Perez-Zoghbi J. F., Karner C., Ito S., et al. Ion channel regulation of intracellular calcium and airway smooth muscle function. *Pulm Pharmacol Ther.* 2009; 22(5): 388–97.

11. Delmotte P., Sanderson M. J. Effects of albuterol isomers on the contraction and $Ca2+$ signaling of small airways in mouse lung slices. *Am J Respir Cell Mol Biol.* 2008; 38(5): 524–31.

12. Rhoden K. J., Meldrum L. A., Barnes P. J. Inhibition of cholinergic neurotransmission in human airways by beta 2-adrenoceptors. *J Appl Physiol (1985).* 1988; 65(2): 700–05.

13. Scola A M., Loxham M., Charlton S. J., Peachell P. T. The long-acting beta-adrenoceptor agonist, indacaterol, inhibits IgE-dependent responses of human lung mast cells. *Br J Pharmacol.* 2009; 158(1): 267–76.

14. Gosens R., Zaagsma J., Meurs H., Halayko A. J. Muscarinic receptor signaling in the pathophysiology of asthma and COPD. *Respir Res.* 2006; 7: 73.

15. Penn R. B., Benovic J. L. Regulation of heterotrimeric G protein signaling in airway smooth muscle. *Proc Am Thorac Soc.* 2008; 5(1): 47–57.

16. Jude J. A., Wylam M. E., Walseth T. F., Kannan M. S. Calcium signaling in airway smooth muscle. *Proc Am Thorac Soc.* 2008; 5(1): 15–22.

17. Barnes P. J., Chung K. F., Page C. P. Inflammatory mediators of asthma: an update. *Pharmacol Rev.* 1998; 50(4): 515–96.

18. Busse W. W., Lemanske R. F. J. Asthma. *N Engl J Med.* 2001; 344(5): 350–62.

19. Barnes P. J. How corticosteroids control inflammation: Quintiles Prize Lecture 2005. *Br J Pharmacol.* 2006; 148(3): 245–54.

20. Mak J. C., Hisada T., Salmon M., Barnes P. J., Chung K. F. Glucocorticoids reverse IL-1beta-induced impairment of beta-adrenoceptor-mediated relaxation and up-regulation of G-protein-coupled receptor kinases. *Br J Pharmacol.* 2002; 135(4): 987–96.

21. Eickelberg O., Roth M., Lorx R., et al. Ligand-independent activation of the glucocorticoid receptor by beta2-adrenergic receptor agonists in primary human lung fibroblasts and vascular smooth muscle cells. *J Biol Chem.* 1999; 274(2): 1005–10.

22. Radmark O., Werz O., Steinhilber D. Samuelsson B. 5-Lipoxygenase: regulation of expression and enzyme activity. *Trends Biochem Sci.* 2007; 32(7): 332–41.

23. Peters-Golden M., Henderson W. R., Jr. Leukotrienes. *N Engl J Med.* 2007; 357(18): 1841–54.

24. Finn D. F., Walsh J. J. Twenty-first century mast cell stabilizers. *Br J Pharmacol.* 2013; 170(1): 23–37.

25. Gould H. J., Sutton B. J., Beavil A. J., et al. The biology of IGE and the basis of allergic disease. *Annu Rev Immunol.* 2003; 21: 579–628.

26. Fahy J. V., Fleming H. E., Wong H. H., et al. The effect of an anti-IgE monoclonal antibody on the early- and late-phase responses to allergen inhalation in asthmatic subjects. *Am J Respir Crit Care Med.* 1997; 155(6): 1828–34.

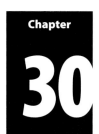
Cardiovascular Physiology

Bhoumesh Patel and Denes Papp

Cardiac Cycle

Consists of electrical and mechanical cycle initiating at the sinoatrial (SA) node

Electrical impulse propagation: SA node → atrial internodal tracts → AV node → Bundle of His → Bundle branches → Purkinje fibers[1]

Action Potential

SA node:

Phase 0: Depolarization inward Ca^{2+} current L-type Ca^{2+} channels

Phase 3: Repolarization outward K^+ current

Phase 4: Spontaneous depolarization inward Na^+ current. The rate of phase 4 depolarization sets the heart rate.

Ventricle:

Phase 0: Depolarization inward Na^+ current

Phase 1: Outward K^+ current

Phase 2: Inward Ca^{2+} current L-type (slow); outward K^+ current

Phase 3: Repolarization outward K^+ current

Phase 4: Resting potential (Figure 30.1)

Intrinsic rates: AV node 40–60, Bundle of His 40, and Purkinje fiber 15–20

SA node: Innervated by right vagus

AV node: Innervated by left vagus

Wiggers diagram

Displays synchronicity between pressure, volume, ECG, valve status, and heart sounds (Figures 30.2 and 30.3)

Systole: Divided into isovolumetric contraction, rapid ejection, and slower ejection phases.

Isovolumetric contraction is the time between mitral valve closure (S_1) and aortic valve opening during which LV volume remains constant.

Ejection occurs when ventricular pressures exceed aortic arterial pressure, the aortic valve opens, and blood is ejected. Systole ends when ventricular pressure falls below aortic pressure leading to closure of the aortic valve that produces S_2. The aortic valve closes slightly before the pulmonic valve during inspiration due to prolonged RV ejection by increased venous return.

Diastole: Divided into isovolumetric relaxation, early ventricular filling, diastasis, and atrial systole.

Isovolumetric relaxation is the time between aortic valve closure and mitral valve opening during which LV volume remains constant. This is an active process that requires energy.

Early filling follows when ventricular pressure falls below atrial pressure, the mitral valve opens, and blood volume enters the ventricle, followed by diastasis (slow ventricular filling) and atrial kick.

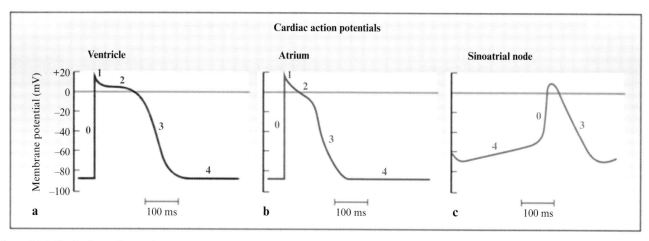

Figure 30.1 Cardiac Action Potentials

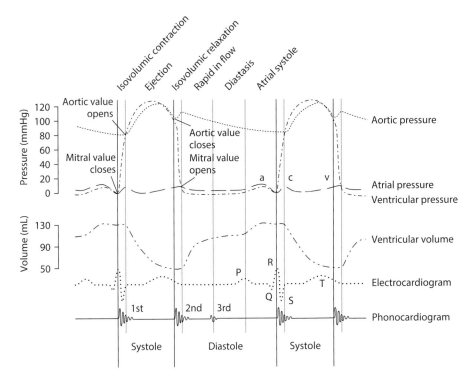

Figure 30.2 Wiggers Diagram

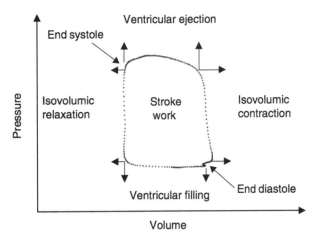

Figure 30.3 Left ventricular pressure volume loop

Early rapid filling provides 70–75 percent of ventricular end-diastolic volume, diastasis (3–5 percent), and atrial systole (15–25 percent).

CVP waveform: Usually measured at the junction of SVC and RA. A normal waveform contains five components – three peaks (a, c, v) and two descents (x, y).

a wave: Atrial contraction

c wave: Tricuspid valve bulging into atrium during isovolumetric contraction

x descent: Atrial relaxation

v wave: Passive filling the RA from venous return

y descent: Atrial emptying into the ventricle

Ventricular Function

CO: Cardiac output

SV: Stroke volume

HR: Heart rate

$$CO = SV \times HR$$

SV = EDV – ESV (end diastolic volume – end systolic volume)

Stroke volume depends on preload (~EDV), contractility, and afterload (~SVR) (Figure 30.4).

Preload: determined by EDV; affects tension of ventricular muscle before contraction[2]

Frank-Starling mechanism = ↑venous return → ↑myocardial fiber stretching → ↑force of contraction → ↑SV

Contractility: The strength of myocardium contraction is determined by coupling of actin–myosin cross-bridge. The coupling process is a major determinant of its contractility.

- Increased inotropy by sympathetic stimulation leads to increase in SV and cardiac output for a given EDV.
- Contractility is increased mainly by raising intracellular calcium[2]

Afterload: Determined mostly by SVR and aortic pressure. Increase in hypertension, aortic stenosis, or by α_1 agonists. Decrease in sepsis, neurogenic shock, or by α antagonists.[2]

Myocardial Oxygen Supply/Demand

Supply – LV myocardium is perfused mostly during diastole; RV perfused during both diastole and systole.

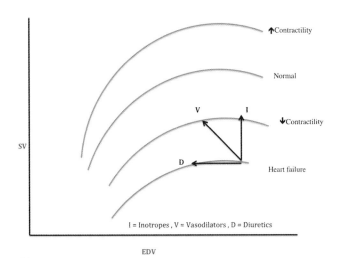

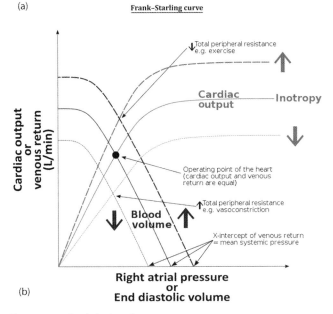

(a)

Frank–Starling curve

(b)

Figure 30.4 Frank–Starling Curve

VR = Venous return

P_V = Venous pressure (increased by limb muscle contractions, sympathetic adrenergic activation)

P_{RA} = Right atrial pressure (increased in CHF, pulmonary HTN, decreased with inspiration)

R_V = Venous vascular resistance (increased by valsalva, pregnancy)[3]

Blood Pressure

SVR: systemic vascular resistance

MAP: mean arterial pressure

PP: pulse pressure

CPP: coronary perfusion pressure

DBP: diastolic blood pressure

CVP: ventral venous pressure

RAP: right atrial pressure

RVSP: right ventricular systolic pressure

RVDP: right ventricular diastolic pressure

PAP: pulmonary arterial pressure

PCWP: pulmonary capillary wedge pressure

$$CO = HR \times SV$$

$$MAP = SVR \times CO = 2/3 \, DBP + 1/3 \, SBP$$

$$PP = SBP - DBP$$

$$PP \propto \frac{SV}{Aortic\ compliance} \text{ Mostly dependent on aortic compliance.}$$

$$CPP = DBP - LVEDP$$

CVP	0–8
RAP	0–8
RVSP	15–25
RVDP	0–8
PAP systolic	15–25
PAP diastolic	8–15
PAP mean	10–20
PCWP	6–14

$SVR = 80*(MAP - CVP)/CO$
Normal = 800−1200 dynes·s·cm^{-5}

$PVR = 80*(MPAP - PCWP)/CO$
Normal = 60−200 dynes·s·cm^{-5}

Resistance $\propto$ viscosity (dependent on hematocrit and plasma proteins)

Cardiac Reflexes

Baroreceptor: Mechanoreceptors located in *carotid sinus and aortic arch* with afferent signals via *Hering's nerve (branch of glossopharyngeal) and vagus nerves* respectively → nucleus tractus solitaries → efferent through vagus nerve

Bainbridge (atrial stretch reflex): Sudden increase in venous return leads to stretching of receptors located in the

Demand – The most important determinants of myocardial oxygen demand are heart rate, contractility, and wall tension. Wall tension is directly proportional to the pressure and radius of the heart and inversely proportional to wall thickness (LaPlace's law).[3]

$$\sigma = (P \times r)/h$$

(σ, wall stress; P, ventricular pressure; r, ventricular radius; h, wall thickness)

Fick principle: Under steady states, the total uptake of a substance by the peripheral tissues is equal to the product of the blood flow to the peripheral tissues and the arterial–venous concentration gradient of the substance.[2]

$$CO = VO_2/CaO_2 - CvO_2$$
$$VO_2 = \text{Oxygen consumption}$$
$$CaO_2 - CvO_2 = \text{The systemic arteriovenous oxygen content difference}$$

Venous Return

Veins are the primary capacitance vessels of the body (60–70 percent of blood volume)

$$VR = (P_V - P_{RA})/R_V$$

wall of the right atrium and cavoatrial junction that travel via the vagus and results in increased heart rate.

Bezold–Jarisch: Chemo and mechanoreceptors in LV sense noxious stimuli with afferent via the vagus nerve and response with the bradycardia, hypotension, and coronary vasodilatation.[3]

Microcirculation

Fluid movement across the capillary membrane is driven by the Starling pressures and is described by the following equation:

Fluid movement = $K(P_c - P_i) - \sigma(\pi_c - \pi_i)$

P_c is the capillary hydrostatic pressure (increased with heart failure, venous constriction, arteriolar dilation)

P_i is the interstitial hydrostatic pressure

π_c is the capillary oncotic pressure (decreased with nephrotic syndrome, liver failure, malnutrition)

π_i is the interstitial oncotic pressure

K is the filtration coefficient (increased with burns, inflammation)

σ is the reflection coefficient

Capillary flow regulation is controlled by arterioles, metarterioles, and a band of smooth muscle called precapillary sphincters.

The Fahraeus–Lindqvist effect is a phenomenon that leads to decrease in blood viscosity by reduction in hematocrit in arterioles and capillaries relative to the hematocrit of large arteries.[3]

Regional Blood Flow and Regulation

Mixed venous saturation (SvO$_2$): Measures oxygen saturation of blood right before returning to heart. Used as a surrogate to interpret oxygen consumption and delivery.

$$SvO_2 = SaO_2 - [(VO_2)/(Hb \times 1.36 \times CO)]$$

VO$_2$: Oxygen consumption

SvO$_2$: Venous oxygen saturation

SaO$_2$: Arterial oxygen saturation

- High SvO$_2$: Either from increased oxygen delivery (i.e., increased inspired oxygen, hyperbaric oxygen) or high flow states (i.e., sepsis, hyperthyroid, high output states) or decreased oxygen consumption (i.e., hypothermia, anesthesia)

- Low SvO$_2$: Either from decreased oxygen delivery (i.e., decreased hemoglobin, decreased oxygen supply, or decreased flow state) or increased oxygen consumption (i.e., sepsis, hyperthermia, shivering, pain, seizures)[3]

Blood flow to an organ is regulated by arteriolar resistance via either local control (intrinsic) or neural control (extrinsic).

Coronary: Blood flow is regulated locally by *adenosine and hypoxia.*

Cerebral: Besides *autoregulation*, cerebral blood flow is regulated by *CO$_2$* which is a *vasodilator*. An increase in cerebral PCO$_2$ causes vasodilation of the cerebral arterioles.

Pulmonary: Blood flow is regulated by the partial pressure of O$_2$ in alveolar gas through *hypoxic pulmonary*

vasoconstriction. Local vasoconstriction shunts blood away from poorly ventilated areas toward well-ventilated areas.

Renal: Blood flow is auto regulated via combination of the myogenic regulation of afferent arterioles and tubuloglomerular feedback.

Hepatic: Blood flow is regulated by *adenosine.* Decreased in hepatic blood flow leads to accumulation of adenosine which causes hepatic artery dilation.

Skeletal muscle: Blood flow is regulated both by local metabolites and by sympathetic. At rest, blood flow is regulated primarily by *sympathetic innervation*. During exercise, blood flow is increased due to metabolites like *lactate, adenosine, and K.*[3]

Uterine: Minimal local autoregulation of blood vessels. Blood flow is strictly dependent on arterial pressure and inversely related to vascular resistance.

Hormonal Control

Renin–angiotensin–aldosterone system: Regulates both *blood pressure* and *volume.*

Low arterial pressure and blood volume causes the release of renin from the kidneys. Renin catalyzes the conversion of angiotensinogen to angiotensin I. Angiotensin I is then converted to angiotensin II by angiotensin-converting enzyme (ACE), primarily in the lungs.

Angiotensin II has the following effects:

- Increased SVR by arteriolar vasoconstriction via AT$_1$ receptors.
- Decreases sodium excretion by increasing sodium reabsorption by proximal tubules of the kidney.
- It causes the release of aldosterone from the adrenal cortex.
- It causes the release of ADH (AVP) from the posterior pituitary gland.
- Augments norepinephrine (NE) release from sympathetic nerves and sensitizes vascular smooth muscle effects of NE.

Arginine vasopressin (AVP): Regulates *blood volume*

AVP is released by the posterior pituitary gland controlled by the hypothalamus. It is released in response to increased plasma osmolality or stress. It acts on renal collecting ducts via V$_2$ receptors to increase water permeability and V$_1$ receptors on vascular smooth muscle to cause vasoconstriction through the IP$_3$ signal transduction pathway.

Atrial natriuretic peptide (ANP): Regulates *blood volume*

ANP is stored in the atrial muscle cells and released into the bloodstream when the atria are stretched. By increasing sodium excretion, it decreases blood volume. It also inhibits renin release as well as aldosterone and AVP secretion.

Erythropoietin: Regulates *blood volume*

Erythropoietin is released by the kidneys in response to hypoxia and reduced hematocrit. It causes bone marrow to increase production of red blood cells, raising the total mass of circulating red cells.

References

1. Crystal G., Heerdt P. Chapter 21: Cardiovascular Physiology: Integrative Function, *Pharmacology and Physiology for Anesthesia*. Hugh Hemmings Jr, Talmage Egan, eds. Elsevier, Philadelphia, PA, 366–89.

2. Costanzo L. Chapter 4: Cardiovascular Physiology, *Physiology*. Linda S. Costanzo, ed. Elsevier, Philadelphia, PA, 113–84.

3. Pagel P., Freed J. Chapter 6: Cardiac Physiology, *Kaplan's Cardiac Anesthesia*. Joel A. Kaplan, John G.T. Augoustides, Gerard R. Manecke Jr., Timothy Maus, David L. Reich, eds. Elsevier, Philadelphia, PA, 143–78.

Basics of Cardiopulmonary Resuscitation, Medications, Defibrillators, and Advanced Cardiac Life Support Algorithms

Agathe Streiff and Tyler Chernin

The initial assessment of an unresponsive patient, the sequence of events, CPR, medications, defibrillation, and post-resuscitative care will be described in this chapter. Unless stated otherwise, all the below recommendations apply to the adult patient.

The Initial Assessment

1. **Scene safety:** You cannot save someone if it is not safe for you or the other rescuers.
2. **Check responsiveness:** In less than 10 seconds, check for breathing and pulse. If the patient is unresponsive, not breathing, and no pulse is detected, proceed as instructed below.
3. **Activate the emergency response system:** Unlike the out-of-hospital cardiac arrest (OHCA) chain of survival, the in-hospital cardiac arrest (IHCA) chain of survival includes surveillance and prevention, such as rapid response teams (RRT) and medical emergency teams (MET), which have been shown to be effective (see Figure 31.1).
   - If you have another rescuer, start CPR right away while they activate the emergency response system and fetch the AED.
   - If you are alone, activate the emergency response system and bring the AED prior to starting CPR. Per 2015 guidelines, it is acceptable to call for help using mobile devices.

Early Defibrillation for Shockable Rhythm[2]

- If cardiac arrest was *witnessed* and an AED is *immediately* available:
  - Defibrillate now
- If cardiac arrest was *unwitnessed* or an AED is *not immediately* available:
  - Two or more rescuers: One rescuer should initiate CPR while another rescuer searches for AED and applies pads, then defibrillate as soon as possible. (Changed from 2010 recommendations, which stated that in unwitnessed cardiac arrest or where an AED was not immediately available, 1.5 to 3 minutes of CPR may be considered prior to defibrillation.)
  - One rescuer without mobile phone: Leave victim to activate emergency response system and obtain AED prior to initiating CPR
- Shock energy for defibrillation in cardiac arrest:
  - **Biphasic:** 120–200 J initial dose or maximum available
  - **Monophasic:** Less common due to newer AEDs. 360 J
- Nonshockable rhythms:
  - Asystole
  - Pulseless electrical activity (PEA)
- Shockable rhythms:
  - Ventricular fibrillation
  - Ventricular tachycardia

In-hospital cardiac arrest sequence

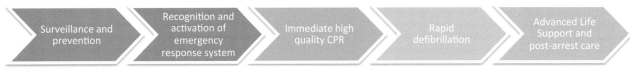

Out-of-hospital cardiac arrest sequence

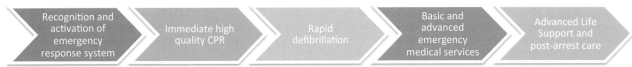

Figure 31.1 Difference between in-hospital and out-of-hospital cardiac arrest algorithm
Adapted from *2010 ACLS Handbook of Emergency Cardiovascular Care for Health Care Providers.*[1]

Table 31.1 ACLS algorithm for the adult, pediatric, and infant patients

Recommendation	Adult patient	Pediatric patient	Infants (<1 year of age)
Witnessed cardiac arrest and *immediately* available AED	Defibrillate then initiate CPR		
Unwitnessed cardiac arrest or AED *not immediately* available with 1 rescuer	1. Leave victim to activate emergency response system and obtain AED 2. Initiate CPR	1. Initiate 2 minutes of CPR 2. Leave victim to activate emergency response system, obtain AED 3. Return to victim, continue CPR	
Unwitnessed cardiac arrest or AED *not immediately* available with 2 or more rescuers	Initiate CPR while other rescuer activates emergency response system, obtains AED		
CPR *with* an advanced airway	1 breath every 6 seconds		
CPR *without* an advanced airway	30:2 compressions to breaths ratio	1 rescuer: 30:2 2 or more rescuers: 15:2	
CPR compression depth	At least 2 inches (5 cm)	At least 1/3 AP diameter About 2 inches (5 cm)	At least 1/3 AP diameter About 1½ inches (4 cm)

Source: Adapted from *2010 ACLS Handbook of Emergency Cardiovascular Care for Health Care Providers.*[1]

- Shock energy for unstable tachyarrhythmias without cardiac arrest:
  - Narrow and regular: Synchronized cardioversion 50–100 J
  - Narrow and irregular: Synchronized cardioversion 120–200 J biphasic or 200 J monophasic
  - Wide and regular: 100 J
  - Wide and irregular: Defibrillation dose (see above)

CPR Sequence: C–A–B

- Prioritize **C**irculation over **A**irway and **B**reathing to avoid delays to first compression
- CPR *without* an advanced airway (advanced airway: endotracheal tube or supraglottic airway)[2] → 30:2 compressions to breaths ratio
- CPR *with* an advanced airway → 1 breath every 6 seconds (10 breaths/minute)

High Quality Chest Compressions

- **Adequate rate:** 100–120 compressions/minute
- **Adequate depth:** In adults, at least 2 inches (5 cm) and no more than 2.5 inches (6 cm)
- **Allow complete chest recoil after each compression:** Do not lean on chest between compressions; allow the heart to refill
- **Minimize interruptions:** Do not interrupt compressions for intubation, application of pads, and keep pulse checks less than 10 seconds
- **Avoid excessive ventilation**: Avoid excessively forceful breaths
- Rotate compressor every 2 minutes.
- EtCO$_2$ >10 mm Hg. Low EtCO$_2$ after 20 minutes of CPR is poor prognostic sign
- Diastolic pressure < 20 mm Hg on intra-arterial pressure reflects inadequate compressions
- Table 31.1 lists the adjustments to these recommendations for the pediatric and newborn patient

Medications

- Epinephrine intravenously (IV) or intraosseous (IO) 1 mg every 3 to 5 minutes
- The combination of vasopressin and epinephrine in cardiac arrest demonstrated no advantage over epinephrine. For simplification, vasopressin has been removed from the 2015 ACLS algorithm (see Figure 31.2)
- Steroids, if given with vasopressin and epinephrine, may provide some benefit for IHCA

Tachyarrhythmias

- Algorithm:
  1. Hemodynamically stable or unstable
  2. QRS wide or narrow
  3. Irregular or regular ventricular rhythm
- Check a pulse:
  - No pulse → see pulseless electrical activity (PEA) algorithm
  - Pulse present →
    - Assessment using C–A–B
    - Provide oxygen
    - Hemodynamically unstable → immediate synchronized cardioversion
    - Hemodynamically stable →
      - 12 lead electrocardiogram (ECG)
      - Frequently check blood pressure
      - See Table 31.2

Unstable Ventricular Tachycardia and Ventricular Fibrillation

- Ventricular fibrillation (VF) is usually more resistant to shocks
- For both, first line treatment is to initiate CPR
- Both VT and VF should be defibrillated as soon as possible with monophasic 360 J or diphasic 200 J
- Ventricular tachycardia (VT) is divided into the following categories, each with different treatment implications:

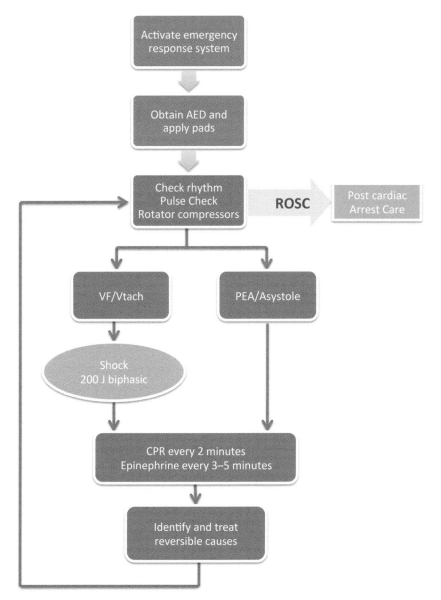

Figure 31.2 Cardiac arrest algorithm
Adapted from *2010 ACLS Handbook of Emergency Cardiovascular Care for Healthcare Providers: Cardiac Arrest Circular Algorithm.*[1]

○ **Monomorphic VT**
  ▪ First line treatment is amiodarone. Lidocaine may also be considered.
○ **Polymorphic** VT, i.e., Torsades de pointes
  ▪ Associated with Wolff–Parkinson–White (WPW) syndrome, baseline prolongation of QT interval
  ▪ Precipitated by electrolyte disturbances and drugs (i.e., tricyclic antidepressants, haloperidol, droperidol, type Ia antiarrhythmics)
  ▪ Treatment: Shorten the QT interval. Magnesium, increasing heart rate with pacing or catecholamines, and for refractory rhythms, phenytoin, and lidocaine
  ▪ Note: Type Ia antiarrhythmics *prolong* the QT and are NOT helpful in Torsades.

Asystole and PEA Arrest
• Defibrillation is *not* helpful since the goal is to obtain any rhythm back
• Treatment depends on the cause:
  ○ Sodium bicarbonate may be helpful in the setting of asystole caused by
    ▪ Severe acidosis
    ▪ Hyperkalemia
    ▪ Tricyclic antidepressant overdose
  ○ Anesthesiologists must consider the context of PEA arrest, such as tension pneumothorax during a jet ventilation case, pericardial tamponade during a cardiac catheterization case, etc.
  ○ Phenytoin, lidocaine, procainamide may be useful in PEA arrest. Atropine is no longer part of the algorithm

Table 31.2 ACLS treatment algorithm for stable tachyarrhythmias

QRS size	Rhythm regularity	Diagnosis	Treatment
Narrow (<0.12 second)	Regular	Sinus tachycardia Aflutter	– Vagal maneuvers – 6 mg adenosine IV push – If needed, follow with 12 mg adenosine – Address underlying causes such as pain, anxiety, and hypovolemia
Narrow	Irregular	Atrial fibrillation (AF) Atrial flutter (note: regular rhythm but similar treatment to atrial fibrillation) Multi-focal atrial tachycardia	– Consider expert consultation – Consider beta-blockers, diltiazem – If becomes unstable, cardioversion
Wide	Regular	Ventricular tachycardia SVT with aberrancy	– Expert consultation – For ventricular tachycardia, consider amiodarone – For SVT with aberrancy, consider adenosine 6 mg
Wide	Irregular	Pre-excited atrial fibrillation Recurrent polymorphic VT Torsades de Pointes	– Expert consultation – For pre-excited atrial fibrillation such as AF and WPW, avoid AV nodal blocking agents such as digoxin, diltiazem, verapamil

Source: Adapted from *2010 ACLS Handbook of Emergency Cardiovascular Care for Health Care Providers.*[1]

Unstable Bradyarrhythmias

- Causes[3]
  - Hypoxemia
  - Vagal stimulation
  - Drug overdose (i.e., beta blocker, calcium channel blocker, cholinergic drugs, digitalis, propofol, dexmedetomidine)
  - Sinus or atrioventricular (AV) node ischemia
  - Increased intracranial pressure
- It is important to *first* assure adequate oxygenation and ventilation, then consider sympathomimetic or vagolytic drugs
- Treatment
  - Narrow complex bradycardia from nodal failure or AV blocks → atropine (1 mg every 3 to 5 minutes)
  - Atropine works by decreasing vagal tone and increasing heart rate, however, for infranodal conduction blocks, it may be ineffective and may increase the degree of block by increasing the atrial rate without increasing the ventricular rate
  - For hemodynamically unstable patients and those with high degree of AV block, initiate transthoracic pacing or transvenous pacing

Reversible Causes

- **H's and T's** Hypovolemia
  - Hypoxia
  - Hydrogen ion (acidosis)
  - Hypo- or hyperkalemia
  - Tension pneumothorax
  - Tamponade, cardiac
  - Toxins. For OHCA, 2015 updated guidelines state that bystander naloxone can be administered intravenously

(IV) or intramuscularly (IM) for suspected life-threatening opioid-associated emergencies.
  - Thrombosis, pulmonary
  - Thrombosis, coronary

Post-Cardiac Arrest Care

- Emergency coronary angioplasty is recommended for patients with ST elevation, hemodynamically unstable or electrically unstable patients without ST elevation with a suspected cardiovascular lesion.
- Mild therapeutic hypothermia is beneficial for out-of-hospital VF arrest, but is unclear for out-of-hospital non-VF arrest and inpatient VF arrest. Additionally, hypothermia may exacerbate bradyarrhythmias.
- All comatose adult patients with return of spontaneous circulation (ROSC) after VF arrest should have a targeted temperature management (TTM) of 32–36°C maintained for at least 24 hours minimum.
- Actively preventing fever after TTM is reasonable.[4]

Other 2015 Updates to the *2010 ACLS Guidelines*

- Extracorporeal CPR (ECPR) may be considered as an alternative to conventional CPR for selected patients with cardiac arrest due to reversible suspected etiology.
- Impedance threshold devices (ITD) are no longer recommended.
- Mechanical piston devices have not demonstrated a benefit over manual chest compressions.

Neonatal Resuscitation

- Neonatal cardiac arrest is mainly due to inadequate ventilation, so assessment of ventilation is key.
- Risk assessment
  1. Term gestation
  2. Good tone
  3. Breathing or crying

- The first minute of life, also known as the **Golden Minute**, continues to be important to assess the neonate and initiate resuscitative efforts.
  - Assess **Apgar score** (see Table 31.3)
    - **Appearance** (color)
    - **Pulse** (heart rate)
    - **Grimace** (reflex irritability to tactile stimulation)
    - **Activity** (muscle tone)
    - **Respiration**
- **Temperature**. Avoid hypothermia, provide warmth, and check temperature
- **Oxygenation**
  - Resuscitation of preterm infants less than 35 weeks should be with low oxygen (up to 30 percent FiO_2) and titrated to oxygen saturations
  - During CPR, use 100 percent FiO_2
- **Heart rate**
  - Above 100 bpm and *no signs* of cyanosis, labored breathing → routine postnatal care
  - Above 100 bpm and signs of cyanosis, labored breathing → clear airway, monitor SpO_2, consider continuous positive airway pressure (CPAP)
  - Below 100 bpm → optimize ventilation as above, reassess
  - Below 60 bpm → initiate chest compressions, consider intubation, positive pressure ventilation (PPV).

Table 31.3 Apgar score

Sign	0	1	2
Appearance	Blue or pale	Pink with blue extremities	Pink
Pulse	Absent	<100/minute	>100/minute
Grimace	None	Grimace only	Cry or active withdrawal
Activity	Limp	Some flexion	Active motion
Respiration	None	Weak cry, hypoventilation	Vigorous cry

Source: Adapted from *2010 ACLS Handbook of Emergency Cardiovascular Care for Health Care* Providers.[1]

If heart rate continues to be low, administer IV epinephrine

- **Special situations**
  - *Delayed cord clamping* for longer than 30 seconds is reasonable for healthy term neonates
  - Meconium: In the presence of meconium-stained amniotic fluid and
    - a vigorous, pink infant → routine postnatal care and reassessment
    - a poor muscle tone, inadequate breathing efforts → place infant in a radiant warmer and begin PPV. Routine intubation for tracheal suctioning is no longer recommended.

References

1. American Heart Association. Highlights of the 2015 American Heart Association – Guidelines Update for CPR and ECC. 2015. https://eccguidelines.heart.org/wp-content/uploads/2015/10/2015-AHA-Guidelines-Highlights-English.pdf (Accessed February 20, 2017).

2. Hazinski M. F., Samson R., Schexnayder S. *Handbook of Emergency Cardiovascular Care for Healthcare Providers*. Dallas: American Heart Association; 2010.

3. Marini J. J., Wheeler A. P. *Critical Care Medicine: The Essentials*, 4th edn. New York: Lippincott Williams & Wilkins; 2010, 361–75.

4. Oropello J. M., Pastores S. M., Kvetan V. *Critical Care*. New York: McGraw-Hill Education; 2016.

32

Chapter

Cardiovascular Anatomy

Claire Joseph and Diana Anca

Coronary Circulation

Coronary Artery Circulation

Space between the aortic valve cusps and ascending aorta are referred to as aortic sinuses. The right and left aortic sinuses contain coronary ostia from which the right and left coronary arteries arise, respectively.

Left coronary artery (LCA) – two branches
- Left anterior descending (LAD) – along inter-ventricular groove and terminates at apex of left ventricle (LV). Supplies apex of right ventricle (RV) and anterior wall of LV
    1. Proximal LAD: From left coronary ostia to first diagonal branch
    2. Mid LAD: From first diagonal branch to distal LAD
       Diagonal branches (supplies anterolateral heart)
           D1 = first diagonal branch of the LAD
           D2 = second diagonal branch of the LAD
    3. Distal LAD: Distal one-third of LAD
       Septal branches (supplies the anterior two thirds of the inter-ventricular (IV) septum, bundle branches, and Purkinje system)

- Left circumflex (LCX) – along the left atrioventricular (AV) groove
    1. Obtuse marginal branches – supplies lateral LV
       OM1 = first obtuse marginal branch of the circumflex
       OM2 = second obtuse marginal branch of the circumflex
    2. AVCx = AV branch of the circumflex artery
       15–25 percent terminates into the left posterior descending artery (PDA) branch[1]
       45 percent SA node blood supply is from the LCX[1]

Right coronary artery (RCA) – Along the right AV groove supplies the inferior and infero-septal walls of the LV
- Proximal RCA: Ostia until right marginal artery
  55 percent sino-atrial (SA) node blood supply from the RCA[2]
- Mid RCA: Proximal half segment, from right marginal artery until PDA take off

  Right marginal artery – acute marginal branches to the anterior RV wall
- Distal RCA: Distal half, after PDA take-off

PDA: Supplies the posterior and inferior aspect of the LV and AV node (typically RCA). Can be co-dominant with supply from both RCA and LCx

AV nodal artery branch 80 percent of population comes off of RCA

Post LV = posterior left ventricular artery
  Supplies most of the anterior and posterior walls of RV, the RA, the upper one-half of atrial septum, the post one-third of the IV septum, and the inferior wall and posterior base of LV

Septum supplied by septal perforator branches from the RCA or the LAD

Coronary circulation is right- or left-dominant based on origin of PDA (RCA versus LCx). Left dominance is more common than right dominance. Approximately 5 percent can be co-dominant (PDA supplied by RCA and LCX)

Papillary muscle blood supply:
- Anterior papillary muscle: LCx (OM1) and LAD (D1)
- Posterior papillary muscle: RCA
    o Posterior papillary infarction/rupture can occur after an RCA MI[3,4]

Anatomical Relationships between Coronary Vessels

Coronary sinus with LCX

Great cardiac vein with LAD and LCX

Middle cardiac vein with PDA

Small cardiac vein with right marginal and RCA[4]

Coronary Venous Circulation

There are two networks of myocardial venous drainage:
1. Epicardial coronary veins: Distributed alongside major coronary arteries and drain into the RA via coronary sinus
   Exception: Anterior cardiac veins drain directly into RA
2. Thebesian venous system: Direct venous drainage from endocardium into chambers of the heart
   Approximately 5–10 percent of venous drainage[1]

Coronary Lymphatic Drainage

Extensive lymphatic plexus in sub-endocardial connective tissue of all chambers of the heart

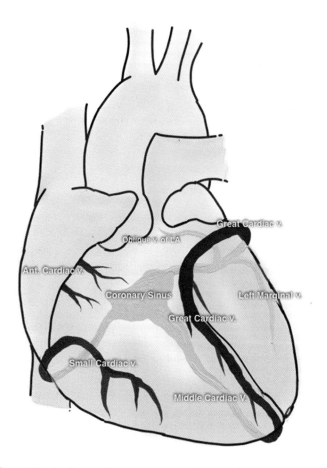
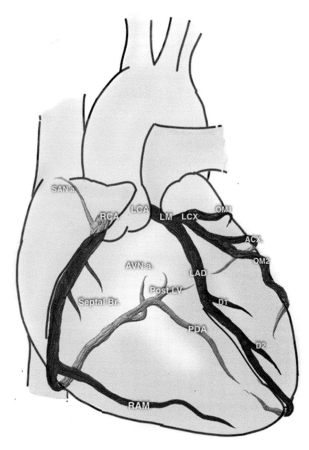

Figure 32.1 Cardiac arterial and venous circulation – anterior view

LCA = left coronary artery, LAD = left anterior descending artery, LCX = left circumflex, LM = left main coronary artery, DM1 = first diagonal, D2 = second diagonal, ACx = atrial circumflex artery, OM1 = first obtuse marginal, OM2 = second obtuse marginal, PDA = posterior descending artery, post LV = posterior left ventricular artery, AVN a = atrioventricular nodal artery, SAN a = sino-atrial nodal artery, RCA = right coronary artery, RAM = right anterior marginal.[6]

Lymphatics confluence into conduit located in AV groove

Coronary lymphatics drain into the mediastinal lymphatic plexus and into the thoracic duct (Figure 32.1)[1–3]

Heart Conduction System

1. SA node: SA node is located at the junction of superior vena cava (SVC) and RA. Located in the sulcus terminals of the RA. The SA node is innervated with post-ganglionic adrenergic and cholinergic nerves.

2. Inter-nodal tracts: Anterior, middle, and posterior inter-nodal tracts, Bachmann's bundle.

3. AV node: Located in the RA at the base of the interatrial septum below the coronary sinus. The AVN and His Bundle are innervated by adrenergic and cholinergic fibers.

4. Bundle of His: Bundle of His with the AVN and goes into the membranous septum then goes into the bundle branches, right and left.

5. Bundle branches
   - Right bundle branch
   - Left bundle branch
     o Left anterior
     o Left posterior division

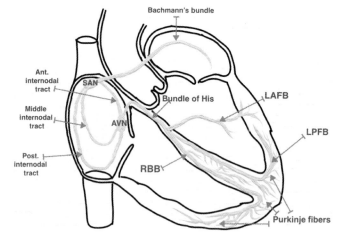

Figure 32.2 Cardiac conduction pathway

LAFB: left anterior fascicular bundle; LPFB: left posterior fascicular bundle; RBB: right bundle branch; AVN: atrioventricular node; SAN: sino-atrial node.[6]

6. Purkinje fibers: The conduction system of the heart initiates impulses and conducts them through the heart to produce the heart cycle and coordinate the contraction of cardiac chambers. It consists of cardiac muscle cells and fibers which conduct the impulses. Purkinje fibers connect with the ends of the bundle branches to form networks on the endocardial surfaces of both ventricles (Figure 32.2).[6–8]

References

1. Miller R. D. *Miller's Anesthesia.* Churchill Livingstone Elsevier, 2015.

2. Kaplan J. A., Reich D. L., Savino J. S. *Kaplan's Cardiac Anesthesia: The Echo Era.* 3rd edn., Elsevier, 2016.

3. Barash P. G. *Clinical Anesthesia.* Lippincott Williams, 2013.

4. Miller R. D., Manuel P., Stoelting R. K. *Basics of Anesthesia.* Philadelphia, PA: Elsevier/Saunders, 2011.

5. Jain A. K., Smith E. J., Rothman M. T. The Coronary Venous System: An Alternative Route of Access to the Myocardium. *J Invasive Cardiol.* 2006 Nov; 18(11): 563–8.

6. Zhu X. *Surgical Atlas of Cardiac Anatomy.* Springer, 2014.

7. Kenny T. *The Nuts and Bolts of Cardiac Pacing,* 1st edn. Wiley-Blackwell, 2008.

8. Iaizzo P. A. *Handbook of Cardiac Anatomy, Physiology, and Devices.* Springer, 3rd edn., 2015.

Cardiovascular Pharmacology

Chapter 33

Edward Mathney and Shane Dickerson

Digoxin

Mechanism of Action
- Inotropy: inhibition of transmembrane Na/K-ATPase resulting in increased intracellular sodium. Intracellular sodium/extracellular calcium exchange via sodium/calcium exchanger results in increased inotropy by increased intracellular calcium.
- Anti-arrhythmic
  - Slowed V_{max} and action potential conduction velocity
  - Increased duration of phase 4 and phase 0 of cardiac action potential
  - Increased vagal tone to heart
    - AV node most sensitive to these effects

Uses
- Atrial fibrillation/flutter
- Congestive heart failure (CHF)

ECG changes
- ST depressions, T-wave inversions
- Prolonged PR interval
- "Salvador Dali moustache" change – a "scoop" after QRS
- In setting of toxicity
  - PVC, bigeminy

Side effects/toxicity
- Narrow therapeutic window
  - Treatment: Digoxin immunoglobulin
- Adverse effects more common in the setting of hypokalemia
- GI upset, visual disturbances (yellow/green hue), AV block[1]

Inotropes and Adrenergic Agents

Epinephrine
- Mechanism of action: Non-selective direct adrenergic agonism (α_1, α_2, β_1, β_1)
  - Increased inotropy, chronotropy, automaticity
  - Systemic vasoconstriction and bronchodilation
  - Endocrine: Increased gluconeogenesis, glycogenolysis, lipolysis; decreased insulin secretion
- Uses
  - Anaphylaxis

  - Heart failure (left and right)
  - Cardiac arrest
- Adverse effects
  - Hyperglycemia
  - Hypokalemia
  - Lactic acidosis
  - Myocardial ischemia

Norepinephrine
- Mechanism of action: α_1, α_2, β_1 agonism
  - Potent vasoconstrictor
  - Increased pulmonary vascular resistance due to α_1 agonism
- Uses
  - Treatment of hypotension
  - Used in septic shock and post-cardiac bypass
- Adverse effects
  - Severe hypertension (HTN), worsening pulmonary HTN
  - Cardiac ischemia due to increased afterload
  - Organ dysfunction and metabolic acidosis

Phenylephrine
- Mechanism of action: α_1 agonist resulting in arterial vasoconstriction
  - Reflex bradycardia mediated by increased baroreceptor firing
- Uses
  - Treatment of mild hypotension
  - Septic shock (not first line)
  - Myocardial ischemia
    - Increased afterload and decreased HR, increased coronary perfusion
- Adverse effects
  - Bradycardia
  - Decreased cardiac output (CO) in the setting of left ventricular (LV) dysfunction – owing to increased afterload
  - Increased peripheral vascular resistance (PVR)

Ephedrine
- Mechanism of action: Indirect sympathomimetic resulting in increased HR, contractility, BP, and CO

Table 33.1 Effects of vasoactive/inotropic agents

Drug	α	β₁	β₂	CO	HR	SVR	MAP	PVR
Epinephrine	++	++	++	↑	↑	↑	↑	0
Norepinephrine	+++	++	0	0	0	↑	↑	↑
Phenylephrine	+++	0	0	0	↓	↑	↑	↑
Ephedrine	+	+	+	↑	↑	↑	↑	0
Dobutamine	0	+++	+	↑	↑	↓	↓	↓
Dopamine	++	++	0	↑	↑	↑	↑	0
Isoproterenol	0	+++	+++	↑	↑	↓	↓	0
Milrinone	0	0	0	↑	0	↓	↓	↓
Vasopressin	0	0	0	↑	0	↑	↑	0

- o Ineffective in patients with decreased sympathetic reserve (i.e., sepsis, chronically ill)
- Uses
  - o Hypotension and bradycardia
- Adverse effects
  - o Tachyphylaxis with repeated dosing
  - o Can cause agitation and insomnia
  - o Concomitant use with MAOIs
    - Exaggerated response to ephedrine
    - Risk for serotonin syndrome

Dopamine
- Mechanism of action: Agonism of α_1, β_1, and D_1 dopamine receptor
  - o Dose-dependent effects
    - 0.5–3.0 mcg/kg/minute → D_1
      - Increased glomerular filtration rate (GFR), renal blood flow (RBF), Na⁺ excretion, and decreased SVR
    - 3–10 mcg/kg/minute → β_1
      - Norepinephrine release → increased CO, BP, increased PVR
    - Over 10 mcg/kg/minute → α_1
      - Increased systemic vascular resistance (SVR)
  - o Diuretic and natriuretic effects
- Uses
  - o Septic shock
    - Better agents available (i.e., norepinephrine, dobutamine)
- Adverse effects
  - o Tachycardia
  - o Arrhythmogenic
  - o Myocardial ischemia
  - o Gut ischemia at high doses
  - o Decreased ventilatory response to hypoxemia

Dobutamine
- Mechanism of action
  - o β1 agonism resulting in increased contractility, HR, and ejection fraction
  - o Decreased SVR owing to β_2-mediated effects

- Uses
  - o Pharmacologic stress testing
  - o Treatment of low output states, including post-cardiopulmonary bypass
- Adverse effects
  - o Tachycardia
  - o Arrhythmia
  - o Myocardial ischemia

Isoproterenol
- Mechanism of action: Non-selective beta agonist
  - o Increased inotropy, chronotropy, and lusitropy
    - Results in increased cardiac output and blood pressure
    - β_2 effects result in net decreased SVR
- Uses
  - o Treatment of symptomatic bradycardia
  - o Used to elicit arrhythmias in electrophysiology lab
- Adverse effects
  - o Arrhythmia
  - o Myocardial ischemia[2] (Table 33.1)

Levosimendan[3]
- Mechanism of action: Sensitizes myocardial myofilaments to the effects of calcium resulting in increased inotropy and CO
- Uses
  - o CHF
- Phosphodiesterase inhibitors[2–5]

Milrinone
- Mechanism of action: Phosphodiesterase type III inhibitor. Results in increased cAMP levels
  - o Increased CO
  - o Decreased SVR, PVR, LV end diastolic pressure (LVEDP)
- Uses
  - o Weaning from cardiopulmonary bypass
    - Secondary benefit: Increases blood flow in CABG grafts
  - o CHF (left and right failure)

- o Reversal of cerebral vasospasm following subarach-noid hemorrhage (SAH)
- Adverse effects
  - o Hypotension
    - May require concomitant use of vasopressor owing to its systemic vasodilatory effects
  - o Arrhythmia: PVCs
  - o Impaired platelet aggregation
- Other agents in same class
  - o Enoximone, inamrinone, olprimone, pироximone[1]
  - o Cilostazol
    - Used in the treatment of claudication
    - Less cardiovascular effects than other drugs in class

Sildenafil

- Mechanism of action: Phosphodiesterase type-V inhibitor with net result of increased cGMP
  - o cGMP-mediated smooth muscle relaxation
- Uses
  - o Management of pulmonary hypertension
    - Efficacy independent of etiology
- Adverse effects
  - o Concomitant use with nitrates can result in severe hypotension and coronary steal
  - o Headache
  - o Dyspepsia
  - o Dizziness
- Other agents in same class
  - o Tadalafil

Anti-arrhythmics

Class I

- Mechanism of action: Inhibit fast inward depolarizing current carried by sodium ions. Decreased V_{max}
- Class Ia
  - o Effects on action potential
    - Phase 0 decreased
    - Depolarization prolonged
    - Conduction decreased
    - Action potential duration increased
  - o Examples
    - Quinidine: Used to treat atrial and ventricular arrhythmias. However, it may increase ventricular response rate in AF/flutter.
      - Risk of prolonged QT interval → asystole
    - Procainamide: Used to treat ventricular arrhythmias, atrial premature contractions, atrial fibrillation/flutter
      - Adverse effects: Prolonged QT (less than quinidine), GI upset, CNS symptoms, agranulocytosis
      - In setting of renal insufficiency, toxic metabolite N-acetylprocainamide may accumulate

- Disopyramide: Effective treatment for SVT/VT
  - Adverse effects: Prolonged QT interval, negative inotropic effects, reflex increase in SVR, anticholinergic side effects (GI upset, visual impairment, urinary retention)
- Class Ib
  - o Effects on action potential
    - Phase 0 minor effects
    - Depolarization minor effects
    - Minor effects on conduction
    - Action potential duration decreased
  - o Examples
    - Lidocaine: Used in the treatment of ventricular arrhythmias. Also exhibits local anesthetic, sedative properties, and broncho-dilatory properties. Decreases sympathetic response to direct laryngoscopy.
      - Adverse effects: CNS (fatigue, disorientation → agitation → seizures) – local anesthetic toxicity
    - Mexiletine/tocainide: Exhibit effects on action potential but neither conduction nor QT interval. Useful in treatment of VT not SVT
      - Adverse effects: Nausea, dysarthria, dizziness, paresthesia
- Class Ic
  - o Effects on action potential
    - Phase 0 significant decrease
    - Depolarization mild effects
    - Conduction significantly slowed
    - Action potential duration minimal effects
  - o Examples
    - Flecainide: Can significantly alter accessory pathway refractory period. Used in SVT/VT and Wolff–Parkinson–White syndrome. Very effective in decreasing PVCs and VT
      - Adverse effects: Rare. Minimal effects on QT interval
    - Propafenone: Use-dependent sodium channel blockade. Blocks beta receptors and potassium channels as well. Used in the treatment of VT/SVT
      - Adverse effects: Worsening of bronchospastic lung disease. GI upset, blurred vision, altered taste
    - Moricizine: Also blocks potassium channels. No effects on atrial tissue. Used in VT/VF
      - Adverse effects: Can be pro-arrhythmic. Tremor, headache

Class II

- Mechanism of action: Beta-adrenergic receptor antagonism resulting in decreased automaticity, increased action potential duration, decreased rate of spontaneous depolarization in SA node, slowed AV nodal conduction, increased effective refractory period

- Examples
  - Propranolol: Non-selective
    - Avoid in patients with diabetes and a history of bronchospasm
    - Withdrawal syndrome can occur with abrupt discontinuation
    - Adverse effects: Hallucinations, depression, insomnia
  - Metoprolol
    - Selective β_1 antagonism. Used in the treatment of SVT/VT
    - Adverse effects: Like propranolol, its use can suppress signs of hypoglycemia
  - Esmolol
    - Selective β_1 antagonism with short (~27 minutes) half-life. Metabolized by red cell esterases

Class III

- Mechanism of action: Potassium channel blockade and prolongation of repolarization. Increased action potential duration/effective refractory period
- Examples
  - Amiodarone
    - Effective in the treatment of SVT/VT/VF. Prolongs repolarization and refractory period in SA node, AV node, His-Purkinje system, and in the myocardium
    - May decrease heart's response to T3
    - Half-life of weeks (14–107 days) with large volume of distribution (1.3–66 L/kg)
    - Adverse effects: Hypotension, prolonged QT (chronic use only), thyrotoxicity, dyspnea, apical pulmonary fibrosis
  - Bretylium
    - Biphasic response: Initially results in release of norepinephrine (increased BP, SVR, automaticity) followed by adrenergic antagonism
    - Prolonged effective refractory period
    - Adverse effects: Orthostasis alleviated by the use of tricyclic compounds
  - Sotalol
    - Prolongs refractory period
    - Has beta blocking qualities
    - Used in the treatment of SVT/AF/VT
    - Patients at increased risk of torsades de pointes and prolonged QT
  - Ibutilide
    - Risk of prolonged QT and torsades de pointes
  - Dofetilide
    - Potassium channel blockade without slowing conduction
    - Major effects on QT interval
    - Greater effects on atrial tissue and thus used in conversion/treatment of AF
  - Dronedarone
    - Like amiodarone with greater effects on atrial tissue

- Methane for iodine substitution that reduces thyrotoxicity compared to amiodarone
  - Shorter half-life and smaller volume of distribution
  - Not as effective as amiodarone in the treatment of AF
  - Vernakalant
    - More effective at higher heart rates
    - Blocks atrial sodium and potassium channels
    - Used in the rapid conversion of AF
    - Approved in Europe but not in the United States

Class IV

- Mechanism of action: Decreased slow-channel calcium conductance; decreased action potential duration; slowed AV nodal conduction
- Examples
  - Verapamil
    - Used in the treatment of SVT, AF, atrial flutter
    - Cardiac depressive effects especially when used in the setting of inhalational anesthesia
    - Little effect on accessory pathways and therefore ineffective with antidromic reentry (e.g., wide complex WPW)
    - Risk of AV block when used in conjunction with beta blockers
    - Prolongation of neuromuscular blockade
  - Diltiazem
    - Similar effects as verapamil
    - Treatment for VF in acute cocaine toxicity[1]

Others

- Adenosine
  - Very short half-life (~2 seconds)
  - Negative chronotropic, dromotropic, and inotropic effects
  - Potent AV nodal blockade used in the treatment of AV nodal reentry
    - Exaggerated response in those with transplanted heart
  - Dosing: 6 mg → 6 mg → 12 mg (q1 minute)

Anti-anginal Drugs

AHA/ACC Non-ST Segment Elevation Acute Coronary Syndrome Guidelines (2014)[6]

- Oxygen therapy in patients with oxygen saturation less than 90 percent, respiratory distress, or high-risk features of hypoxemia (Class I recommendation)
- Nitrates
  - Sublingual nitroglycerin every five minutes for up to three doses (0.3–0.4 mg) to relieve chest pain. If pain is not alleviated and there are no contraindications, intravenous nitroglycerin may be administered (Class I recommendation)
  - Do not implement nitrates if a phosphodiesterase inhibitor has been administered within 24 hours (Class III harm)

- Analgesics
  - Morphine sulfate may be administered if chest pain persists despite maximal anti-ischemic medical therapy (Class IIb evidence)
  - Aside from aspirin, do not administer NSAIDS as this class of drugs has been associated with major adverse cardiac events (Class III harm)
- Beta-blockers
  - Administer beta-blockers (metoprolol, carvedilol, or bisoprolol) within 24 hours if no contraindications exist (Class I recommendation)
    - Contraindications include decompensated CHF, low-output states, and reactive airway disease
  - Continue beta blocker therapy after ischemic event
- Calcium channel blockers
  - A non-dihydropyridine calcium channel blocker may be substituted for a beta blocker as initial therapy if a contraindication to beta blockade exists (Class I recommendation)
  - Third-line agents after beta blockers and nitrates. If however, contraindications to latter two medications exist, calcium channel blockers are appropriate for long-term use (Class I recommendation)
  - Recommended for use in patients with coronary spasm (Class I recommendation)
- ACE inhibitors
  - These agents should be started and continued in patients with ejection fraction less than 40 percent and in patients with hypertension, diabetes, or CKD (Class I recommendation)
  - ARBs are a suitable substitute in patients who experience significant side effects of ACE inhibitors (Class I recommendation)
  - Aldosterone antagonism is recommended in patients post myocardial infarction on both ACE inhibitors and a beta blocker without renal insufficiency.
- Antiplatelet/antithrombotic agents
  - Aspirin therapy should be initiated in patients presenting with ACS and continued indefinitely. Initial dose 162 or 325 mg followed by 81 mg daily thereafter (Class I recommendation)
    - Clopidogrel load followed by daily dose is recommended if a contraindication to aspirin therapy exists (Class I recommendation)

Specific Agents[7]

- Statins
  - Benefits extend beyond lipid lowering effects
    - Anti-inflammatory properties
    - Improved endothelial function
    - Plaque-stabilizing effects
- Nitrates[8]
  - Mechanism of action: Release of nitric oxide facilitates activation of guanylyl cyclase which results in increased levels of cGMP and both arteriolar and venous vasodilation.

- Coronary arteries are subject to vasodilatory effects with resultant increased oxygen supply to myocardium.
- Decreased preload, left ventricular wall tension, and thus myocardial oxygen demand.
  - Specific agents
    - Isosorbide dinitrate
      - Tolerance and decreased efficacy occur with chronic use
    - Isosorbide mononitrate
      - Bypasses first pass metabolism with 100 percent oral bioavailability
      - Better tolerance profile than isosorbide dinitrate
  - Tolerance and withdrawal symptoms occur in the setting of prolonged use of nitrates
- Ranolazine[9,10]
  - Mechanism of action
    - Inhibition of late myocardial sodium current thus decreasing both intracellular sodium and calcium in ischemic myocardium
    - Little to no effect on hemodynamics
  - Adverse effects
    - Constipation
    - Nausea
    - Weakness

Vasodilators

Nitroprusside

- Mechanism of action: Nitric oxide donor
- Physiologic effects
  - Potent arterial and venous vasodilation (including pulmonary vasculature)
  - Easily titratable
- Adverse effects
  - Severe hypotension
  - Cyanide/thiocyanate toxicity with prolonged use especially in the setting of renal insufficiency

Nitroglycerin

- Mechanism of action: Upon entry into smooth muscle, nitrates are converted to nitric oxide (or S-nitrosothiols) leading to production of cyclic GMP (cGMP) by way of activation of guanylyl cyclase. Ultimately, smooth muscle relaxation occurs as a consequence of myosin light chain dephosphorylation.
- Physiologic effects
  - Preferential systemic venodilation
  - Coronary vasodilation (without coronary steal)
  - Decreased PVR
  - Increased venous pooling leading to decreased venous return and decreased preload
- Adverse effects
  - Hypotension

- o Headache
- o Nausea

Hydralazine

- Mechanism of action: Activation of ATP-dependent potassium channels leading to arterial vasodilation
- Physiologic effects
  - o Arterial vasodilation
- Adverse effects
  - o Reflex sympathetic activation manifesting as tachycardia, headache, flushing

Nesiritide

- Mechanism of action: Analog of brain natriuretic peptide (BNP) that produces both arterial and venous vasodilation via increased cGMP
- Physiologic effects
  - o Arterial and venous vasodilation
  - o No effects on heart rate or contractility
  - o To be administered to in-hospital patients only
- Adverse effects
  - o Hypotension
  - o Renal failure

Calcium Channel Blockers

- Mechanism of action: Binding to sites on the α-1 subunit of L-type voltage-dependent calcium channel
- Physiologic effects
  - o Arterial vasodilation
  - o Coronary vasodilation (nifedipine most potent)
- Adverse effects
  - o Negative inotropy, dromotropy, and chronotropy
    - Hypotension, AV block, heart failure. All more likely in setting of combination therapy with beta blockade, digitalis, or in setting of hypokalemia
  - o Headache
  - o Flushing
  - o Nausea
- Specific calcium channel blockers
  - o 1,4-Dihydropyridine (DHP) derivatives (amlodipine, nifedipine, nimodipine, nicardipine)
    - Potent arterial dilators
    - Reflex activation of sympathetic nervous system
    - Nimodipine can cross blood–brain barrier and is indicated for cerebral vascular spasm
    - Nicardipine has selectivity for coronary and cerebrovascular vessels compared to other DHPs
    - Clevidipine is inactivated by ester hydrolysis with a half-life of one minute
  - o Phenylalkyl amines (verapamil)
    - Less potent arterial dilator than DHPs
    - Less reflex sympathetic activation than DHPs
    - Myocardial depression
  - o Benzothiazipines (diltiazem)
    - Less potent than verapamil with respect to arterial vasodilation

- o Diarylaminopropylamine ester (bepridil)[1]

Alpha-adrenergic Antagonists (Phentolamine – Reversible Antagonism, Phenoxybenzamine – Irreversible Antagonism)

- Mechanism of action: Non-selective alpha-adrenergic antagonism
- Physiologic effects
  - o Decreased PVR
  - o Positive inotropic and chronotropic effects (presynaptic α$_2$ antagonism)
- Adverse effects
  - o Orthostatic hypotension
  - o Reflex tachycardia

Central Acting Alpha-Agonists (Clonidine, Methyl-dopa)

- Mechanism of action: Reduce sympathetic outflow and SVR via agonism of central α$_2$-adrenergic receptors. Pre-synaptic α$_2$ agonism results in decreased release of norepinephrine at synaptic cleft.
- Physiologic effects
  - o Decreased SVR
  - o Decreased sympathetic outflow
- Adverse effects
  - o Rebound hypertension
  - o Sedation
  - o Dry mouth
  - o Autoimmune hemolytic anemia (methyl-dopa)

Endothelin Antagonists (Bosentan, Ambrisentan)

- Mechanism of action: Antagonism of endothelin receptor which is responsible for vasoconstriction

Angiotensin-Converting Enzyme Inhibitors and Angiotensin Receptor Blockers

ACE Inhibitors

- Mechanism of action
  - o Prevents cleavage of angiotensin I to angiotensin II via inhibition of ACE. Angiotensin II mediates vasoconstriction, release of aldosterone, sodium retention, ventricular remodeling, and increases in sympathetic tone.
  - o ACE involved in the breakdown of kinins, including bradykinin.
    - Bradykinin facilitates vasodilation via inducing release of nitric oxide by endothelial cells.
- Uses
  - o Management of hypertension
    - Increased RBF via dilation of afferent and efferent arterioles
    - Protective against development of diabetic nephropathy
  - o CHF
    - Decreased PVR and increased CO
    - Decreased sodium retention and ventricular remodeling in setting of CHF and post-MI (confers a mortality benefit)

- Adverse effects
  - Cough
    - Effect of increased bradykinin
  - Hypotension
  - Hyperkalemia
    - Due to decreased circulating aldosterone
  - Renal insufficiency
  - Angioedema
  - Agranulocytosis

Angiotensin Receptor Blockers (ARB)

- Mechanism of action: Blockage of the AT_1 receptor
  - Greater inhibition of renin–angiotensin–aldosterone system (RAAS) than ACEI
  - No effect on bradykinin levels
- Uses: Same as ACE
- Adverse effects: Same as ACE with exception of cough[11]

Other Agents

- Aldosterone antagonists
  - Spironolactone
    - Mechanism of action
      - Potassium-sparing diuretic that acts as an inhibitor of the renal aldosterone-dependent Na^+/K^+ channel
    - Uses
      - Hypertension
      - CHF
        - Inhibits cardiac remodeling
        - Confers mortality benefit in patients with CHF
    - Adverse effects
      - Hyperkalemia
      - Endocrine side effects
        - Gynecomastia in men and menstrual irregularities in women
  - Eplerenone
    - Mechanism of action
      - Aldosterone receptor inhibition
    - Uses
      - Hypertension
      - CHF
        - Survival benefit
    - Adverse effects
      - Hyperkalemia
- Renin inhibitor (Aliskiren)[12]
  - Mechanism of action: Occupies active site of renin thus preventing cleavage of ATI into AT2
  - Uses
    - Hypertension

Cardiovascular Effects of Electrolytes

Calcium

- Roles

  - Ubiquitous second messenger
  - Important role in coagulation. Links platelets to coagulation factors.
  - Positive inotrope
    - Drugs that increase contractility all result in a net increase in intracellular calcium
  - Peripheral vasoconstriction
- Pathologic states
  - Hypercalcemia
    - Effects
      - Weakness → lethargy → coma
      - Constipation, nausea/vomiting
      - Nephrogenic diabetes insipidus
      - Worsening of digitalis toxicity
    - ECG changes
      - Shortened QTc
      - Prolonged PR interval
    - Causes
      - Increased parathyroid hormone
      - Malignancy
      - Excess vitamin D
      - Decreased renal excretion
        - Thiazides
      - Increased Ca^{2+} intake
        - Milk-alkali syndrome
    - Treatment
      - Non-calcium containing crystalloid
      - Loop diuretics
      - Bisphosphonates
  - Hypocalcemia
    - Effects
      - Decreased myocardial contractility
      - Paresthesia
      - Tetany
      - Seizures
      - Chvostek sign: Facial twitching from tapping on facial nerve
      - Trousseau sign: Forearm spasm from inflating NIBP cuff
      - Heart block
    - ECG changes
      - Prolonged QTc
      - T-wave inversions
      - Osborn waves
      - V fib
    - Causes
      - Hypoparathyroidism
      - Ca^{2+} chelation
        - Commonly seen in setting of blood product transfusion
      - Increased bone deposition
      - Hypoalbuminemia
    - Treatment
      - Calcium supplementation

- Ensure there are no coexisting electrolyte abnormalities, especially magnesium – magnesium depletion can lead to hypoparathyroidism, PTH resistance, and vitamin D deficiency

Magnesium
- Roles
  - Involved in ion channel activity
    - Antagonist of Ca^{2+}
  - Vital to production of ATP, nucleotides, and proteins
    - Cofactor in DNA transcription/translation
  - NMDA antagonist
  - Arteriolar vasodilator
  - Bronchial smooth muscle dilator
  - Tocolytic
  - Anticonvulsant
- Pathologic states
  - Hypermagnesemia
    - Effects
      - Prolonged effect of non-depolarizing neuromuscular blocking agents
        - Use with caution in patients with myasthenia gravis and Eaton–Lambert syndrome
      - Side effects based upon serum level
        - 5–7 mg/dL: Therapeutic in treatment of pre-eclampsia
        - 5–10 mg/dL: Impaired cardiac conduction, nausea
        - 20–34 mg/dL: Sedation, reduced deep tendon reflexes, muscle weakness
        - 24–48 mg/dL: Hypotension
        - 48–72 mg/dL: Areflexia, coma, respiratory paralysis
    - ECG changes
      - Widened QRS interval
      - Prolonged PR interval
    - Causes
      - Iatrogenic in majority of cases
    - Treatment
      - Non-magnesium containing crystalloid administration
      - Diuretic therapy
      - Renal replacement therapy in setting of renal failure
  - Hypomagnesemia
    - Effects
      - Vertigo → weakness → seizure
      - Hypocalcemia
      - Hyperinsulinemia
      - Atherosclerosis
      - Osteomalacia
    - ECG changes
      - Widened QRS interval
      - Prolonged PR interval

- T-wave inversion
- Ventricular arrhythmias
  - Causes
    - Inadequate intake
    - Renal losses
  - Treatment
    - Magnesium supplementation
    - Correction of other electrolyte abnormalities, particularly calcium and potassium[3,13,14]

Phosphorus
- Roles
  - Building block
    - Found in DNA, RNA, ATP, phospholipids, hydroxyapatite (bone), 2,3-DPG
  - Phosphate buffer system
- Pathologic states
  - Hyperphosphatemia
    - Effects
      - Mimic those of hypocalcemia on account of increased bone deposition in setting of hyperphosphatemia
      - Vascular calcification leading to increased afterload and left ventricular hypertrophy[15]
    - ECG changes[16]
      - Prolonged QT interval
      - Ventricular tachycardia
      - Torsades de pointes
    - Causes
      - Tumor lysis syndrome
      - Rhabdomyolysis
      - Reduced excretion
        - Renal failure
        - Hypoparathyroidism
      - Pseudohyperphosphatemia
        - Multiple myeloma
    - Treatment
      - Dialysis
      - Crystalloid infusion
      - Phosphate binders
  - Hypophosphatemia[17]
    - Effects
      - Decreased cardiac contractility
      - Impaired respiratory function
      - Left-shift in oxygen dissociation curve due to paucity of 2,3-DPG
      - Seizures
      - Central pontine myelinolysis
    - ECG changes
      - Ventricular arrhythmia post MI
      - SVT
      - Ectopy
    - Causes
      - Impaired uptake
      - Renal excretion

- Bone shifts
- Hyperventilation can unearth symptoms in patients with chronic deficiency
- Refeeding syndrome
  - Treatment
    - Replete cautiously as there exists a risk of causing severe hypocalcemia

Potassium

- Roles
  - K^+ gradient vital to resting membrane potential
    - Large intracellular to extracellular gradient maintained by $Na^+/K^+/ATPase$
- Pathologic states
  - Hyperkalemia
    - Effects
      - Slowed conduction through AV node
      - Muscle weakness
      - Paralysis
      - Altered cardiac conduction
        - Increased automaticity
        - Enhanced repolarization
    - ECG changes based on serum concentration:
      - 5.5–6.5 mEq/L → tall, peaked T-waves
      - 6.5–7.5 mEq/L → prolonged PR interval
      - Greater than 7.5 mEq/L → widened QRS
      - Greater than 9.0 mEq/L → sine waves, bradycardia, ventricular tachycardia, cardiac arrest
    - Causes
      - Increased intake
      - Renal insufficiency
      - Hypoaldosteronism
      - Drugs including:
        - Potassium-sparing diuretics
        - ACEI/ARB
      - Reperfusion of ischemic tissues
      - Acidosis
    - Treatment
      - Calcium to stabilize cardiac membranes
      - Increased intracellular fluid K to extracellular fluid ratio
      - Increased excretion
        - Insulin
        - Bicarbonate/hyperventilation
        - β_2 agonists
      - Dialysis
      - Gastrointestinal resins (e.g., Kayexalate [polystyrene sulfonate])
  - Hypokalemia
    - Effects
      - Prolonged repolarization
      - Muscle weakness

- ECG changes
  - T-wave flattening or inversion
  - U waves
  - ST segment depression
  - Enlarged P waves
  - Prolonged PR interval
  - Atrial and ventricular arrhythmias
    - AF
    - Ventricular extrasystoles
- Causes
  - Inadequate intake
  - GI losses
  - Mineralocorticoid/glucocorticoid excess
  - Diuretics
  - Hypomagnesemia
  - Intracellular shifts caused by
    - β_2 agonists
    - Insulin therapy
    - Lithium overdose
    - Acute alkalosis
- Treatment
  - Oral and intravenous supplementation
    - Slow IV infusion
    - Utilize central venous catheter when using solutions with concentration >40 mEq/L
      - Highly concentrated solutions can irritate veins

Non-adrenergic Vasoconstrictors

Vasopressin[18]

- Mechanism of action: Synthesized in posterior pituitary gland endogenously and elicits effects via binding of V_1, V_2, and V_3 receptors all of which are G-coupled protein receptors. Vasopressin is released in response to increased serum osmolality and hypovolemia. In addition, vasopressin is released in response to pain, nausea, hypoxia, and pharyngeal stimulation.
- Receptor effects
  - V_1 receptor: Activation of these vascular receptors results in systemic vasoconstriction with relative sparing of the pulmonary vasculature.[19]
    - Additionally, activation of V_1 receptors results in platelet aggregation by way of both von Willebrand Factor and Factor VIII from vascular smooth muscle.
  - V_2 receptor stimulation: Located in distal tubules and collecting ducts of kidney, specifically the basolateral membrane of principal cells. Receptor activation commences cascade leading to increased cAMP with resultant insertion of aquaporin channels in collecting ducts. The net result is water retention.
  - V_3 receptor stimulation: Receptors are located in anterior pituitary and result in increased synthesis of adrenocorticohormone (ACTH).

- Uses
  - Hypovolemic shock
  - Septic shock
    - Vasopressin deficiency in patients in prolonged septic shock
  - Hepatorenal syndrome
  - Bleeding esophageal varices
- Adverse effects
  - Skin necrosis
  - Hyponatremia
  - Bronchospasm
  - Gut ischemia

Terlipressin: Vasopressin Analogue with Longer Half-life (6 hours versus 24 minutes)

Methylene Blue[20]

- Mechanism of action: inhibition of guanylyl cyclase resulting in decreased cGMP
- Uses
  - Post-cardiac bypass vasoplegia
- Adverse effects
  - Association with methemoglobinemia
  - Blue urine
  - Inaccuracies with pulse oximetry readings

References

1. Royster R. L., Groban L., Locke A. Q., Morris B. N., Slaughter T. F. Cardiovascular pharmacology. In: Kaplan J. A., Augoustides J. G. T., Maneck G. R., Maus T., Reich D. L. (eds), *Kaplan's Cardiac Anesthesia: In Cardiac and Noncardiac Surgery*. Philadelphia, PA: Elsevier; 2017, 292–354.

2. Zimmerman J., Cahalan M. Vasopressors and inotropes. In: Hemmings H. C., Egan T. D. (eds), *Pharmacology and Physiology for Anesthesia: Foundations and Clinical Application*. Philadelphia, PA: Elsevier; 2013, 390–404.

3. Levy J. H., Ghadimi K., Bailey J. M., Ramsay J. G. Postoperative cardiovascular management. In: Kaplan J. A., Augoustides J. G. T., Maneck G. R., Maus T., Reich D. L. (eds), *Kaplan's Cardiac Anesthesia: In Cardiac and Noncardiac Surgery*. Philadelphia, PA: Elsevier; 2017, 1327–57.

4. Gold Standard, Inc. Milrinone. Clinical Pharmacology [database online]. Available at http://clinicalpharmacology.com. Accessed 03/08/2017.

5. Gold Standard, Inc. Sildenafil. Clinical Pharmacology [database online]. Available at http://clinicalpharmacology.com. Accessed 03/08/2017.

6. Amsterdam E. A., et al. AHA/ACC guideline for the management of patients with non-ST-elevation acute coronary syndromes. *Circulation*. 2014; 130(25): 2354–94.

7. Tarkin J. M., Kaski J. C. An overview of treatment guidelines: ESC/ACC-AHA/NICE. In: Avanzas P., Kaski J. C. (eds), *Pharmacological Treatment of Chronic Stable Angina Pectoris*. Ebook. Springer; 2015, 33–56 (OVERVIEW).

8. Carro A., Avanzas P. Nitrates. In: Avanzas P., Kaski J. C. (eds), *Pharmacological Treatment of Chronic Stable Angina Pectoris*. Ebook. Springer; 2015, 87–114.

9. Rosano G. M. C., Vitale C., Volterrani M. Ranolazine. In: Avanzas P., Kaski J. C. (eds), *Pharmacological Treatment of Chronic Stable Angina Pectoris*. Ebook. Springer; 2015, 173–88.

10. Gold Standard, Inc. Ranolazine. Clinical Pharmacology [database online]. Available at http://clinicalpharmacology.com. Accessed 03/08/2017.

11. Dolinko A. V., Kuntz M. T., Antman E. M., Strichartz G. R., Lilly L. S. Cardiovascular drugs. In: Lilly L. S. (ed.), *Pathophysiology of Heart Disease: A Collaborative Project of Medical Students and Faculty*. China: Wolters Kluwer; 2016, 400–55.

12. Drago J., Williams G. H., Lilly L. S. Hypertension. In: Lilly L. S. (ed.), *Pathophysiology of Heart Disease: A Collaborative Project of Medical Students and Faculty*. China: Wolters Kluwer; 2016, 310–33.

13. Edwards M. R., Grocott M. P. W. Perioperative fluid and electrolyte therapy. In: Miller R. D., Cohen N. H., Eriksson L. I., et al. (eds), *Miller's Anesthesia*. Philadelphia, PA: Elsevier; 2015, 1767–810.

14. Freudzon L., Akhtar S., London M. J., Barash P. G. Electrocardiographic monitoring. In: Kaplan J. A., Augoustides J. G. T., Maneck G. R., Maus T., Reich D. L. (eds), *Kaplan's Cardiac Anesthesia: In Cardiac and Noncardiac Surgery*. Philadelphia, PA: Elsevier; 2017, 357–89.

15. Hruska K. A., Mathew S., Lund R., Qiu P., Pratt R. Hyperphosphatemia of chronic kidney disease. *Kidney International*. 2008; 74: 148–57.

16. Shiber J. R., Mattu A. Serum phosphate abnormalities in the emergency department. *Journal of Emergency Medicine*. 2002; 23(4): 395–400.

17. Geerse D. A., Bindels A. J., Kuiper M. A., et al. Treatment of hypophosphatemia in the intensive care unit: a review. *Critical Care*. 2010; 14: R147.

18. Kam P. C. A., Williams S., Yoong F. F. Y. Vasopressin and terlipressin: pharmacology and its clinical relevance. *Anaesthesia*. 2004; 59: 993–1001.

19. Currigan D. A., Hughes R. J. A., Wright C. E., Angus J. A., Soeding P. F. Vasoconstrictor responses to vasopressor agents in human pulmonary and radial arteries. An *in vitro* study. *Anesthesiology*. 2014; 121: 930–6.

20. Nguyen L., Roth D. M., Shanewise J. S., Kaplan J. A. Discontinuing cardiopulmonary bypass. In: Kaplan J. A., Augoustides J. G. T., Maneck G. R., Maus T., Reich D. L. (eds), *Kaplan's Cardiac Anesthesia: In Cardiac and Noncardiac Surgery*. Philadelphia, PA: Elsevier; 2017, 1291–310.

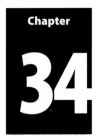

Chapter

34

Gastrointestinal Systems

Bryan Hill, Brian Chang, and Jeron Zerillo

Gastrointestinal System

- The primary role of the gastrointestinal (GI) tract is processing of nutrients via digestion and absorption.
- Digestion and absorption are regulated by the enteric mucosal membrane, the enteric nervous system, and the autonomic nervous system.[1]
- The wall of the GI tract consists of serosa, muscularis, submucosa, and mucosa. There are both longitudinal and circular muscular layers in the muscularis. An individual layer of epithelial cells, the lamina propria, and the muscularis mucosae comprise the mucosal layer.
- There are two main nerve plexuses:
  1. Absorption, secretion, and mucosal blood flow are controlled by the submucosal plexus
  2. Tonic regulation and contractions of the intestinal wall are regulated by the myenteric plexus.[2]
- Intestinal motility regulates nutrient absorption via modulation of transit time and contact with the mucosal brush border.[2]
- Postoperative ileus is most commonly induced by physical manipulation of the intestines and the resultant cascade of neural and inflammatory interactions.[3,4]
- The typical course of uncomplicated ileus lasts ~4 postoperative days. This process consists of a neurogenic phase (mediated by adrenergic innervation) and an inflammatory phase.[5]
- GI system blood flow accomplishes many functions including delivering nutrients and hormones, removing metabolic waste, and helping to maintain the mucosal barrier which prevents transepithelial migration of harmful chemicals and pathogens.[2]
- 25% of cardiac output is delivered to the splanchnic system and contains approximately one third of total blood volume. A reservoir of blood is maintained in the venous system which is mobilized during periods of acute blood loss.[2]
- Hemodynamic variability during laparoscopic surgery is caused by a complex interaction between anesthetic agents,[2] surgical manipulation, patient position,[2] fluid management,[2] insufflation pressure,[2] and carbon dioxide absorption.[2] These factors may influence postoperative GI function.[2]
- The stomach consists of anatomic and functional areas.
  - Anatomic: Fundus, corpus or body, and antrum
  - Functional: Oxyntic and pyloric gland

- Gastrointestinal cells:
  - Parietal cell – dominates the oxyntic gland area[2]
  - Gastric (G) cell - dominates the pyloric gland area.[2]
  - Foveolar cells – secrete mucus and HCO_3 in the stomach.[2]
  - Chief cells – produce pepsinogen, the inactive zymogen of pepsin.[2]
- The stomach is protected against the caustic agents HCl and pepsin via mucus and bicarbonate. Bicarbonate production is increased via prostaglandin production, but this process is inhibited by NSAIDs.[2]
- Some critically ill patients who are coagulopathic and/or on mechanical ventilation for more than 48 hours have an increased incidence of stress ulcers of the stomach. Many other risk factors that may be associated with gastric ulcers include respiratory failure, sepsis, heart failure, hepatic encephalopathy, jaundice, renal failure, stroke, hypertension, previous GI disease and treatment with corticosteroids, NSAIDS, heparin or Warfarin use.[6,7]

Hepatic System

- The liver dual blood supply receives ~30% of the total cardiac output. The portal vein provides ~75% of hepatic blood flow; the hepatic artery provides the other ~25%. The liver oxygen supply is equally distributed (~50%) from each of these vessels.[2]
- Exchange of arterial and venous blood occurs in the hepatic sinusoids, the "capillaries of the liver".[2]
- Hepatic vascular resistance is generally driven by the resistance in postsinusoidal vessels.[2]
- Hepatic vascular tone allows for a significant reservoir of blood to be stored in the liver which may be mobilized in periods of intravascular volume loss.[2]
- The immunologic Kupffer cells are present in hepatic sinusoids and act as a filter by removing bacteria and other harmful substances from portal blood, preventing the entry of these into systemic circulation.[2]
- Acini are the units of liver parenchyma. Each is composed of three progressive circulatory zones. Zone 1 (blood perfusing zone) receives blood rich in O_2 and nutrients. The blood then passes through zone 2 and zone 3. In zone 3, the hepatocytes receive relatively O_2-poor blood, making tissue in this zone susceptible to hypoxic injury.[2]

- The hepatic arterial buffer response (HABR) refers to a compensatory increase in hepatic arterial flow when portal vein flow is decreased. This process is mediated, in part, by adenosine washout. When portal vein flow is impaired, adenosine buildup results in compensatory hepatic arterial vasodilation and increased blood flow. Disruptions in the HABR increase the possibility of hypoxic liver injury.[2]

- The liver is central to metabolism and maintenance of energy for the body. Glycogen is the main component of stored energy in the liver. When glycogen stores are depleted, hepatic gluconeogenesis occurs, enabling the liver to deliver glucose to glucose-dependent tissues such as the brain. Oxidation of fatty acids into ketoacids increases with starvation. These compounds are released from the liver and used as energy substrates by many of the extrahepatic cells.[2]

- Hepatocytes oxidize substances and conjugate substances via the cytochrome P450 system. The products of these reactions are typically more hydrophilic and are more readily excreted.[2]

- Ammonia is highly toxic to many systems including the central nervous system and, without exogenous substances such as lactulose, can be eliminated only by the liver. Hepatocytes metabolize ammonia to urea, which is less toxic.[2]

- The only means of eliminating cholesterol from the body is via liver metabolism of cholesterol to bile acids. Hepatocytes produce bile acids, which are amphipathic molecules that emulsify lipophilic substances, promoting their absorption. The bile acids drain into the duodenum via the common bile duct. The terminal ileum ultimately absorbs bile acids and returns them to hepatocytes through the portal vein. This is called the enterohepatic circulation.[2]

- The liver produces many of the plasma proteins including albumin, which is the most abundant plasma protein. Hepatocytes also synthesize components vitamin K-dependent proteins (factors II, VII, IX, X, protein C, and protein S).[2]

- Cirrhosis-induced portal hypertension leads to a decrease in Total peripheral resistance and systemic blood pressure decrease with compensatory increases in cardiac output. This also results in the bypassing of the hepatic filtering of drugs, nitrogenous waste, and toxins, thus allowing these compounds to enter the central circulation.[2]

- Gradients between the inferior vena cava and the portal vein of greater than 5 mmHg qualify as portal hypertension. Gradients greater than 10 mmHg lead to chronic liver injury, necrosis, fibrosis, and finally cirrhosis. Nonselective beta-blockers such as propranolol decrease hepatic artery blood flow which decreases congestion in the liver, transmitting back to the portal vein, reducing portal pressure. The only definitive treatment for end-stage hepatic disease is liver transplantation.[2,8]

- Large volume ascites can impede ventilation and reduce functional reserve capacity. LVP can quickly and safely reduce abdominal mass in those patients with large volume ascites. In some patients, hemodynamic instability can occur following LVP due to intravascular depletion secondary to rapid re-accumulation of the ascites; so albumin (12.5 g of albumin is given per liter of ascites removed) is commonly given to offset this response, preventing sequelae such as increased creatinine and electrolyte abnormalities.[2]

- *Hepatopulmonary syndrome* results from the formation of microscopic intrapulmonary arteriovenous dilatations in patients with both chronic and acute liver failure. The mechanism is unknown but is thought to be due to increased liver production or decreased liver clearance of vasodilators, possibly involving nitric oxide. The dilation of these blood vessels causes overperfusion relative to ventilation, leading to ventilation–perfusion mismatch and hypoxemia. There is an increased gradient between the partial pressure of oxygen in the alveoli of the lung and adjacent arteries (alveolar-arterial [A–a] gradient) while breathing room air. Additionally, late in cirrhosis, it is common to develop high output failure, which would lead to less time in capillaries per red blood cell, exacerbating the hypoxemia.[2,9,10]

- *Hepatorenal syndrome* is "prerenal" condition, likely due to decreased intravascular tone leading to the inadequate volume status perceived by the juxtaglomerular apparatus, leading to the secretion of renin and the activation of the renin–angiotensin system, which results in the vasoconstriction of vessels systemically and in the kidney specifically. However, the effect of this is insufficient to counteract the mediators of vasodilation in the splanchnic circulation, leading to persistent "underfilling" of the kidney circulation and worsening kidney vasoconstriction, leading to kidney failure. Diagnosis is one of exclusion after other causes of renal failure have been ruled out. Hepatorenal syndrome is often rapidly fatal (<1 month).[2]

References

1. Nicholl, C. G., Polak, J. M., Bloom, S. R. The hormonal regulation of food intake, digestion, and absorption. *Annu Rev Nutr.* 5:215, (1982).
2. Miller, R. D. *Miller's Anesthesia*. Philadelphia, PA: Elsevier, 2015.
3. Mattei, P., Rombeau, J. L. Review of pathophysiology and management of postoperative ileus. *World J Surg.* 30:1382, (2006).
4. Kehlet, H., Holte, K. Review of postoperative ileus. *Am J Surg.* 182:3S, (2001).
5. Boeckxstaens, G. E. Neuroimmune mechanisms in postoperative ileus. *Gut.* (2009).
6. Rosenstock, S., Jørgensen, T., Bonnevie, O. et al. Risk factors for peptic ulcer disease: a population based prospective cohort study comprising 2416 Danish adults. *Gut.* 52:186, (2003).
7. Kurata, J. H., Nogawa, A. N. Meta-analysis of risk factors for peptic ulcer. Nonsteroidal antiinflammatory drugs, Helicobacter pylori, and smoking. *J Clin Gastroenterol.* 24:2, (1997).

8. Arthur, M. J., Tanner, A. R., Patel, C. et al. Pharmacology of propranolol in patients with cirrhosis and portal hypertension. *Gut.* 26:14, (1985).

9. Swanson, K. L., Wiesner, R. H., Krowka, M. J. Natural history of hepatopulmonary syndrome: Impact of liver transplantation. *Hepatology.* 41:1122, (2005).

10. Fallon, M. B., Abrams, G. A., Luo, B. et al. The role of endothelial nitric oxide synthase in the pathogenesis of a rat model of hepatopulmonary syndrome. *Gastroenterology.* 113:606, (1997).

Renal Anatomy and Physiology

Ryan Barnette and Michael D. Lazar

Water: Distribution, Balance, Compartments

Body Fluid

- Body compartments: **60-40-20 rule**
  - Total body water (TBW): 60 percent of body weight
  - Intracellular fluid (ICF): 40 percent of body weight
  - Extracellular fluid (ECF): 20 percent of body weight
- TBW percent: ↑ in babies and ↓ in elderly and obesity
- TBW 40 L, 60 percent body weight
- Average adult male
  - Extracellular fluid volume 15 L = 20 percent of body weight (Table 35.1)
- **Plasma osmolality**: 285–95 mosm/kg = 2 (plasma Na^+) + glucose/18 + BUN/2.8

*Glucose and BUN contributions are minimal and thus osmolality can be approximated by serum Na^+

- **Osmoreceptors**: In the hypothalamus respond to changes in the *tonicity* of body fluid
- **Baroreceptors**: In the right atria and great veins respond to changes in intravascular volume. These receptors prompt the inhibition or stimulation of antidiuretic hormone (ADH or vasopressin) release from the posterior pituitary. ADH acts at *V1 receptors* on *vascular smooth muscle* resulting in *vasoconstriction* and *V2 receptors* on the *renal collecting tubule cells* to increase aquaporin channels and the *reabsorption of H_2O.*
- **Strong ion difference (SID)**: Used to assist in categorizing disorders of acid–base balance. Cations predominate in plasma resulting in net positive +40 charge.[1]

SID = [strong cations] – [strong anions] = [Na^+ + K^+ + Ca^{2+} + Mg^{2+}] – [Cl^- + $lactate^-$]

- Decrease SID → acidosis
  - Free water excess secondary to hyponatremia
  - Diarrhea
  - Increase in anions such as lactic acid or ketoacids

- Increase SID → alkalosis
  - Dehydration resulting in contraction alkalosis
  - Anion loss (i.e., chloride ions via emesis)
- SID of normal saline (NS) = 0 → resuscitation with NS can cause hyperchloremic metabolic acidosis

Electrolytes

Sodium

- Hyponatremia (Na < 135 mEq/L)
  - Symptoms: Neurologic symptoms due to cerebral swelling such as headache, vomiting, gait disturbance, seizures
  - Causes: Evaluation begins with assessment of TBW
    - Hypovolemic hyponatremia → renal versus extrarenal losses
    - Euvolemic hyponatremia → adrenal/thyroid insufficiency, SIADH, medications
    - Hypervolemic hyponatremia → congestive heart failure, liver cirrhosis, renal failure, nephrotic syndrome
  - Treatment: Typically asymptomatic when Na^+ > 125 mEq/L. Conservative correction indicated with normal saline, salt tabs, fluid restriction. If associated with seizures or severe neurologic symptoms correction can be made with hypertonic saline.
  - Goal correction: 4–6 mEq/L increase over 24 hours, not to exceed 8–9 mEq/L in 24-hour period; more rapid correction results in risk of osmotic demyelination
- Hypernatremia (Na > 145 mEq/L)
  - Symptoms: Lethargy, seizures, coma
  - Causes: Pure water loss, hypotonic fluid loss (water loss exceeds Na^+ loss)
  - Treatment: Begin by calculating water deficit.
    - Acute hypernatremia can be corrected at 1 mEq/L/h for the first 6–8 hours to prevent the potential cerebral dehydration and demyelination.
    - Chronic hypernatremia can be corrected by 8 mEq/L/day.[2]

$$\text{Water deficit} = \text{Total body water}[L] \times \left(\frac{\text{Serum } Na^+}{140} - 1 \right)$$

Table 35.1 Breakdown of Total Body Water

Intracellular fluid (ICF) volume	Interstitial fluid	Plasma
40 percent of body weight	80 percent of ECF	20 percent of ECF

ICF: cations = K^+, Mg^{2+} anions = phosphates, proteins; ECF: cation = Na^+, anions = Cl^-, bicarbonate.

Potassium

- Hypokalemia (<3.5 mEq/L)
  - Signs/symptoms: Severe muscle weakness, flattened T-waves/U-waves on ECG
  - Causes: Medications (aminoglycosides, thiazide/loop diuretics, laxative abuse), GI losses (diarrhea, suctioning), renal tubular acidosis, magnesium deficiency
  - Treatment: Potassium chloride – maximum of 60 mEq/L infused through peripheral vein. Up to 200 mEq/L through central veins in critical care setting.[3]
- Hyperkalemia (>5.1 mEq/L)
  - Signs/symptoms: May manifest as muscle weakness and paralysis
    - 6–7 mEq/L → peaked T-waves
    - 10–12 mEq/L → prolonged PR, widening QRS, Vfib, and asystole.[4]
  - Causes: Most K^+ exists intracellularly, therefore increases are likely due to transcellular shifts such that occur in acidotic states. Other causes include aldosterone antagonism, reperfusion of ischemic vascular beds, and renal failure.
  - Treatment: (1) *Stabilize cardiac membranes* with calcium; (2) promote intracellular shift of potassium with alkalosis (i.e., hyperventilation, bicarbonate), insulin with glucose, and beta-agonism; (3) promote K^+ excretion with loop diuretics, resin exchange; (4) hemodialysis

Calcium

- Hypocalcemia (total serum calcium < 8.5 mg/dL, ionized calcium < 4.6 mg/dL)
  - 40 percent serum calcium is ionized → metabolically active
  - 60 percent serum calcium is complexed with albumin
  - Signs/symptoms: Paresthesias, muscle spasms, cardiac dysrhythmias, seizures, QT prolongation on ECG
  - Chvostek's sign – Tapping facial nerve elicits facial muscle contraction
  - Trousseau's sign – Carpal spasm
  - Causes: Vitamin D deficiency, hypoparathyroidism, chronic renal failure
  - Treatment: Calcium gluconate/chloride[5]
- Hypercalcemia (total serum calcium > 14 mg/dL, ionized Ca > 5.8 mg/dL)
  - Signs/symptoms: Lethargy, weakness, nausea, vomiting, abdominal pain, urinary stones, QT shortening, hypertension, psychiatric symptoms, polyuria
  - Causes: Most common are malignancy or hyperparathyroidism. Others include medications such as diuretics and lithium
  - Treatment: Intravenous fluids, loop diuretics, and bisphosphonates

Magnesium

- Hypomagnesemia (serum magnesium < 1.7 mg/dL) – May cause concomitant hypokalemia, hypocalcemia

- Causes: Poor intake (i.e., chronic alcoholics, malnutrition), medication-induced (i.e., diuretics, laxatives), hypercalcemia
- Signs/symptoms: Fatigue, cardiac arrhythmia, nystagmus, athetosis, muscle weakness/cramps, confusion, nervous system irritability
- Treatment: Raise serum levels > 2 mg/dL, also replace potassium and calcium
- Hypermagnesemia (serum magnesium > 2.3 mg/dL)
  - Causes: Intake (i.e., diuretics, laxatives), renal insufficiency, magnesium administration, rhabdomyolysis, lithium toxicity, adrenal insufficiency
  - Signs/symptoms: Hyporeflexia, weakness, vomiting, flushing, urinary retention, respiratory and myocardial depression (>10 mEq/L), heart block, potentiation of neuromuscular blocker by impaired release of acetylcholine at neuromuscular junction
  - Treatment: Stop intake, calcium to antagonize action, loop diuretic

Phosphorus

- Hypophosphatemia (serum phosphate < 2.5 mg/dL)
  - Causes: Chronic alcoholism, intravenous hyperalimentation (TPN), urinary phosphate wasting (i.e., Fanconi syndrome), chronic antacid use
  - Signs/symptoms: Metabolic encephalopathy, delirium, seizures, cardiac arrhythmias, respiratory weakness due to diaphragm weakness, dysphagia, ileus, decreased red- and white-blood cell function
  - Energy source for ATP; therefore, hypophosphatemia results in muscle weakness, leftward shift of the oxyhemoglobin curve (due to decrease in 2,3-DPG (diphosphoglycerate) levels
- Hyperphosphatemia (serum phosphate > 4.5 mg/dL)
  - Causes: Excessive intake, tumor lysis syndrome, rhabdomyolysis, acute/chronic kidney disease, hypoparathyroidism, acromegaly, bisphosphonates, vitamin D toxicity
  - Signs/symptoms: Also causes hypocalcemia; therefore, similar signs and symptoms as hypocalcemia such as cardiac arrhythmias, muscle spasms, acute renal failure
  - Acute severe hyperphosphatemia associated with symptomatic hypocalcemia can be life threatening
  - Treatment:
    - Acute: Normal saline (although may worsen hypocalcemia), hemodialysis
    - Chronic: Low phosphate diet, phosphate binders

Anatomy of the Kidney

- The kidneys are located in the retroperitoneum and are made up of three regions. The outer cortex, the inner medulla, and the innermost papilla, which empties into calyces that forms the ureter.
- The functional unit of the kidney is the nephron, which is made up of the glomerulus and the renal tubule.

The glomerulus contains a group of capillaries intimately involved with the Bowman's capsule and is the site of plasma filtration. The renal tubule is made up of Bowman's capsule, proximal convoluted tubule, descending and ascending loop of Henle, distal convoluted tubule, and the collecting ducts.

Renal Cortex

1. Receives the majority of blood flow
2. Shorter loops of Henle
3. Most specialized for filtration

Renal Medulla

1. Low flow
2. Longer loops of Henle associated with powerful concentration gradient for optimal reabsorption and secretion
3. Most susceptible to ischemia

Renal Physiology

Renal blood flow (RBF) $\approx$ 20 percent of cardiac output. O_2 consumption is dependent on perfusion.

Right and left renal arteries $\rightarrow$ interlobar a. $\rightarrow$ arcuate a. $\rightarrow$ interlobular a. $\rightarrow$ afferent arteriole enters the glomerulus where ultrafiltrate is formed $\rightarrow$ exit the glomerulus as the efferent arteriole which contributes a network of capillaries that surround the tubule throughout its length allowing for the continued secretion and reabsorption of substances based on a variety of direct and indirect influences.

Renal plasma flow (RPF) = RBF $\times$ (1 – Hct)

Filtration fraction = the percentage of filtrate in the Bowman's space relative to the renal plasma flow = GFR/RPF $\times$ 100 $\simeq$ 20 percent

- Afferent arteriole: Dilated by *prostaglandins,* so increases RPF and GFR
- Efferent arteriole: *Constricted* by *angiotensin,* so decreases RPF but increases GFR
- Catecholamines increase FF by constricting afferent and efferent arterioles

GFR is directly proportional to RPF and dependent on the glomerular filtration pressure. As RPF decreases below a critical point GFR decreases substantially, thus the relationship is *not linear.*

Control of RBF

1. Autoregulation occurs between MAPs 80 and 180 mmHg. MAPs < 50 mmHg result in sharp decline in GFR.
2. Tubuloglomerular feedback: Macula densa cells sense decreased $[Cl^-]$ at distal tubule, low BP, or sympathetic stimulation of B_1 receptors $\rightarrow$ secrete renin
3. Cardiac atria cells sense increased volume $\rightarrow$ secrete atrial natriuretic peptide (ANP) $\rightarrow$ relaxes smooth muscle in the afferent arteriole $\rightarrow$ $\uparrow$GFR
4. Angiotensin II, prostaglandins, and catecholamines affect GFR
5. Neuronal and paracrine regulation via sympathetics from levels T4–L1 and dopamine

GFR is a reflection of overall renal function. Through the passive ultrafiltration of plasma across the glomerular membrane, the kidney is able to regulate total body salt and water content, electrolyte composition, and eliminate waste products of protein metabolism. Alterations in GFR can occur either with changes to any aspect of the Starling forces or through a change in RPF. The forces responsible for glomerular filtration are similar to the forces that operate in systemic capillaries – the Starling forces. GFR can be calculated by inulin clearance (completely filtered and not secreted or reabsorbed). However, in clinical practice creatinine clearance is measured as an estimate of GFR.

Starling Equation

$$GFR = K_f[(P_{GC} - P_{BS}) - \pi_{GC}]$$

Net filtration = $K_f([P_c - P_i] - \sigma[\pi_c - \pi_i])$

K_f = filtration coefficient

P_{GC} = hydrostatic pressure in glomerular capillary

P_{BS} = hydrostatic pressure in Bowman's space

π_{GC} = oncotic pressure in glomerular capillary

P_c = capillary hydrostatic pressure

P_i = interstitial hydrostatic pressure

σ = reflection coefficient

π_c = capillary oncotic pressure

π_i = interstitial oncotic pressure

Tubular Resorption

- Proximal tubule
  - 65–75 percent Na^+, water, and Cl^- are reabsorbed
  - Secretion of hydrogen and reabsorption of bicarbonate ions
  - Secretes organic cations like creatinine
  - As glucose clearance exceeds >160–200 mg/dL exceeds proximal tubules ability/threshold for reabsorption resulting in glucosuria
  - Drugs: Carbonic anhydrase inhibitors (i.e., acetazolamide)
- Loop of Henle (LOH)
  - 25–35 percent ultrafiltrate makes its way to the LOH
  - 15–20 percent Na^+, Ca^{2+}, and Mg^{2+} reabsorbed
  - Drugs: Loop diuretics
- Distal tubule
  - PTH regulated Ca^{2+} reabsorption
  - Aldosterone mediated Na^+ reabsorption
  - Drugs: Thiazides and thiazide-like diuretics (i.e., hydrochlorothiazide, metolazone)
- Collecting duct
  - Site of sodium and H_2O reabsorption mediated by aldosterone
  - Drugs: potassium sparing diuretics (i.e., spironolactone, amiloride)

*Vasopressin receptor inhibitors (i.e., conivaptan) work at both distal tubule and collecting duct

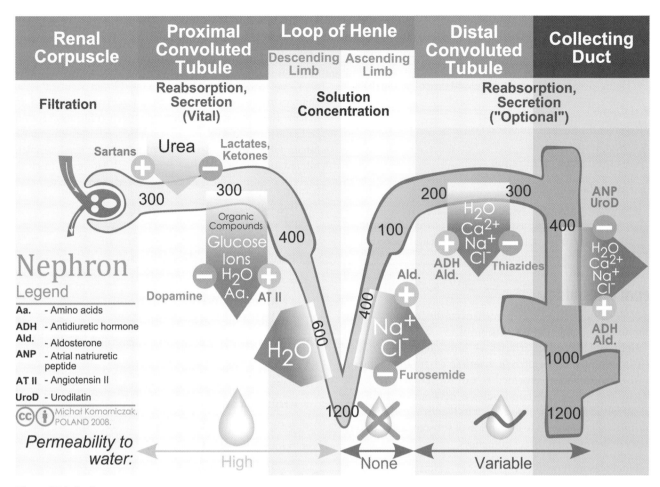

Figure 35.1 Nephron system

The kidneys secrete the following hormones:

- Erythropoietin (EPO)
- Renin
- Prostaglandins
- 1,25-OH$_2$ Vitamin D (Figure 35.1)

Renin–Angiotensin–Aldosterone System (RAAS)

Release of renin depends on beta-adrenergic stimulation, changes in afferent arteriolar wall pressure, and changes in Cl$^-$ flow past the macula densa. Renin acts on angiotensinogen (made in the liver) to form angiotensin I (ATI) (in the lungs). Angiotensin converting enzyme (ACE) acts on AT-I to form angiotensin-II (AT-II), which is responsible for blood pressure regulation and aldosterone secretion.

ADH – produced in hypothalamus → transported to posterior pituitary for release in response to increased serum osmolarity → increases water resorption via aquaporin channel insertion in cells of the collecting tubule.[6]

- **Diabetes insipidis:**
  - Central – decreased secretion of ADH
  - Nephrogenic – kidneys unresponsive to ADH
    - Associated with chronic renal disease, lithium toxicity, hypercalcemia, hypokalemia[7]
- **SIADH (syndrome of inappropriate ADH):** Excessive ADH secretion by the posterior pituitary
  - Euvolemic hyponatremia – Increased diuresis secondary to atrial natriuretic peptide, inhibition of RAAS
  - Urine Na > 20 mEq/L, low serum uric acid

Drug Clearance

Three mechanisms

- Glomerular filtration
- Active secretion by the renal tubules
- Passive reabsorption by the tubules

Drugs may be metabolized by the liver into water-soluble molecules for excretion by the kidney. Alkalinization or acidification of urine can ionize and trap molecules within the tubule for excretion.

- Weak bases → trapped in acidic environments
  - Treatment: ammonium chloride
- Weak acids (e.g., aspirin) → trapped in basic environments
  - Treatment: bicarbonate

Renal Function Tests

BUN (Blood–Urea–Nitrogen)

Protein digestion in the liver produces urea, which aids in the excretion of nitrogenous waste products such as ammonia in the kidneys. It is a surrogate of renal health and is partially reabsorbed at the proximal tubule. When flow to the kidneys is reduced in conditions, such as hypovolemia, the reabsorption is increased and BUN levels rise. Besides intravascular volume status, the BUN levels are *altered with nutritional status, pregnancy, hepatic disease, GI hemorrhage, among others.*

Azotemia = increased BUN and creatinine

Creatinine Clearance

Cockcroft–Gault equation

$$= \frac{(140 - \text{age}) \times \text{wt (kg)}}{\text{Serum} \times \text{creatinine(mg/dL)} \times 72} \times (\times 0.85 \text{ for women})$$

Creatinine is secreted by the renal tubules. Therefore, *Creatinine clearance* is an overestimation of GFR.

Urinalysis

1. RBC – indicates glomerular filtration dysregulation (e.g., trauma, infections, tumors)
2. WBC – infection
3. Proteinuria – parenchymal disease
4. Fatty casts – nephrotic syndrome
5. Ketones – DKA, starvation
6. Urine specific gravity: (range: 1.003–1.03) indirect measure of hydration
7. Urine osmolality: (350–500 mOsm) indirect measure of hydration
8. Urine sodium: (20–40 mEq) indirect measure of sodium excretion

Oliguria = urine output < 0.5 mL/kg/hour

Anuria = UOP < 100 mL/day (Table 35.2)

Fractional excretion of sodium (FENa$^+$): Utilized to assist in differentiating pre-renal, intrarenal, and post-renal etiologies of acute renal failure.

$$\text{FENa}^+ = \text{Na}_{\text{urine}} \times \text{creatinine}_{\text{plasma}} \times 100$$

$$\text{Na}_{\text{plasma}} \times \text{creatinine}_{\text{urinary}}$$

<1% = prerenal
>1% = intrarenal or postrenal

Renal Pathology

Acute kidney injury = Abrupt loss of kidney function resulting in retention of urea and other nitrogenous waste products and in the dysregulation of extracellular volume and electrolytes.

AKI defined according to KDIGO (kidney disease improving global outcomes)

- Increase in serum creatinine by >0.3 mg/dL within 48 hours;

Table 35.2

Test of glomerular function	Normal values	Causes of pathology
BUN	8–20 mg/dL	Dehydration, protein intake, GI bleeding, catabolism
Serum creatinine	0.5–1.2 mg/dL	Age, muscle mass, catabolism
Creatinine clearance	120 mL/minute	Age, medications

Table 35.3

Test	Postrenal	Renal	Prerenal
BUN:creatinine	<15	<15	>20
FENa	>4%	>1%	<1%
Urine Na	>40	>20	<20
Urine osmolality	<350	<350	>500

- Increase in serum creatinine to >1.5× baseline which is known to have occurred within the prior 7 days; or
- Urine volume <0.5 mL/kg/hour for 6 hours (Table 35.3)

Pre-renal kidney injury occurs with decreased perfusion to the kidneys, which may occur due to hypotension, blood loss, heart failure, and liver disease.

Contrast-Induced Nephropathy (CIN)

- Injury to the kidneys is multifactorial
- Risk factors: diabetes mellitus, chronic kidney failure, concomitant exposure to other nephrotoxic agents, dehydration, advanced age
- Prevention: normal saline infusion 100 mL/hour × 12 hours prior to exposure is the only intervention supported by most literature. The literature is inconclusive on the effectiveness of N-acetylcysteine and bicarbonate.

Chronic Kidney Disease (CKD)

CKD is divided into different stages of disease according to the GFR and the presence of albuminuria:

1. Stage 1 disease is defined by a normal GFR (>90 mL/minute/1.73 m^2) and persistent albuminuria
2. Stage 2 disease is a GFR between 60 and 89 mL/minute/1.73 m^2 and persistent albuminuria
3. Stage 3 disease is a GFR between 30 and 59 mL/minute/1.73 m^2
4. Stage 4 disease is a GFR between 15 and 29 mL/minute/1.73 m^2
5. Stage 5 disease is a GFR of <15 mL/minute/1.73 m^2 or ESRD[8]
   - Causes: diabetes mellitus, chronic hypertension, glomerulonephritis, obstructive, toxicity, hepatitis B/C, and HIV

- Signs and symptoms of chronic kidney insufficiency typically manifest when GFR < 15 mL/minute, and when present may indicate end-stage renal disease (ESRD)

End-Stage Renal Disease

Hyperkalemia, hypocalcemia, metabolic acidosis, uremia (a cause of platelet dysfunction), hyperphosphatemia, anemia (decreased erythropoietin and iron deficiency)

- Treatment → dialysis versus continuous veno-venous hemofiltration (CVVH)
- Indications (AEIOU)

  Acidosis (pH < 7.1)

  Electrolyte abnormalities (Hyperkalemia > 6.5)

  Ingestion of toxic substance that can be dialyzed

  Overload (volume)

  Symptomatic **U**remia (>30 mg/dL)

- CVVH: Convection and ultrafiltration, reserved for critically ill patients that would not tolerate cardiovascular stress associated with dialysis. Greater overall clearance and volume removal compared to hemodialysis (24-hour removal compared to 3–4 hours)
- Hemodialysis – Diffusion of substances across a semipermeable membrane
  - Adverse effects: Hypotension (too much fluid removed), "dialysis disequilibrium" (rapid fluid and urea shifts resulting in cerebral edema, headache, coma), hypocalcemia, fever, hypokalemia-induced arrhythmias, bleeding (due to heparinization)[9]
  - Electrolyte disturbances: Hypokalemia/magnesemia/calcemia, increased pH due to bicarbonate infusion, hyper or hyponatremia[9]

Acid–Base Balance and the Kidney

The kidneys are essential in the management of acid–base balance in the body through the reabsorption of HCO_3^- and the excretion of H^+ (or NH_4^+).

HCO_3^- reabsorption (primarily at the proximal tubule)

- Na^+/H^+ exchanger at the luminal membrane of cells pumps H^+ ions into the lumen → combines with filtered HCO_3^- → forms $H_2CO_3^-$ → breaks down into CO_2 and H_2O which are reabsorbed into the cell where they are converted via carbonic anhydrase back to HCO_3^- and H^+. The bicarbonate is reclaimed and the H^+ is used to repeat the cycle.
- Contraction alkalosis – activation of renin–angiotensin system results in angiotensin-II-mediated stimulation of the Na^+/H^+ exchanger → increase reabsorption of HCO_3^-.[10]
  - Seen with diuretic use and as a complication of vomiting

H^+ Excretion (primarily at the distal tubule and collecting duct) hydrogen combines with HPO_4^{2-}, NH_3, and Cl^-.

- H^+ ATPase – stimulated by aldosterone
- H^+/K^+ ATPase

Respiratory Alkalosis

- Initial change: ↓PCO_2 due to increased alveolar ventilation
- Compensatory response: ↓HCO_3
  - Acute → intracellular buffering, for every 10 mmHg change in PCO_2 bicarbonate will fall 2 mEq/L
  - Chronic → decreased renal reabsorption of bicarb, for every 10 mmHg change in PCO_2 bicarb will fall 5 mEq/L
- Causes: Hyperventilation secondary to pneumonia, pulmonary edema, PE, salicylates, pregnancy, sepsis, anxiety

Respiratory Acidosis

- Initial change: ↑PCO_2
- Compensatory response: ↑HCO_3^-
  - Acute → intracellular buffering, 1 mEq/L ↑HCO_3^- for every 10 mmHg change in PCO_2
  - Chronic → generation of new bicarb due to the excretion of ammonium, 4 mEq/L ↑HCO_3^- for every 10 mmHg change in PCO_2
- Causes: Hypoventilation secondary to sedatives, neuromuscular pathology, airway obstruction, COPD/asthma

Note: "1-2-4-5" rule: change of 1, 2, 4, 5 mEq/L for acute acidosis, acute alkalosis, chronic acidosis, chronic alkalosis, respectively

Metabolic Alkalosis

- Initial change: ↑HCO_3^-
- Compensatory response: ↑ PCO_2 via decreased ventilation
- Causes: GI suctioning, vomiting, loop/thiazide diuretics, primary aldosteronism

Metabolic Acidosis

- Initial change: ↓HCO_3^-
- Compensatory response: ↓PCO_2 via increased ventilation, $PCO_2 = (1.5 \times [HCO_3^-]) + 8 \pm 2$ = expected compensation
- Causes: "MUDPILES" and "HARDUPS"
  - Causes of anion gap metabolic acidosis (*MUDPILES*): methanol, uremia, diabetic ketoacidosis, propylene glycol, infection/isoniazid, lactic acid, ethylene glycol, salicylates[11]
  - Causes of non-anion gap metabolic acidosis (*HARDUPS*): hyperalimentation (TPN), acetazolamide/topiramate, renal tubular acidosis/CKD, diarrhea, ureterosigmoid conduit, pancreatico-enteric fistula, saline[11]
- Treatment: Alkalinize urine to trap ionic species for excretion, correct acidemia, hemodialysis in critical cases
  - Salicylate poisoning: Tinnitus, tachypnea (CNS stimulation → respiratory alkalosis), tachycardia, sweating, nausea/vomiting, hyperthermia, altered mentation
  - Ethylene glycol poisoning: Ingredient in antifreeze, ingestion symptoms include altered mentation, seizures, pulmonary edema, kidney failure associated with calcium oxalate crystals. Metabolism by alcohol dehydrogenase generates toxic formic acid

- Methanol: Metabolized by alcohol dehydrogenase into toxic formaldehyde resulting in symptoms that include nausea/vomiting
  - Treatment: EtOH and fomepizole compete for alcohol dehydrogenase limiting metabolism of methanol and ethylene glycol

Acid–Base Tips

- Henderson–Hasselbach equation $pH = pKa + \log [A^-]/[HA]$
- Winters formula $P_{CO_2} = 1.5\,(HCO_3^-) + 8 \pm 2$
  - Estimates expected change in CO_2 in metabolic acidosis.

- Anion gap $(AG) = Na^+ - (Cl^- + HCO_3^-) = 10{-}15$ (normal value)

  Acidemia $= pH < 7.36$

  Alkalemia $= pH > 7.44$

  Acid–base disorder workup? Obtain pH, PCO_2, HCO_3

- First, determine primary disorder
- Second, calculate anion gap
- Third, determine whether compensation is expected

The respiratory system compensates for acid–base disturbances rather quickly, whereas the renal systems response is delayed.

References

1. Neligan P. J. (2012). Chapter 35. Monitoring and Managing Perioperative Electrolyte Abnormalities, Acid–Base Disorders, and Fluid Replacement. In: Longnecker D. E., Brown D. L., Newman M. F., Zapol W. M., eds. *Anesthesiology*, 2nd edn. New York, NY: McGraw-Hill.
2. Liamis G., Filippatos T. D., Elisaf M. S. Pages 299–306. Published online: February 23, 2016.
3. Wee T., Goldberg M., Gulati A., Schleyer A. (2010, September 15). Hypokalemia. Retrieved March 3, 2017, from https://eresources .library.mssm.edu:2073/#!/content/ medical_topic/21-s2.0-1014738

4. "Hyperkalemia." Open Anesthesia. (n.d.). Retrieved March 10, 2017, from https://selfstudyplus.openanesthesia .org/kw/entry/14128
5. Regmi, S., Silva, P., Pollak, E., Lash, R. (2012, May 3). Hypocalcemia. Retrieved March 3, 2017, from https:// eresources.library.mssm.edu:2073/#!/ content/medical_topic/21-s2.0-1014736
6. SIADH Electrolytes. (n.d.). Retrieved March 7, 2017, from https:// selfstudyplus.openanesthesia.org/kw/ entry/14051
7. Diabetes Insipidus Intracranial Surgery. (n.d.). Retrieved March 7, 2017, from https://selfstudyplus .openanesthesia.org/kw/entry/13547

8. Cohen, D., Goldberg, M., Gulati, A., & Ferri, F. (2014, March 5). Chronic Kidney Disease. Retrieved March 8, 2017, from https://eresources .library.mssm.edu:2073/#!/content/ medical_topic/21-s2.0-1014826
9. Hemodialysis Effects. (n.d.). Retrieved March 7, 2017, from https://selfstudyplus.openanesthesia .org/kw/entry/14051
10. Costanzo, L. S. (2014). *Physiology*, 5th edn. Philadelphia, PA: Saunders/ Elsevier.
11. Metabolic Acidosis: Etiology. (n.d.). Retrieved March 5, 2017, from https:// selfstudyplus.openanesthesia.org/kw/ entry/-KJIGu7f9QcFZFfOJ-A7

Chapter 36

Renal Pharmacology

Jonah Abraham, Douglas Adams, Marshall Bahr, and Sanford Littwin

Diuretics[1,2,5]

Carbonic Anhydrase Inhibitors: Acetazolamide, Methazolamide
- Site of action: Proximal tubule
- Mechanism: Inhibits the activity of carbonic anhydrase (enzyme that converts $CO_2 + H_2O \rightleftharpoons HCO_3 + H^+$)
  - Reduces hydrogen ion secretion at renal tubule, with increased excretion of sodium, potassium, bicarbonate, and water
- Adverse drug reactions: Inhibits sodium resorption, interferes with hydrogen excretion
  - Chronic administration may lead to hyperchloremic, hypokalemic acidosis
  - Alkalinized urine may lead to nephrolithiasis
  - Peripheral neuropathy, sulfa allergy

Loop Diuretics: Furosemide, Torsemide, Ethacrynic Acid, Bumetanide
- Site of action: Thick ascending limb of the loop of Henle
- Mechanism: Inhibits Na^+, K^+, 2 Cl^- transport system
  - Blocks more ions, therefore produces more diuresis in comparison to other diuretics
- Adverse drug reactions: Inhibits sodium and chloride resorption, augments secretion of potassium
  - Chronic administration may lead to hypochloremic, hypokalemic metabolic alkalosis
  - Ototoxicity, hypokalemia, sulfa allergy, gout
  - Hyperuricemia (gout), hypocalcemia, hypomagnesemia, hyperglycemia, pancreatitis, hypokalemia, ototoxicity

Thiazides: Hydrochlorothiazide, Chlorthalidone, Metolazone
- Site of action: Distal tubule and connecting segment
- Mechanism: blocks Na^+/Cl^- co-transporter
  - Leads to increase in urinary sodium and eventual diuresis
- Adverse drug reaction: Inhibits sodium resorption, augments secretion of potassium
  - Leads to hypokalemia (through acceleration of sodium–potassium exchange)
  - May lead to hyperglycemia, hyperlipidemia, hyperuricemia (gout), hypomagnesemia, hypercalcemia
  - Chronic administration may lead to hypochloremic, hypokalemic metabolic alkalosis

Potassium-Sparing Diuretics: Spironolactone, Trimaterene, Amiloride, Eplerenone
- Site of action: Cortical collecting tubule
- Mechanism: Aldosterone-sensitive sodium channels. Works via two different mechanisms:
  - Spironolactone: Competitively inhibits the mineralocorticoid receptor aldosterone which increases the synthesis and activity of the Na^+/K^+ pump
  - Amiloride and triamterene: Directly decrease sodium channel activity
- Adverse drug reactions: Inhibits sodium resorption and sodium–potassium exchange (preventing loss of potassium)
  - Chronic administration may lead to hyperkalemia, gynecomastia, hirsutism

Osmotic Diuretics: Mannitol, Glycerin
- Site of action: Proximal tubule
- Mechanism: Freely filtered, non-reabsorbable, non-metabolized sugar alcohol
  - Remains in the tubular lumen creating osmotic gradient of water into lumen
- Adverse drug reactions: Hyperosmolality which reduces cellular water, increased excretion of water, volume depletion, and hypernatremia
  - High doses lead to hyperosmolar plasma, extracellular volume expansion, dilutional *hyponatremia, hyperkalemia*, and metabolic acidosis

Dopaminergic Agents[3]

Dopamine
- Mechanism: Mixed agonist effects with dopaminergic, α and β receptors
  - *Dopaminergic*: Effects mediated by increased cAMP
    - Low infusion rate (1–5 mcg/kg/min): Increased renal blood flow and urine output
    - Intermediate dosage (5–15 mcg/kg/min): Increased renal blood flow, heart rate, cardiac output, and blood pressure
    - High dosage (>15 mcg/kg/min): Alpha-adrenergic effects predominate, vasoconstriction, increased blood pressure

- ○ **α-*Alpha***: (>5 mcg/kg/min)
  - α$_1$ stimulation leading to vasoconstriction
  - Theoretically decreased renal blood flow
- ○ **β-*Beta***: (3–5 mcg/kg/min dosing)
  - Direct and indirect β$_1$ and β$_2$ stimulation
  - Increased cardiac contractility and cardiac output

Fenoldopam[4]
- Mechanism: Selective D$_1$ receptor agonist
  - ○ Decreases blood pressure
  - ○ Increases renal blood flow, creatinine clearance, urinary flow, and sodium excretion
  - ○ Does not directly cause increased cardiac contractility but may lead to reflex tachycardia

References

1. Hropot M., Fowler N., Karlmark B., Giebisch G. Tubular action of diuretics: distal effects on electrolyte transport and acidification. *Kidney Int.* 1985; 28: 477.
2. Rose B. D. Diuretics. *Kidney Int.* 1991; 39: 336.
3. Jain, A. Chen, H. ROSE-AHF and Lessons Learned. *Curr Heart Fail Rep.* 2014 Sep; 11(3):260–5. doi: 10.1007/s11897-014-0208-6.
4. Weber RR, McCoy CE, Ziemniak JA, Frederickson ED, Goldberg LI, Murphy MB. Pharmacokinetic and pharmacodynamic properties of intravenous fenoldopam, a dopamine1-receptor agonist, in hypertensive patients. *Br J Clin Pharmacol.* 1988; 25: 17–21.
5. Sica D. A., Carter B., Cushman W., Hamm L. Thiazide and loop diuretics. *J Clin Hypertens. (Greenwich).* 2011; 13(9): 639–43. doi: 10.1111/j.1751-7176.2011.00512.x.

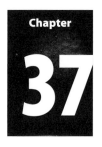
Hematologic System: Coagulation, Anticoagulation, Antiplatelet, and Thrombolytics

Katelyn O'Connor and Raj Parekh

Hemostasis

- **Primary Hemostasis:** Formation of the platelet plug (Figure 37.1)
  - Injured endothelium exposes procoagulant subendothelial matrix which *binds to platelets*
  - Platelet adhesion: Occurs via *von Willebrand Factor* (*vWF*) and transmembrane glycoproteins (GP)
  - Platelet activation: Platelets become activated by exposed subendothelium and *thrombin*, leading to conformational changes causing multiple events
    - ADP-rich granules released, allowing ADP to bind platelet receptors (i.e., P2Y$_{12}$) to recruit more platelets
    - Arachidonic acid produced and converted to thromboxane A$_2$ by COX-1
  - Platelet plug: Fibrinogen cross-links with GP IIb/IIIa receptors on platelets to form the *platelet plug*

- **Secondary hemostasis:** Coagulation factors *produce fibrin* which cross-links to stabilize the platelet plug (Figure 37.2)
  - Extrinsic pathway: Exposed tissue factor in the endothelium will *activate thrombin* (factor IIa) and factor IXa

  - Intrinsic pathway: Thrombin activates *factor X, XI, factor VIIIa*
  - Common pathway: Thrombin also activates *factor V*

Three common groups of drugs (anticoagulants, antiplatelet agents, and thrombolytic agents) are used to treat and prevent particular vascular diseases. Older anticoagulants include unfractionated heparin (UFH), low molecular weight heparin (LMWH) and warfarin whereas newer oral anticoagulants include direct thrombin inhibitors and factor Xa inhibitors. Indications for newer drugs are continually changing as new data is published and reviewed by the FDA. The same is true for antiplatelet agents where more effective drugs are being discovered and used in every day practice.

Anticoagulants

Unfractionated Heparin

- Mechanism:
  - *Binds antithrombin III* and induces conformational change that facilitates its ability to primarily inactivate thrombin (factor IIa) and factor Xa but also *inactivates factors VII, IX, XI, and XII*

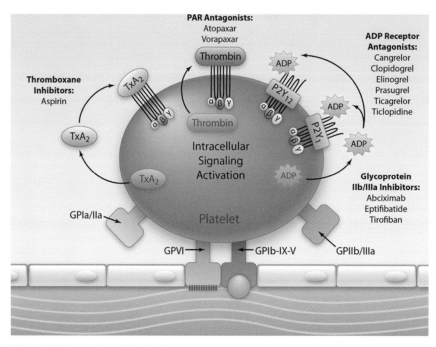

Figure 37.1 Formation of platelet plug

The three pathways that makeup the classical blood coagulation pathway

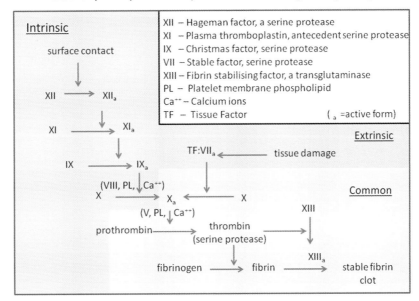

Figure 37.2 Coagulation cascade
Data from Pallister and Watson (2010)[1]

Table 37.1 Types of HIT

HIT type-I:
- *Non-immune-mediated*
- Rapid onset (2–5 days)
- *<50% decrease in platelets*
- Resolves on its own

HIT type-II:
- *IgG reaction* to platelet factor 4-heparin (PF4) complexes
- Onset 5–14 days
- *Systemic thrombosis* (venous and arterial)
- Discontinue heparin and start alternative IV anticoagulant (i.e., direct thrombin inhibitor)

- o Inactivating thrombin prevents the conversion of fibrinogen to fibrin
- Advantages: Preferred in renal failure
- Disadvantages: Hereditary or acquired antithrombin III deficiency can result in heparin resistance, such that normal doses of heparin fail to provide adequate anticoagulation
  - o Risk of heparin-induced thrombocytopenia (HIT) – Two types are discussed in Table 37.1
    - Bleeding
    - Rapid bolus → moderate ↓ SVR and BP (unclear reason)
- Reversal: With protamine
  - o **Mechanism of action:** *acid–base neutralization* – protamine (+) antagonizes heparin (−)
  - o Common reversal dose is 1 mg of protamine per 100 units of heparin
  - o **Protamine reactions:**
    - Type 1: *systemic hypotension* secondary to rapid administration causing *mast cell and histamine release*
    - Type 2: *anaphylaxis from IgE-mediated* dose-independent reaction in a patient with *previous exposure*

- Type 3: *pulmonary hypertensive crisis* via protamine–heparin complex stimulation of *thromboxane A2 release*[2-5]

Low Molecular Weight Heparin

- Mechanism:
  - o Binds and *enhances* effects of *antithrombin III*
  - o LMWH-antithrombin III complex binds to and preferentially *inactivates factor Xa*
  - o Has shorter saccharide units than UFH and so make LMWH ineffective in inhibiting thrombin directly
- Advantages: Does not require regular PTT screening and so can be used for outpatient treatment.
- Disadvantages:
  - o Increased risk of bleeding with long-term use
  - o Risk of HIT, monitor platelet count periodically (lower risk compared to UFH)
  - o Decreased kidney function could significantly increase plasma level[2-5]

Warfarin

- Mechanism:
  - o Inhibits *vitamin K epoxide reductase* in the liver which reduces the *gamma carboxylation of vitamin K-dependent coagulation factors*
  - o Decreases the amount of vitamin K-dependent clotting proteins: *Factors II, VII, IX, and X and anticoagulant proteins C+S* (hence a transient pro-coagulant effect)
- Drug interactions:
  - o CYP450 inducers: St. John's Wort, barbiturates, carbamazepine, phenytoin, rifampin → *decreased warfarin effects*

185

Table 37.2 Heparin, LMWH, and warfarin[2–7]

Type	Onset	Half-life	Metabolism	Monitoring	Reversal
Heparin IV, SQ	IV: immediate SQ: 20–30 min	30–60 min	Inactivated in liver and kidney	PTT ACT (high dose)	Protamine
LMWH SQ	20–60 min	3–6 h	Renal clearance	Factor Xa assay[a]	Protamine[b]
Warfarin PO, IV	90 min	35–40 h	Hepatic (CYP450)	PT/INR	Non-urgent: Vitamin K Urgent: FFP, prothrombin complex concentrate (PCC)

[a]Routine monitoring typically unnecessary.
[b]Less reliable reversal agent than for heparin.

Table 37.3 Direct thrombin inhibitors[2,3,8,9]

Type	Mechanism	Half-life	Metabolism	Monitoring	Notes
Argatroban IV	*Reversible* binding to catalytic site of thrombin	45 min	Hepatic	PTT, ACT	– Preferred in renal insufficiency
Dabigatran PO	*Prodrug* converted in liver; binds *reversibly* to thrombin	12–14 h	Renal clearance	Dilute thrombin time, PTT	– Peak effect in 2 hrs – Dose adjustment in renal insufficiency – Reversal with Idarucizumab (Praxbind) – Activated charcoal and hemodialysis can also aid in non-emergent reversal
Hirudin IIV, topical	Binds *irreversibly* to thrombin	40–80 min	Renal clearance	ECT (ecarin clotting time)	– Naturally occurring peptide found in leeches
Bivalirudin IV	Binds *reversibly* to thrombin	25 min	Peptidase degradation, renal excretion	Low dose: PTT High dose: ACT	– Studied for use as heparin substitute in cardiac surgery with HIT type II
Lepirudin IV (infusion)	Binds *irreversibly* to thrombin	60 min	Renal	PTT	– Recombinant form of hirudin – Accumulates in renal failure – *Fatal anaphylaxis* (if treated again within 3 months of exposure)

- CYP450 inhibitors: Levofloxacin, omeprazole, amiodarone → *increased warfarin effects*
- Disadvantages:
  - Bleeding
  - Warfarin-induced skin necrosis: Protein C with a half-life of 6 hours has quick decline in plasma, resulting in initial shift toward clotting
  - Crosses the placenta (Table 37.2)[2,3,7]

Direct Thrombin Inhibitors

- Mechanism: Bind directly to thrombin (factor IIa) which:
  - Prevent the conversion of fibrinogen to fibrin
  - Prevent the activation of factors V, VIII, IX, and XIII
  - Prevent the activation of platelets
- Indications: Include treatment and prevention of venous thromboembolism (VTE), atrial fibrillation, acute coronary syndrome, and HIT (Table 37.3)[2,3]

Factor Xa Inhibitors

- Mechanism: Binds to factor Xa which prevents it from converting prothrombin to thrombin

- Same potential indications as direct thrombin inhibitors
- No FDA-approved reversal agent (Table 37.4)

Antiplatelet Agents

Aspirin

- Mechanism:
  - Irreversible *inhibitor of COX-1 and COX-2*
  - Prevents formation of thromboxane (potent platelet aggregator)
- Indication: Secondary prevention of cardiovascular events in patients with coronary artery disease, peripheral vascular disease, cerebrovascular disease
- Disadvantages (dose-related): dyspepsia → peptic ulcers with bleeding/perforation

Dipyridamole

- Weak antiplatelet agent on its own, but extended-release formulation combined with low dose aspirin is used for prevention of stroke in patients with transient ischemic attacks (TIA)

Table 37.4 Factor Xa inhibitors[2,3,9-11]

Type	Mechanism	Half-life	Metabolism	Monitoring	Notes
Fondaparinux IV	Pentasaccharide unit binds and activates antithrombin III	21 h	Cleared unchanged by kidneys	*Not required	– Does NOT cause HIT – Increased risk of bleeding with long-term use
Rivaroxaban PO	*Reversibly* binds and inhibits factor Xa, preventing conversion of prothrombin to thrombin	5–9 h	33% renal clearance 66% fecal/biliary	– Anti-Xa assay – Dilute PT assay	– Peak effect 2.5–4 h – Emergent reversal with PCC4 or PCC3 plus FFP – Avoid with CrCl < 15 mL/min
Apixaban PO	*Reversibly* binds and inhibits factor Xa, preventing conversion of prothrombin to thrombin	15 h	25% renal clearance 75% fecal/biliary	– Anti-Xa assay – Dilute PT assay	– Peak effect 1–2 h

- Mechanism:
  - *Inhibits phosphodiesterase* → blocks the breakdown of cAMP
  - Increased cAMP → reduce intracellular calcium → inhibits platelet activation

GP IIB/IIIA Inhibitors

- Mechanism: Prevents binding of fibrinogen and vWF to GP IIb/IIIa receptors, causing *inhibition of platelet aggregation*
- Reversal: None (control by discontinuation of drug)

ADP Receptor Antagonists

- Mechanism: Interferes with fibrinogen binding to platelets and thus *inhibits ADP-induced primary and secondary platelet aggregation* (Table 37.5)[3]

Antithrombotic Agents

Tissue Plasmin Activators (tPa)

- Also serves as *anticoagulant*: Fibrinolysis generates increased amounts of circulating fibrin degradation products → *inhibit platelet aggregation* by binding to platelet surfaces
- Avoid surgery or puncture of noncompressible vessel within 10-day period after use
- Native:
  - Streptokinase, urokinase
  - Potent activators of plasmin
  - Mechanism: Cleave bond from plasminogen to form plasmin
- Exogenous:
  - Alteplase, tenecteplase
  - Mechanism: More fibrin selective; less selectivity for circulating plasminogen

Alternatives to Transfusion

- Normovolemic hemodilution[12]
  - Principle: If RBC concentration is decreased, total RBC loss is reduced when a large amount of blood is lost and cardiac output is maintained because intravascular volume is maintained
  - Mechanism:
    - 1–2 units removed just prior to surgery via large bore IV
    - Replace with crystalloid/colloids: Patient remains normovolemic, but now with Hct 21–25%
    - Blood stored in CPDA (citrate–phosphate–dextrose–adenine) bag at room temperature (up to 6 hours) to preserve platelet function
    - Blood should be infused in reverse order of removal: First unit has highest Hct, platelets, and clotting factors and is preferably transfused last
  - Effects:
    - Decrease in blood viscosity → increase in tissue perfusion and reduced intraoperative RBC loss
    - Decreased arterial O_2 content → compensatory tachycardia and increased cardiac output → increased myocardial O_2 consumption → potential risk of myocardial ischemia
- Sequestration[12]
  - Principle: Pooling of blood in vascular space until it is needed
  - Mechanism:
    - Tourniquets placed on the upper and lower extremities allow blood to be isolated from the general circulation
    - Sequestered volume replaced with crystalloid/colloid
    - When tourniquets released, blood bolus returns to circulation

Table 37.5 Antiplatelet drugs[3]

Type	Mechanism	Half-life	Metabolism	Monitoring	Notes
Abciximab IV	GP IIB/IIIA inhibitor	30 min	Proteolytic cleavage (unbound)	*Not recommended*	– 24–48 h for platelets to normalize
Eptifibatide IV	GP IIB/IIIA inhibitor	2.5 h	Renal clearance/urinary excretion	*Not recommended*	– 8 h for platelets to normalize
Tirofiban IV	GP IIB/IIIA inhibitor	2 h	Negligible metabolism (excreted in urine unchanged)	*Not recommended*	– 8 h for platelets to normalize
Clopidogrel PO	Prodrug metabolized by P450 to irreversibly inhibit platelet $P2Y_{12}$ receptors	6 h	Hepatic (active and inactive metabolites)	*Not recommended*	– Steady state in 7 days – 60% platelet inhibition – Preferred to ticlopidine (better safety profile) – Higher incidence of heightened platelet reactivity (HPR) and hence treatment failure then prasugrel
Ticlodipine PO	Inhibits ADP receptor-mediated platelet activation	13 h	Hepatic (active metabolite)	*Not recommended*	– Steady state in 14–21 days – Black Box Warning: agranulocytosis, TTP, aplastic anemia – Not available in United States
Prasugrel PO	P2Y-12 receptor irreversible inhibitor	4 h	Rapid intestinal and serum metabolism via ester hydrolysis, then CYP450 to active metabolite	$P2Y_{12}$ assay, TEG	– Peak effect 1 h – 90% platelet inhibition – Contraindicated if prior TIA/stroke
Ticagrelor PO	*Reversible* ADP analog on P2Y-12 receptor	7–9 h	Hepatic via CYP34A	p2y-12assay, TEG	– Peak effect 2–4 h

- o Effects:
  - Volume overload may occur with tourniquet release
  - Greater tourniquet time → greater amount of acidic blood returned to circulation
  - Risk of stasis and thrombosis in sequestered extremities
- Autotransfusion[12]
  - o Preoperative:
    - Collection 4–5 weeks prior to procedure
    - Minimum requirement is to donate 1 unit: Hct $\geq$ 34% or Hgb $\geq$11 g/dL
    - Requires concurrent iron supplementation and erythropoietin therapy
    - Advantages:
      - Reduced risk of infection and transfusion reaction
      - Conservation of blood resources
      - Blood can be frozen indefinitely for later use
    - Disadvantages:
      - Expensive
      - Does not necessarily reduce the need for allogenic transfusion
      - Does not reduce certain risks: Immunological reactions due to clerical errors, bacterial contamination, improper storage

- Intraoperative (Cell Saver)
  - o Estimated blood volume needs to be >1,000–1,500 mL to be effective
  - o Mechanism:
    - Blood loss aspirated into reservoir and mixed with heparin
    - RBCs are concentrated and washed to remove debris and anticoagulant
    - Salvaged blood concentrate reinfused to patient contains RBC and normal saline with Hct 50–60%
  - o Advantages:
    - Often accepted by Jehovah's Witnesses
    - Valuable in patients with alloantibodies
    - Limits exposure to pathogens
  - o Disadvantages:
    - Contraindications: Septic contamination, malignancy
    - Complications: Dilutional coagulopathy (coagulation factors, platelets, and calcium are not salvaged), hemolysis, air embolism, DIC, reinfusion of excess anticoagulant

Blood Substitutes[12]
Can carry and release oxygen and offer benefit for short periods. There is still a lack of evidence of their safety and efficacy for longer periods (30 days).

Table 37.6 Immunosuppressive and antirejection drugs[13,14]

Type	Mechanism	Side effects	Notes
Prednisone	Inhibit T-cell interaction	*Cushing's disease*, poor wound healing, bone disease, glucose intolerance, hypertension, cataracts	– Useful in treatment and prevention of acute rejection
Muromonab-CD3	Inhibit T-cell interaction	Fever, anaphylactic reactions, and pulmonary edema, cytokine release syndrome	– Primarily used for induction therapy for solid organ transplant
Antithymocyte globulin	Inhibit adhesion molecules	*Anaphylaxis*, leukopenia, fever, nausea, chills	– Used for induction therapy and treatment of acute kidney rejection
Cyclosporine	Inhibit cytokine synthesis	*Nephrotoxicity*, hepatotoxicity, *hypertension*, and neurotoxicity	– Induction and maintenance – *P450 interactions*: CYP3A – Alters barbiturate, benzodiazepine, fentanyl, and isoflurane requirements – Enhance neuromuscular blockade (NMB) – *Require monitoring of drug level* (renal and hepatic function can be affected)
Tacrolimus	Inhibit cytokine synthesis	*Nephrotoxicity*, neurotoxicity, hypertension, glucose intolerance, *lowers seizure threshold*	– Maintenance and rescue therapy for refractory acute rejection of liver transplant – *P450 interactions*: CYP3A – *Require monitoring of drug level* (renal and hepatic function can be affected)
Sirolimus	Inhibit cytokine synthesis	Myelosuppression, hyperlipidemia	– Used for maintenance, combined with other drugs to avoid permanent renal damage – Long half-life – *P450 interactions*: CYP3A4
Azathioprine	Inhibit DNA synthesis	Myelosuppression, hepatic dysfunction, pancreatitis	– Used for maintenance – Antagonizes NMB in renal failure
Mycophenolate mofetil	Inhibit DNA synthesis	Myelosuppression, diarrhea, vomiting	– Used for maintenance and chronic rejection – Never combine with azathioprine (risk of myelosuppression)

- Polymerized hemoglobin-based oxygen carriers
  - Hemoglobin molecules polymerized for longevity
  - Advantage: Ability to load hemoglobin at physiologic PaO_2 (just like normal Hgb)
  - Disadvantage:
    - Hypertension: Complication of clinical trials due to inhibition of endogenous NO
    - Toxicity to myocardium, liver, and kidneys documented (currently offered on a compassionate use basis)
- Perfluorocarbon emulsions
  - Hydrophilic liquids with fluoride and carbon atoms
  - Advantage: Can dissolve significant amounts of gases, including O_2 and CO_2
  - Disadvantage: Linear O_2 dissociation curve, thus supplemental O_2 and supraphysiologic PaO_2 required to maximize oxygen delivery
- Neither type has been released for clinical use

Erythropoietin[12]
- GP hormone produced by peritubular cells of the kidney
- Mechanism: Acts as a cytokine for RBC production in the bone marrow by *promoting blast cell maturation*
- Use:
  - Preoperative anemia for elective, non-cardiac surgery → decreases need for intraoperative blood transfusions, and overall morbidity and mortality rates
  - Jehovah's Witnesses (off-label)
  - Stimulate erythropoiesis in CKD patients
- Typically takes 2 weeks or more to gain as much as 2 gm/dL of Hgb concentration
- Recombinant erythropoietin is very expensive
- Black box warning: Death, MI, stroke, venous thromboembolism
- Must dose with supplemental iron (Table 37.6)

References

1. Pallister C. J., Watson M. S. *Haematology*, 2 edition. Kent, UK: Pallister and Watson Scion Publishing Ltd.; 2010.
2. Badr R. Hematologic System: Anticoagulants: Mechanism of Action, Comparison of Drugs, Drug Interactions, Monitoring of Effects, Side Effects and Toxicity. In: *Learnly: Online Anesthesia Basic Science Curriculum*. Stanford, CA: Stanford AIM Lab; 2017.
3. Oprea A. D. Hematologic System: Pharmacology: Antithrombotic and Anti-Platelet Drugs: Mechanism of Action, Comparison of Drugs, Drug Interactions, Monitoring of Effects, Side Effects and Toxicity. In: *Learnly: Online*

Anesthesia Basic Science Curriculum. Stanford, CA: Stanford AIM Lab; 2017.

4. Miller R.D. *Miller's Anesthesia.* 6th edn. Philadelphia, PA: Churchill Livingstone/Elsevier; 2010, 357–9.

5. Heparin (unfractionated). In: Lexi-Comp Online™, Lexi-Drugs Online™. Hudson (OH): Lexi-Comp, Inc.; Accessed via UpToDate Feb 27, 2017.

6. Enoxaparin. In: Lexi-Comp Online™, Lexi-Drugs Online™. Hudson (OH): Lexi-Comp, Inc.; Accessed via UpToDate Feb 27, 2017.

7. Warfarin. In: Lexi-Comp Online™, Lexi-Drugs Online™. Hudson (OH): Lexi-Comp, Inc.; Accessed via UpToDate Feb 27, 2017.

8. Dabigatran. In: Lexi-Comp Online™, Lexi-Drugs Online™. Hudson (OH): Lexi-Comp, Inc.; Accessed via UpToDate Feb 27, 2017.

9. Leung L. L. K. Direct Oral Anticoagulants: Dosing and adverse effects. In: *UpToDate*, Post T. W. (Ed.), UpToDate: Waltham, MA. Accessed Feb 27, 2017.

10. Apixiban. In: Lexi-Comp Online™, Lexi-Drugs Online™. Hudson (OH): Lexi-Comp, Inc.; Accessed via UpToDate Feb 27, 2017.

11. Rivaroxaban. In: Lexi-Comp Online™, Lexi-Drugs Online™. Hudson (OH): Lexi-Comp, Inc.; Accessed via UpToDate Feb 27, 2017.

12. Peiris P. *Hematologic System: Alternatives to Transfusion.* In: *Learnly: Online Anesthesia Basic Science Curriculum.* Stanford, CA: Stanford AIM Lab; 2017.

13. Cox Williams E., McFayden G. Hematologic System: Pharmacology: Immunosuppressive and Anti-Rejection Drugs. In: *Learnly: Online Anesthesia Basic Science Curriculum.* Stanford, CA: Stanford AIM Lab; 2017.

14. Freeman B., Berger J. *Anesthesiology Core Review*, New York, NY: McGraw-Hill Education, 2014; 503–5.

Chapter

38

Transfusions

Christy Anthony and Michal Gajewski

Indications for Transfusion

- Excessive blood loss (>30 percent blood volume)
  - Healthy patients may lose up to 20 percent of their blood volume before signs of hypovolemia occur due to compensatory vasoconstriction.[1]
    - When anemia develops, there is
      - Cardiac output (CO) secondary to ↓ systemic vascular resistance (SVR)
      - Redistribution of blood flow to organs with greater oxygen requirements (e.g., brain, heart)
        - Oxygen delivery remains constant until the hematocrit (Hct) drops below 30 percent[1]
      - An increase in oxygen extraction that allows O_2 delivery despite the lower O_2 tension
        - This usually begins to occur when the Hct < 25 percent[1]
- Maximum allowable blood loss (MABL)
  - MABL = estimated blood volume (EBV) × (initial Hct − minimum acceptable Hct)/initial Hct (Table 38.1)[1]
- Signs of inadequate perfusion[2]
  - Unstable vital signs (e.g., hypotension, tachycardia)
  - Signs of end-organ dysfunction (e.g., rise in lactate, increasing base deficit)
- Laboratory indicators
  - Morbidity and mortality does not increase until hemoglobin (Hgb) falls below 7 g/dL. Thus, unless there is ongoing or expected blood loss, transfusion goals are typically[1,2]:
    - In healthy adults transfuse when Hgb < 7 g/dL
    - In patients with cardiac disease transfuse when Hgb < 10 g/dL

Table 38.1 Estimated blood volume[1,2]

Age group	Blood volume (mL/kg)
Premature infant	**90–105**
Full term newborn	80–90
Infant (3 months–1 year)	70–80
Child (1–12 years)	70–75
Adult female	60–65
Adult male	65–70

Blood Collection and Processing

- Whole blood collection[1]
  - Centrifugation is used to separate whole blood into various components.
  - Blood may also be separated via *apheresis*, where one component is collected and the remaining components are returned to the donor (Figure 38.1).
- Leukoreduction[1,2]
  - Removes white blood cells (WBC) from the red blood cells (RBC) and platelets
  - Reduces risk of human leukocyte antigen (HLA) allo-immunization preventing *febrile reactions*
  - Reduces risk of cytomegalovirus (CMV) transmission to less than 0.1 percent
- Washing[1]
  - Washing cellular components with saline is mostly done to remove plasma in patients with *allergic transfusion reactions,* particularly patients with *IgA deficiency*
    - The prevalence of IgA deficiency is estimated to be 1:600–800 in the general population
- Irradiation[1]
  - Units are exposed to gamma irradiation to damage donor WBC DNA and prevent cellular immune response to recipient tissue
  - Used to prevent transfusion-related *graft versus host disease* (GVHD)

Blood Products, Preservation, and Storage

- Packed red blood cells (PRBCs)
  - One unit PRBCs = 250–300 mL and Hct 70–80 percent
  - Transfusion of 1 unit PRBCs = roughly 1 g/dL increase in adult hemoglobin concentrations
  - Can be stored at 1–6°C for 21–35 days or up to 42 days with additive solution
    - If frozen at ≤65°C, can be stored up to 10 years
  - Administration of younger blood (i.e., stored < 14 days) has been associated with better outcomes (e.g., decreased mortality rate and fewer postoperative complications, especially with major surgery)
  - RBC preservation solution: CPDA
    - Citrate: anticoagulation effect by binding calcium and inhibiting initiation of coagulation cascade

191

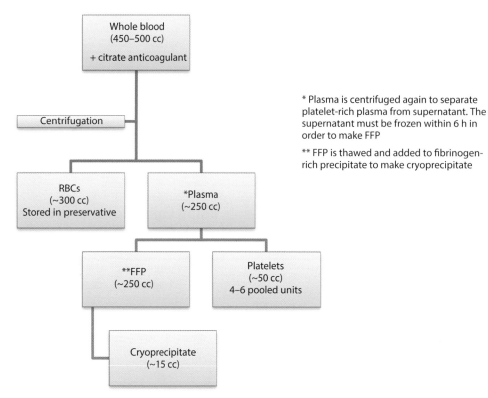

Figure 38.1 Processing and separation of whole blood[1]

- ▪ Phosphate: Buffer
- ▪ To maintain ATP levels and RBC integrity
  - • Dextrose
  - • Adenine
- • Storage of blood products can result in the following derangements:
  - ○ Depletion of 2,3-DPG within 2 weeks → Leftward shift of oxygen dissociation curve
  - ○ Increased K⁺ secondary to hemolysis
  - ○ Citrate toxicity
    - ▪ Will occur if the transfusion rate exceeds approximately 1 unit per 5 minutes
    - ▪ Can cause a reduction in ionized calcium levels
      - • Signs of citrate toxicity include hypotension, narrow pulse pressure, elevated intraventricular end diastolic pressure, prolonged QT interval, widened QRS complexes, and flattened T waves
    - ▪ Likely to occur in the setting of hypothermia, liver disease, and pediatric patients
    - ▪ Citrate is metabolized into bicarbonate → can cause metabolic alkalosis
    - ▪ Worsened by hyperventilation due to decreased CO_2 causing decreased calcium ion concentration
    - ▪ Fresh frozen plasma (FFP) and platelets contain the highest citrate content
    - ▪ Treatment: Calcium[1,2]
- • Platelets
  - ○ Blood preservation and storage[2]
    - ▪ Stored at room temperature for up to 5 days in order to preserve function of clotting factors

- ▪ This increases risk of bacterial growth
- ▪ Platelet-related sepsis can be fatal and occurs as frequently as 1 in 5,000 transfusions
- ○ Preparation for transfusion[1]
  - ▪ A platelet concentrate derived from a single unit of donor blood will have an approximate volume of 50 mL and will raise the platelet count by 5,000 to 10,000
    - • These single units can be pooled from different donors however this increases recipient risk
  - ▪ More typically multiple units of platelets are derived from a single donor via plasmapheresis
    - • The expected increase in platelet count after receiving a "pack" is 30,000 to 60,000
  - ▪ Does not require compatibility testing
- ○ Indications for platelet transfusion: Transfuse if platelet count is[1,2]
  - ▪ <100,000/μL
    - • If patient is to undergo surgery at a critical site (e.g., spine, ophthalmological procedures, etc.)
  - ▪ <75,000/μL
    - • If patient is undergoing massive transfusion
  - ▪ <50,000/μL
    - • If patient is in disseminated intravascular coagulation (DIC)
    - • Prophylactically, if patient is undergoing an invasive procedure (e.g., lumbar puncture, endoscopy, neuraxial anesthesia, etc.)
    - • In a stable patient with coagulopathy or other signs of active bleeding

- <10,0000/μL
  - In any patient, even if stable and without any signs of active bleeding or coagulopathy
- Fresh frozen plasma
  - Blood preservation and storage[2]
    - FFP is the fluid portion obtained from a single unit of whole blood that is frozen within 6 h of collection
      - Can also be separated via apheresis
    - All coagulation factors (except platelets) are present in FFP
      - Factors V and VIII are the most labile, and thus freezing within 6 h is required
  - Preparation for transfusion[2]
    - Initial therapeutic dose of FFP is 10–15 mL/kg to obtain at least 30 percent factor activity
      - One bag contains approximately 250 mL
    - Repeat dosing should depend on PT and aPTT
    - ABO compatibility testing is necessary with FFP
  - Indications[2]
    - Liver dysfunction with clinical signs of bleeding
    - DIC with clinical signs of bleeding
    - Bleeding associated with massive transfusion and estimated blood loss > one blood volume
    - Emergent reversal of vitamin K antagonists, such as warfarin
    - Heparin resistance secondary to antithrombin (AT) deficiency when AT concentrate is not available
    - Correction of inherited factor deficiencies when there is no specific factor concentrate (e.g., factor V)
    - Correction of acquired multi-factor deficiencies with evidence of bleeding or in anticipation of major surgery or an invasive procedure
    - Treatment of thrombotic microangiopathies (thrombotic thrombocytopenic purpura, HELLP syndrome, or hemolytic uremic syndrome)
    - Treatment of hereditary angioedema when C1-esterase inhibitor is not available
- Cryoprecipitate (Cryo)
  - Blood preservation and storage[1]
    - The fraction of plasma that precipitates when FFP is thawed that is then centrifuged is called cryoprecipitate
    - This product contains fibrinogen, fibronectin, vWF, factor VIII, and factor XIII
  - Preparation for transfusion[1]
    - One unit = 10–20 mL, and a usual adult dose is about 4–6 bags
    - Contains more fibrinogen per volume than FFP
    - Does not require ABO compatibility testing
  - Indications[1]
    - Hemophilia A (cryo contains high concentrations of factor VIII in a small volume)
    - Hypofibrinogenemia because cryo contains more fibrinogen than FFP

Preparation for Transfusion

- Compatibility testing[1,2]
  - Type and screen (T&S)
    - ABO compatibility determines which antigens and antibodies are present on the patient's red blood cell and serum, respectively
    - RBCs are also checked for the presence of "Rh factor" in order to avoid anti-D alloimmunization
      - Blood that has been typed and screened has been typed for A, B, and Rh antigens and screened for common antibodies
        - Universal PRBC donor: O−
        - Universal PRBC recipient: AB+
        - Universal FFP donor: AB+
        - Eighty-five percent of the population is Rh+
        - Female patients of the parturient age should receive only Rh− blood, in order to minimize the risk of developing antibodies to the Rh+ antigen (Rh sensitivity), as this can result in erythroblastosis fetalis in a future pregnancy
    - T&S is ordered when the scheduled surgical procedure is unlikely to require transfusion of blood but the blood will be screened for antibodies which could complicate obtaining blood if a transfusion is needed
      - More cost-efficient as no unit of blood has been designated for the patient and may therefore be available for use by others
    - The chance of a significant hemolytic reaction related to the use of T&S blood is approximately 1 in ~40,000 units transfused
  - Type and cross (T&C)[1,2]
    - Major: Donor's erythrocytes are incubated with the recipient's plasma
      - The major cross-match checks for IgG antibodies (Kell, Kidd, Duffy)
    - Minor: Incubation of the donor's plasma with the recipient's erythrocytes
    - Agglutination occurs if either the major or minor cross-match is incompatible
    - Delayed hemolytic transfusion reactions commonly involve these antibodies

Blood Donation and Salvage

- Autologous blood[1]
  - Two primary reasons for the use of autologous blood
    - To decrease or eliminate complications from allogeneic blood transfusions
    - To conserve blood resources
  - Autologous blood donation
    - Current indications: Patients in whom it would be difficult to find compatible blood types, patients who refuse allogenic blood transfusion, and adolescent scoliosis surgery

- Contraindications: Children < 10 years of age, active infection, aortic stenosis, recent myocardial infarction or stroke, uncontrolled hypertension
  - Criteria: Patient-donors must have a hemoglobin of at least 11 g/dL
  - Most patients can donate 10.5 mL/kg of blood approximately every 5–7 days (maximum, 2–4 units), with the last unit collected at least 72 h before surgery to permit restoration of plasma volume
  - Oral iron supplementation or preoperative erythropoietin is recommended when blood is withdrawn within a few days preceding surgery
- Uncrossmatched blood[1]
  - In emergency situations where blood compatibility testing cannot be completed, the option is to administer O-negative (universal donor) PRBCs
  - The incidence of a serious reaction without a crossmatch is <1 percent
  - Note that if the patient's blood type becomes known and available after 2 units of type O-negative PRBCs have been transfused, subsequent transfusions should continue with O-negative blood
    - This is because O-negative whole blood may contain high titers of anti-A and anti-B hemolytic antibodies
- Perioperative blood cell salvage[1]
  - Acute normovolemic hemodilution (ANH)
    - This is the process of extracting multiple units of blood in the early intraoperative period and replacing the volume with crystalloid solution
    - The formula for MABL is used to calculate the volume that can be safely removed down to a target Hct of 27 percent (depending on the cardiovascular status of the patient)
    - By hemodiluting the patient, fewer RBC will be lost per milliliter of blood loss during surgery
    - At the end of surgery, the patient's concentrated, undiluted blood, which is high in Hct and oxygen-carrying capacity, clotting factors, and functional platelets, is reinfused
    - Blood must still be anticoagulated with citrate
  - Cell saver
    - An external semi-automated device that collects blood from the surgical field into a reservoir that contains anticoagulant (heparin or citrate)
      - The blood is then filtered and centrifuged
      - The remaining RBCs are washed from other blood components, surgical debris, and remaining anticoagulant, and delivered to a saline reservoir for future administration
      - The blood can be stored for up to 6 h at 4°C
    - Most modern day cell savers provide RBC concentrates with Hct of 60–70 percent
    - Has reduced the need for allogenic blood transfusion in major surgeries (e.g., orthopedic, spine

fusion, and off-pump high-risk cardiac surgery) in patient with blood loss greater than 20 percent blood volume (or 1 L)
  - Complications: Dilutional coagulopathy, reinfusion of excessive anticoagulant (heparin), hemolysis, air embolism, and DIC
  - Contraindications: Microbial contamination of surgical field or malignant disease at operative site
- Designated donor[1]
  - Directed donations can be made by family or friends for a specific patient
  - This method can potentially decrease the number of donor exposures by using the same donor
  - Risk of infection is still considered the same, and so blood is still processed and tested as with any other blood donation
  - Cellular components from blood relatives must be irradiated to prevent the risk of GVHD from closely matched donor lymphocytes that are not rejected by the recipient
- Special considerations[1,2]
  - Jehovah's Witness patients do not accept blood transfusion nor do they store their own blood for either autologous or allogeneic donation
    - Albumin is accepted among certain patients, and a discussion is usually made with regards to this product
    - Intraoperative blood salvage is sometimes a possible form of blood conservation, so long as the machine utilized maintains continuity of blood with the patient

Volume Expanders

- Crystalloids: Solutions that contain water and electrolytes that distribute freely within intravascular (33 percent) and interstitial compartments (67 percent)[2]
  - Balanced salt solutions[1,2]
    - Salt solution with electrolyte composition similar to extracellular fluid (ECF) (e.g., lactated ringers (LR), plasmalyte, normosol)
    - HYPOtonic with regards to sodium
    - Buffer is usually included; generated bicarbonate in vivo
    - Includes small quantities of other electrolytes
    - Plasmalyte is acceptable for dilution of PRBCs; however, LR should be avoided due to its calcium content, as well as its hypotonicity which can cause cell lysis
  - Normal saline (0.9 percent NaCl)[1,2]
    - Slightly HYPERtonic
    - Contains more chloride than the ECF in large quantities, can result in mild hyperchloremic (nonanion gap) metabolic acidosis
    - No buffers or other electrolytes
    - Ideal solution for dilution of PRBCS given it is almost isotonic

Table 38.2 Fluid composition

Fluid	pH	Osmolarity	Na$^+$	K$^+$
NaCl (0.9 percent)	6.0	308	154	0
Lactated ringers	6.5	273	130	4
Plasmalyte	7.4	294	140	5
Five percent albumin	7.4	330	145	2

- Preferred solution in patients with brain injury, hypochloremic metabolic alkalosis, or hyponatremia
  - ○ Hypertonic salt solutions[2]
    - Na$^+$ concentration ranges from 250 to 1,200 mEq/L
    - Create an osmotic gradient that helps move water from extravascular to intravascular space
    - Useful in minimizing tissue edema in patients with prolonged bowel surgery, burns, brain injuries
    - Not used for resuscitation measures given the short intravascular half-life and the potential for hemolysis at the point of injection from high osmolality
  - ○ Five percent dextrose[2]
    - Functions as free water, since dextrose is metabolized
    - Iso-osmotic
    - Used to correct hypernatremia
    - May be used to prevent hypoglycemia in diabetic patients who have been given insulin (Table 38.2)
- Colloids: Solutions composed of large molecular weight (MW) substances that remain intravascular longer than crystalloids
  - ○ Five percent albumin[2]
    - Oncotic pressure of ~20 mmHg, half-life of about 16 h, but can be as short as 2–3 h in pathologic conditions
    - Minimal risk of infection with appropriate preparation methods
    - No effects on coagulation
  - ○ Dextran[2]
    - Water-soluble glucose polymers synthesized from sucrose
    - MW of dextran 40 is 40,000 Daltons and Dextran 70 is 70,000 Daltons
    - Not used as a volume expander
    - Dextran 40 is used in vascular surgery to prevent thrombosis
    - Both solutions eventually become degraded to glucose
    - Side effects: Anaphylaxis or anaphylactoid reactions (1/3,300), increased bleeding time secondary to decreased platelet adhesiveness, Rouleaux formation, noncardiogenic pulmonary edema from direct toxicity to pulmonary capillaries

  - ○ Hydroxyethyl starch (HES)[1,2]
    - Synthetic colloid solution that is a modification of natural polysaccharide
    - HES preparations are described by their concentration, average molecular weight, molar substitution, and C2 to C6 ratio
      - MW: Low (<70 kDa), medium (130–270 kDa), or high (>450 kDa)
      - Molar substitution: Refers to the number of hydroxyethyl residues per 10 glucose subunits
        - ○ HES preparations with 7 hydroxyethyl residues per 10 glucose subunits (a ratio of 0.7) are called hetastarches
      - C2:C6 ratio: The pattern of hydroxyethyl substitution on specific carbon atoms of the HES glucose subunits
    - Generally, the higher the MW and molar substitution, the more prolonged the volume effect, but with more potential side effects
    - Six percent solutions are isotonic
    - Side effects vary with different HES preparations. They can include
      - Coagulation disturbances: HES interferes with vWF, factor VIII, and platelet function
      - Renal toxicity: Usually with the older, high MW preparations
      - Tissue storage: Manifests as pruritus in up to 22 percent of patients

Blood Filters and Pumps

- Blood filters are utilized during transfusion to remove clots and cell aggregates that form during collection and storage[1,3]
  - ○ All blood products should be administered through a filter
  - ○ Standard blood infusion sets contain 170–260 μm filters to siphon debris
  - ○ Leukocyte filters are available for transfusion when leukocyte-reduced red cells or platelets are not available
  - ○ Platelets should be administered through large-pore filters (>150 μm); they should not be transfused though sets which have already been used for blood due to aggregation[3]
  - ○ FFP and cryoprecipitate can be transfused via a standard blood filter
  - ○ Filters should be changed at least every 12 h or when flow rate decreases
- Mechanical pumps are available to help with appropriate transfusion rates for special populations, particularly neonates and pediatric patients[1,2]
  - ○ Pressure bags should be used with rapid transfusion (5 minutes/unit) if needed
    - Inflating the bag to about 200 mmHg is usually sufficient
    - Pressure of 300 mmHg can cause lysis of the RBCs

Effects of Cooling and Heating: Blood Warmers

- Blood warmers
  - Administration of cooled blood products can result in hypothermia, especially during rapid infusion[1,2]
    - The infusion of 1 unit of RBCs at 4°C can decrease the core body temperature by 0.25°C
    - This can result in platelet and coagulation factor dysfunction, arrhythmias, myocardial depression, as well as increased blood loss and risk of postoperative infections
  - Specially designed warmers are used to rewarm the blood prior to entry into the patient's intravascular system
    - Note that each blood warmer is designed to warm the blood to normal body temperature of 37°C; some have been manufactured to operate up to 43°C
    - Instructions for each manufacturing company should be read carefully and followed precisely for appropriate use
  - Unrecognized malfunction of warmers may result in hemolysis of the erythrocytes, especially when overheating occurs

Synthetic and Recombinant Hemoglobin

- Blood substitutes
  - Hemoglobin-based oxygen carrying solutions (e.g., Hemopure)[1,4]
    - Several hemoglobin solutions have been made from pools of human or bovine hemoglobin, or from recombinant hemoglobin, all of which are chemically modified to facilitate O_2 offloading
    - This however is still under investigation and no FDA-approved Hb-substitute has been approved for clinical use
- Stimulants of erythropoiesis
  - Erythropoietin[5-8]
    - For surgery scheduled in >3 weeks: subcutaneous injection 600 U/kg weekly for 3 weeks prior, for a total of four doses, the last being the day of surgery
    - For surgery scheduled in <3 weeks: 300 U/kg daily for a total of 15 doses
  - Iron[5,7,9]
    - Oral supplementation: 100–200 mg/day for 2–4 weeks
    - Intravenous formulations: 3–4 weeks prior to surgery
  - Vitamin B_{12}[5,9]
    - 1 mg IM daily × 7 days, or 1–2 mg PO daily × 4 months
  - Folate[5,9]
    - 1 mg/day for up to 4 months, or until the patient's anemia is corrected
  - Can be used in conjunction with autologous blood transfusion, or in patients who refuse any type of blood products, such as Jehovah's Witnesses

References

1. Barash P., Cullen B., Stoelting R., et al. *Clinical Anesthesia*, 7th edn. Philadelphia, PA: Lippincott Williams & Wilkins; 2013.
2. Miller R., Pardo M., Jr. *Basics of Anesthesia*, 6th edn. Philadelphia, PA: Elsevier Saunders; 2011.
3. Team NTL. Blood Administration 2009. Available from: www.transfusionguidelines.org/ ...to...sets...blood...blood.../rtc-sw_ news-jan_3.pdf (accessed on January 17, 2017).
4. Varnado C. L., Mollan T. L., Birukou I., et al. Development of recombinant hemoglobin-based oxygen carriers. *Antioxid Redox Signal*. 2013; 18(17): 2314–28.
5. Koury M. J., Ponka P. New insights into erythropoiesis: the roles of folate, vitamin B12, and iron. *Annu Rev Nutr*. 2004; 24: 105–31.
6. Elliott S. Erythropoiesis-stimulating agents and other methods to enhance oxygen transport. *Br J Pharmacol*. 2008; 154(3): 529–41.
7. Munoz M., Gomez-Ramirez S., Campos A., Ruiz J., Liumbruno G. M. Pre-operative anaemia: prevalence, consequences and approaches to management. *Blood Transfus*. 2015; 13(3): 370–9.
8. Products J. PROCRIT® Prescribing Information 2015. Available from: www.procrit.com/professionals/ elective_surgery.html (accessed on January 17, 2017).
9. Patel M. S., Carson J. L. Anemia in the preoperative patient. *Med Clin North Am*. 2009; 93(5): 1095–104.

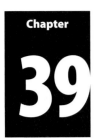

Chapter 39

Reactions to Transfusions

Marc Sherwin, Natalie Smith, and Sang Kim

Complications of Transfusions

Infections (Table 39.2)

- Hepatitis
  - Most cases are anicteric
  - Hepatitis B is most common
  - Hepatitis C is more serious: Progresses to chronic hepatitis, cirrhosis in 20 percent of carriers, hepatocellular carcinoma in 5 percent of carriers[5]
  - Treatment: Ledipasivir–Sofosbuvir (Harvoni) >96 percent cure rate for some genotypes[6]
- Cytomegalovirus (CMV)
  - Most common infection of blood transfusion[5]
  - Patients at risk: Pregnant, premature neonates; immunosuppressed, allograft recipients; splenectomy[7]
  - CMV safe products: Plasma components, seronegative donors, leuko-reduced components
- Bacterial
  - Incidence: More common with platelets than packed red blood cells (PRBC)
    - Positive bacterial cultures in *PRBC* – 1:7,000[5]
    - Sepsis from PRBC transfusion – 1:250,000[5]
    - Positive bacterial cultures in *platelets* – 1:2,000[5]
    - Sepsis from platelet transfusion – 1:25,000[5]
  - Prevention: Transfuse blood within 4 hours[5]
- Other infectious diseases: Theoretical transmission but no available tests:
    - Malaria, chagas, severe acute respiratory syndrome (SARS), Creutzfeldt-Jakob disease[6]

Citrate Intoxication

- Citrate is added to PRBC as citrate–phosphate–dextrose–adenine (CPDA)[8]
- Prevents clot formation by chelating calcium
- Most commonly seen in massive transfusion, especially when giving fresh frozen plasma (FFP)
  - Transfusion rate > 1mL/kg/min which is equivalent to 1 PRBC every 10 min[8]
- Signs and symptoms
  - Liver metabolizes citrate into *bicarbonate*
    - In patients with liver dysfunction, citrate will chelate recipient calcium causing hypocalcemia[8]
  - Hypocalcemia, metabolic alkalosis, hypotension, narrow pulse pressure, increased left ventricular end diastolic pressure and central venous pressure (CVP), and EKG changes:
    - Prolonged QT, widened QRS, flattened T wave
- Risk factors
  - Massive transfusion, hypothermia (metabolism halved when temperature decreases from 37°C to 31°C), hyperventilation, impaired hepatic blood flow, and pediatric patients[8]
- Treatment
  - Intravenous calcium gluconate or chloride

Electrolyte and Acid Base Abnormalities

- Blood storage leads to: ↓ pH, ↓ 2,3 DPG, and ↑ K+
- Hyperkalemia:
  - As high as 19–50 mEq/L in blood stored for 21 days[8]
  - Risks for hyperkalemia: Trauma, impaired renal function, and neonates[8]
- Hypocalcemia:
  - Associated with citrate intoxication – see above
- Acidosis:
  - Storage media very acidotic (e.g., CPDA = pH 5.5)[8]
  - Lactate and pyruvate accumulate with storage
  - pH of blood stored for 21 days ~6.9[8]
- Alkalosis:
  - Citrate metabolized to bicarbonate leading to metabolic alkalosis

Massive Transfusion

- Massive transfusion occurs when greater than 20 units of PRBCs are given within 24 hours (approximately 1 blood volume in a 70 kg patient)
  - Alternative definitions: >50 percent blood volume in 4 hours, 150 mL/min blood loss, 4 units in 1 hour[9]
- Complications:
  - Coagulopathy
    - 35 percent of coagulation factors remain after replacement of 1 blood volume with PRBCs due to dilution[9]
    - Platelets decrease to 50,000/μL after 2 blood volumes[9]
    - Fibrinogen decreases to 100 g/dL after 2 blood volumes[9]
  - Hypothermia

Table 39.1 Types of Reactions[1–4]

	Febrile non-hemolytic transfusion reaction	Allergic transfusion reaction (ATR)	Acute hemolytic transfusion reaction (AHTR)	Delayed hemolytic transfusion reaction (DHTR)
Presentation	– Fever and/or chills, head-ache, nausea, and vomiting – Occurs *during or within 4 hours* after transfusion completion[1]	– Mild: Isolated, pruritic, urticarial lesions – Severe: Anaphylaxis; acute, life threatening, systemic reactions with respiratory compromise, hypotension, and GI symptoms – Anaphylactoid: Systemic reaction that is not mediated by IgE – Occurs within *seconds to 45 minutes*[2]	– Widely varying clinical manifestation, from minimal hemolysis without clinical signs and symptoms to brisk hemolysis with DIC, hypotension, renal failure, shock, and death – Early signs and symptoms of AHTR include fever and chills, which occur within minutes of transfusion – In anesthetized patients, hemoglobinuria may be the only sign[3]	– Fever, chills, jaundice, malaise, back pain, and, infrequently, renal failure – Occurs *3–10 days* after transfusion
Mechanism of action	– Non-immune pathway: Passive transfusion of donor cytokines – *Immune pathway: Donor leukocytes + recipient antibodies* – Final pathway to febrile reaction: *Release of cytokines*: IL-1β, IL-6, and TNF-α from *activated monocytes and macrophages* – Cytokines lead to prostaglandin E2 → acts on the hypothalamus to increase body temperature[1]	– *Donor allergen* binds to pre-formed *recipient antibodies* – IgE-mediated, type-1 hypersensitivity reactions – The allergen or antibody can be transferred via transfusion – i.e., donor who consumed peanuts transfer allergen to recipient who has peanut allergies – i.e., donor with peanut allergy transfer their antibodies to recipient who consumed peanuts[2]	– Transfusion of ABO incompatible RBCs into patients with antiA and/or B antibodies. Can also involve minor antigens (Kell, Rh, Duffy, and Kidd). – IgM and IgG → bind C1q → complement cascade C3a & C5b → RBC lysis → vasoconstriction, activate platelets and coagulation cascade, histamine, bradykinins, IL-8 and TNA-α[3]	– Exposure to a *minor RBC antigen* after history of transfusion or pregnancy – Primary immune response: Not clinically significant – Anamnestic response: The offending antigen is re-exposed → rapid increase in IgG antibody production leads to hemolysis[4]
Diagnosis/ test	– No specific tests available for diagnosis (diagnosis of exclusion) – Exclude hemolytic reactions, ABO incompatibility, septic transfusion reactions (obtain culture), TRALI, medication reactions[1]	– Test for *anti-IgA* if severe allergic reaction – If diagnosed with IgA deficiency, patient should receive products from IgA-deficient donors or washed products – Anaphylactic reactions reported in deficiencies of haptoglobin, C3 and C4[2]	– Positive direct anti-globulin test (DAT) – Signs of hemolysis: ↑ LDH ↑ bilirubin ↓ haptoglobin ↓ hemoglobinuria – Signs of DIC: low fibrinogen and platelets[3]	– DAT – DAT done with anti-IgG and anti-C3 reagents – Laboratory findings: reticulocytosis, unconjugated hyper-bilirubinemia, and urine urobilinogen[4]
Incidence	– Historically was most common transfusion reaction (43–75 percent) – Incidence decreased to < 0.2% with pre-storage leukocyte reduction (RBC and platelets) – Risk factors: hematologic malignancies, frequent transfusions, older platelets (4–5 days) higher incidence than ≤3 day old (4.6 vs. 1.1 percent)[1]	– Approximately 1:20,000-47,000 transfusions – Four percent of transfusion-related death is due to anaphylaxis – With RBC transfusion: 0.03–0.61 percent – With platelet transfusion: 0.3–0.6 percent – With plasma transfusion: 1–3 percent – Factor VIII, IX, vWF, and other recombinant concentrates: 1 in 5,000 doses[2]	– Among transfusion related deaths, 9 percent were from ABO-incompatible transfusion – Risk of ABO incompatible transfusion: 1:38,000–100,000 – 50 percent asymptomatic – Risk of death from: 1:1.5 million[3]	– Occurs in 1 in 1,500[4]
Treatment	– Immediately stop the transfusion – Administer acetaminophen for anti-pyretic effect (avoid aspirin and NSAIDs) – Meperidine (20–50 mg IV) for severe rigor if not on monoamine oxidase inhibitor (MAOI) or have end stage renal disease (ESRD) due to risk of seizures from normeperidine metabolite[1]	– Mild allergic reaction: Stop transfusion temporarily and administer antihistamine – may resume if symptoms cease – Severe allergic reaction: Stop transfusion and prepare to intubate, administer epinephrine 100 μg IV bolus every 3–5 minutes, anti-histamine, H2 receptor antagonist, and glucocorticoid[2]	– Check clerical work to ensure correct blood type, product, and patient – Send the transfused product back to blood bank along with sample from recipient – Check for: Hemolysis, DAT, ABO type – Stop the transfusion – Intravenous fluid, diuretic to maintain urine output, consider dopamine infusion for hypotension[3]	– Treatment usually unnecessary without symptomatic anemia – If minor antigen is not identified and transfusion is required, the benefit/risk should be weighed[4]

(cont.)

Table 39.1 *(cont.)*

	Febrile non-hemolytic transfusion reaction	Allergic transfusion reaction (ATR)	Acute hemolytic transfusion reaction (AHTR)	Delayed hemolytic transfusion reaction (DHTR)
Prevention	– Leukoreduction (pre- or post-storage) – Removal of plasma supernatant in platelets – Premedication (e.g., acetaminophen or diphenhydramine) is ineffective; leuko-reduced blood products[1]	– Patients *without* history of ATR: Majority of clinical studies show no benefit to prophylaxis – Patients *with* history of ATR to *platelets*: Concentrating platelets via plasma reduction led to 75% reduction in incidence while washing them led to 95% reduction – Washing platelets reduces incidence by 95 percent[2] – Patients *with* history of ATR to other blood products: Premedication does not prevent reactions, however, may reduce symptoms	– Give ABO-compatible products and follow guidelines for checking products prior to transfusion – Perform root cause analysis and corrective action plans[3]	– Permanent record-keeping of all clinically significant antibodies – "Active" RBC type and screen in those possibly requiring transfusion[4]

Table 39.2 Infection risk with blood transfusions

Human T-lymphotropic virus (HTLV-II)	1:2,993,000
Human immunodeficiency virus-1 and -2 (HIV)	1:1,476,000
Hepatitis C virus (HCV)	1:1,149,000
Hepatitis A virus (HAV)	1:1,000,000
Hepatitis B virus (HBV)	1:280,000

Data from AABB: *AABB technical manual,* ed 17, 2011, AABB; and Fiebig ER, Busch MP. Infectious risks of transfusions. In: Spiess BD, Spence RK, Shander A (eds). *Perioperative Transfusion Medicine,* Philadelphia, PA: Lippincott Williams & Wilkins; 2006.

- Unwarmed blood products will decrease patient's temperature
- Prevent by warming blood through plastic coils or cassettes in warm water[9]

Pulmonary Complications
- Transfusion-related acute lung injury (TRALI)
  - Definition
    - New acute lung injury (ALI) within 6 hours of transfusion[10,11]
    - Rule out preexisting ALI etiology and other risk factors for ALI[10,11]
  - Diagnosis[11]
    - Evidence of hypoxemia:
      - $PaO_2/FiO_2 < 300$ or $SaO_2 < 90$ percent on room air
    - New diffuse bilateral infiltrates on chest radiograph
    - Lack of evidence of circulatory overload
      - i.e., PCWP < 18 mmHg, lack of improvement with diuretics, etc.
    - Rapid development of tachypnea, cyanosis, dyspnea, fever, and frequently hypotension[12]
    - Physical exam findings include diffuse crackles, decreased breath sounds on auscultation, hypoxemia, acute decrease in pulmonary compliance

(increase peak and plateau airway pressures in mechanically ventilated patients)[12]
  - Mechanism of action
    - Direct antigen–antibody mediated reaction[10,13]
      - Donor alloantibodies cause activation of recipient's immune system leading to inflammatory cascade
      - Alloantibodies lead to recipient neutrophil and monocyte activation leading to increased lung vasculature permeability[12,14]
    - "Two-hit" and "Multi-causal" Models[12,15]
      - HLA and HNA antibodies have NOT been identified in at least 15 percent of TRALI cases[13]
      - Patient-specific risk factors may prime the patient's immune system leading to neutrophil "priming", which leads to enhanced neutrophil response
    - Final common pathway
      - Neutrophil activation → release of inflammatory mediators → endothelial activation and breakdown of the endothelial-cell lung barrier → pulmonary edema and lung injury[16]
      - *Neutropenia* is a common, early finding in TRALI secondary to neutrophil sequestration within the lungs[12]
  - Blood products implicated in TRALI
    - Plasma containing products carry the highest risk of TRALI (i.e., FFP and platelets)[13]
      - All blood products, including RBCs, have been implicated[2,3]
    - Previously parous female donors are more likely
      - Exposed to paternal HLA from the fetus during pregnancy[16–18]
      - Plasma and whole blood transfusions in the United States now primarily come from males and nulliparous females[19]

- o Incidence
  - ▪ Most common cause of transfusion-related death accounting for 37 percent of transfusion related mortality[20]
  - ▪ Estimated incidence of 1 in 5,000 blood products[12,14]
- o Treatment
  - ▪ Stop transfusion, supportive care, resolves within 72–96 hours[13,20,21]
  - ▪ Treatment strategies virtually identical to ARDS protocol
    - • Low tidal volumes, low plateau pressures, high FiO_2, and PEEP
- o Prevention
  - ▪ Decrease unnecessary transfusions
  - ▪ Utilizing point of care testing (i.e., thromboelastography (TEG)) to guide transfusion management[21,22]
- Transfusion-associated circulatory overload (TACO)
  - o Definition
    - ▪ Development of at least four of the following symptoms:
      - • Acute respiratory distress, acute or worsening pulmonary edema on CXR, positive fluid balance, increased blood pressure, tachycardia[23,24]
  - o Presentation
    - ▪ Increased CVP, evidence of left heart failure on echocardiogram, increased brain natriuretic peptide (BNP), CXR evidence of pulmonary edema[24–26]
    - ▪ Physical exam findings: Tachycardia, hypertension, hypoxemia, diaphoresis, anxiety, dyspnea, jugular venous distension, rales, rhonchi and/or wheezing, use of accessory muscles
  - o Mechanism of action
    - ▪ Volume overload
  - o Incidence
    - ▪ Second most common cause of transfusion-related death accounting for 18 percent of all transfusions-related mortality[23]
    - ▪ Incidence: 1 in 356–10,000
    - ▪ More common in elderly (70–85 years old), pregnant patients, infants, patients with cardiac disease, renal disease, or chronic obstructive pulmonary disease (COPD)[23,25,27]
  - o Treatment
    - ▪ Most cases resolve within 24–72 hours[27]
    - ▪ Stop the transfusion, administer supplemental oxygen, make the patient sit upright, consider diuretic therapy[25,27]
  - o Prevention
    - ▪ Decreased risk with slower transfusion rate[23]
    - ▪ Consider splitting future transfusions into smaller aliquots[25]

Immunosuppression
- Transfusion can reduce immunoresponsiveness and propagate inflammation
  - o Increased risk of postoperative bacterial infection, cancer recurrence, and mortality with transfusions[5]
  - o Renal transplant patients with preoperative blood transfusion have post-transfusion immunosuppression which improves graft survival[5]

References

1. Maramica I. K. Transfusion medicine and hemostasis. In: Shaz, Hillyer, Roshal, Abrams (eds), 2nd ed. *Febrile Non-Hemolytic Transfusion Reactions*; 2013. Chapter 59, 389–94.

2. Savage W. Transfusion medicine and hemostasis. In: Shaz, Hillyer, Roshal, Abrams (eds), 2nd ed. *Allergic Transfusion Reactions*; 2013. Chapter 60, 395–9.

3. Bellone M., Hillyer C. D. Transfusion medicine and hemostasis. In: Shaz, Hillyer, Roshal, Abrams (eds), 2nd ed. *Acute Hemolytic Transfusion Reactions*; 2013. Chapter 61, 401–7.

4. Josephson C. Transfusion medicine and hemostasis. In: Shaz, Hillyer, Roshal, Abrams (eds), 2nd ed. *Delayed Hemolytic Transfusion Reactions*; 2013. Chapter 62, 409–12.

5. Butterworth J. F., IV, Mackey D. C., Wasnick J. D. (eds). Fluid management & blood component therapy. 5th ed. *Morgan & Mikhail's Clinical Anesthesiology*; 2013. Chapter 51.

6. Tong M. J., El-Farra N. S., Reikes A. R., et al. Clinical outcomes after transfusion-associated hepatitis C. *N Engl J Med*. 1995; 332: 1463–6.

7. Preiksaitis J. K., Brown L., McKenzie M. The risk of cytomegalovirus infection in seronegative transfusion recipients not receiving exogenous immunodepression. *J Infect Dis* 1988; 157: 523–9.

8. Katherine T. F., Edward C. N. Patient blood management: transfusion therapy. 8th ed. *Miller's Anesthesia*, 2015; Chapter 61.

9. Shaz B. Transfusion medicine and hemostasis. In: Shaz, Hillyer, Roshal, Abrams (eds), 2nd ed. *Massive Transfusion*; Elsevier, 2013. Chapter 56.

10. Toy P., Gajic O., Bacchetti P., et al. Transfusion-related acute lung injury: incidence and risk factors. *Blood*. 2012; 119: 1757–67.

11. Kleinman S., Caulfield T., Chan P., et al. Toward an understanding of transfusion-related acute lung injury: statement of a consensus panel. *Transfusion*. 2004; 44: 1774–89.

12. Silliman C. C., McLaughlin N. J. D. Transfusion-related acute lung injury. *Blood Rev*. 2006; 20: 139–59.

13. Triulzi D. J. Transfusion-related acute lung injury: current concepts for the clinician. *Anesth Analg*. 2009; 108: 770–6.

14. Sachs U. J. H., Wasel W., Bayat B., et al. Mechanism of transfusion-related acute lung injury induced by HLA class II antibodies. *Blood*. 2011; 117: 669–77.

15. Middelburg R. A., Van Der Bom J. G. Transfusion-related acute lung injury not a two-hit, but a multicausal model. *Transfusion*. 2015; 55: 953–60.

16. Bux J., Sachs U. J. H. The pathogenesis of transfusion-related acute lung injury (TRALI). *Br J Haematol*. 2007; 136: 788–99.

17. Eder A. F., Herron R., Strupp A., et al. Transfusion-related acute lung injury surveillance (2003–2005) and

the potential impact of the selective use of plasma from male donors in the American Red Cross. *Transfusion*. 2007; 47: 599–607.

18. Gajic O., Rana R., Winters J. L., et al. Transfusion-related acute lung injury in the critically Ill: Prospective nested case-control study. *Am J Respir Crit Care Med*. 2007; 176: 886–91.

19. Sher G., Markowitz M. A. TRALI risk mitigation for plasma and whole blood for allogeneic transfusion-association bulletin #14-02. *AABB*. 2014; 1–14.

20. Spencer Yost C., Matthay M. A., Gropper M. A. Etiology of acute pulmonary edema during liver transplantation: A series of cases with analysis of the edema fluid. *Chest*. 2001; 119: 219–23.

21. Tsai H.-I., Chou A.-H., Yang M.-W. Perioperative transfusion-related acute lung injury: A retrospective analysis. *Acta Anaesthesiol. Taiwanica*. 2012; 50: 96–100.

22. Morita Y., Pretto E. A. Increased incidence of transfusion-related acute lung injury during orthotopic liver transplantation: a short report. *Transplant Proc*. 2014; 46:3593–7.

23. Bolton-Maggs P. H. B, Cohen H. Serious Hazards of Transfusion (SHOT) haemovigilance and progress is improving transfusion safety. *Br J Haematol*. 2013; 163: 303–14.

24. Clifford L., Jia Q., Subramanian A., et al. Characterizing the epidemiology of postoperative transfusion-related acute lung injury. *Anesthesiology*. 2015; 122: 12–20.

25. Hendrickson J. E., Hillyer C. D. Transfusion medicine and hemostasis. In: Shaz, Hillyer, Roshal, Abrams (eds), 2nd ed. *Transfusion Associated Circulatory Overload*; Elsevier, 2013. Chapter 63.

26. Raval J. S., Mazepa M. A., Russell S. L., et al. Passive reporting greatly underestimates the rate of transfusion-associated circulatory overload after platelet transfusion. *Vox Sang*. 2015; 108: 387–92.

27. Roubinian N. H., Hendrickson J. E., Triulzi D. J., et al. Incidence and clinical characteristics of transfusion-associated circulatory overload using an active surveillance algorithm. *Vox Sang*. 2017; 112: 56–63.

Endocrine and Metabolic Systems

Chapter 40

Daniel R. Mandell and Kathirvel Subramaniam

Hormone Physiology and Common Pathology

- **Thyroid gland**
  - Physiology
    - Thyroid releases T4 and T3 which are iodine-containing hormones that control the body metabolic rate. T4 is secreted more than T3, and most T3 are formed peripherally by conversion of T4 by deiodinases. T3 is more potent.[1]
    - T3 *increases carbohydrate and fat metabolism.* Increased metabolism will increase O_2 consumption, CO_2 production, and minute ventilation[2]
  - Hyperthyroidism
    - Most common etiology – Grave's disease and adenoma[3]
    - Signs and symptoms: Weight loss, diarrhea, weakness, stiffness, heat intolerance, nervousness, increased LV contractility, tachycardia, hypertension, atrial fibrillation in elderly patients[1]
    - Anesthetic management
      - Goal is euthyroid state prior to elective anesthetic
      - Thyroid storm is triggered by stress of surgery
      - Signs/symptoms of thyroid storm are hyperthermia, tachycardia, dysrhythmia, myocardial ischemia, heart failure. Treat with *IV Fluids, sodium iodide, propylthiouracil, hydrocortisone, propranolol, cooling blanket, acetaminophen*[4]
  - Hypothyroidism
    - Incidence in ~5 percent of the population, 95 percent cases from primary thyroid gland failure[3]
    - Signs and symptoms: Lethargy, slow mental function, cold intolerance, bradycardia, decreased cardiac output, decreased ventilatory response to hypoxia and hypercapnia, anemia, coagulopathy, risk of postoperative ileus[4]
    - Anesthesia management
      - Patients are sensitive to most anesthetics and opioids
      - Only implement thyroid replacement in preparation for anesthesia if severe hypothyroidism or myxedema coma
      - Myxedema coma is characterized by stupor, hypoventilation, hypothermia, hyponatremia, hypotension. Treat with *ventilator support,*

levothyroxine, hydrocortisone, IV Fluids, and electrolyte therapy[3]

- **Parathyroid gland**
  - Plays significant role in calcium homeostasis along with vitamin D. Parathyroid hormone increases blood calcium levels in response to hypocalcemia.[1]
  - Primary hyperparathyroidism can occur due to adenoma/hyperplasia of the parathyroid gland, secondary to hypocalcemia, or chronic renal disease.[4]
  - Hypoparathyroidism can occur due to systemic causes or surgical removal of the parathyroid glands.
  - Primary anesthetic consideration is maintenance of serum calcium levels in the perioperative period. In hypocalcemia, follow the Rule of 10: *10 cc of 10 percent calcium gluconate over 10 minutes.* In hypercalcemia, *hydration with isotonic saline then furosemide.*[3]
- **Adrenal medulla**
  - Basic physiology
    - Releases primarily epinephrine, some norepinephrine.
    - Stimulated by sympathetic preganglionic fibers, therefore stimulated by surgery, hypotension, hypovolemia, pain, fear, hypoglycemia, hypoxemia, hypercapnia[1]
  - Pheochromocytoma
    - Catecholamine secreting tumor, rare etiology of secondary hypertension
    - Signs and symptoms: Hypertension, headaches, palpitations, tremor, sweating, flushing
    - Elevated 24-hour urinary *vanillylmandelic acid (VMA),* unconjugated norepinephrine/epinephrine, and plasma catecholamine levels[4]
    - Definitive treatment is tumor resection
    - Prior to resection, initiate alpha antagonist such as phenoxybenzamine. Note: Do not give beta blocker until after establishing alpha blockade due to risk of massive vasoconstriction causing uncontrollable hypertension[3]
- **Adrenal cortex**
  - Mineralocorticoids
    - Aldosterone is the primary mineralocorticoid
    - Stimulated by angiotensin II (therefore secreted secondary to hypotension, hypovolemia), ACTH secretion, hyperkalemia

- Mechanism is Na^+ reabsorption and K^+/H^+ secretion in renal distal tubule
- Results in expansion of extracellular volume, decrease serum K^+, metabolic alkalosis[2]
  - Glucocorticoids
    - Physiology
      - Cortisol is the primary glucocorticoid
      - Stimulated by ACTH
      - Enhances gluconeogenesis, inhibits peripheral glucose utilization → raised blood glucose
      - Required for vascular and bronchial smooth muscle to respond to catecholamines
      - Most glucocorticoids promote Na^+ retention and K^+ excretion (mineralocorticoid effect)[1]
    - Glucocorticoid excess (Cushing's Disease)
      - Overproduction cortisol or exogenous glucocorticoid
      - Signs and symptoms: Truncal obesity, hypertension, hyperglycemia, increased intravascular volume, hypokalemia, fatigue, osteoporosis, weakness, hyperglycemia, emotional lability, immunosuppression, hypokalemic alkalosis[3]
    - Adrenal insufficiency (Addison disease)
      - Etiology include autoimmune, sepsis, hemorrhage
      - Relative adrenal insufficiency common in critically ill surgical patients with hypotension
      - Signs and symptoms: Fatigue, weakness, anorexia, nausea, vomit, diarrhea, hypotension, hyperkalemia
      - Note: When the body is under stress, the adrenal gland makes approximately 250–300 mg of cortisol in 24 hours
      - Anesthetic management of stress-dose steroids[3]
- **Pancreas**
  - Basic physiology: Alpha cells secrete glucagon, beta cells secrete insulin
    - Rate of insulin secretion primarily determined by plasma–glucose concentration
    - Insulin has multiple metabolic effects
      - Glucose and potassium entry into adipose and muscle cell → decrease plasma glucose and serum K^+
      - Increase glycogen and fatty acid synthesis
      - Decrease glycogenolysis, gluconeogenesis, ketogenesis, lipolysis, and protein metabolism[2]
  - Perioperative management of diabetes
    - Goals are to determine degree of end organ complications, glucose lowering regimen, and need for perioperative glycemic control
    - Consider anesthetic effects of early atherosclerosis in regards to coronary, cerebral, peripheral, and renovascular disease
    - Autonomic neuropathy increases risk of intraoperative hypotension

- Potential airway difficulty with poorly controlled diabetes from *decreased atlanto-occipital joint mobility*
- Management of diabetic ketoacidosis
  - Insulin bolus + insulin infusion
  - IV fluids, anticipate severe total body water deficit
  - Give potassium 10–40 mEq/hour when urine output > 0.5 mL/kg/hour
  - When glucose < 250, add 5 percent dextrose at 100 cc/hour
  - Consider bicarbonate infusion if pH < 6.9
  - Major surgery in diabetic patients increases mortality/morbidity[3]
- **Anterior pituitary**
  - Acromegaly: Excessive growth hormone production
    - Signs and symptoms: Skin and soft tissue changes, bony/cartilage growth, compression of optic nerve and chiasma causing visual field defects, sleep apnea, difficult airway, compression of normal pituitary causing hypopituitarism, visceromegaly[3]
- **Posterior pituitary**
  - Syndrome of inappropriate antidiuretic hormone secretion (SIADH):
    - Signs and symptoms: Hyponatremia, water retention, hypervolemia
    - Treatment: Treat the cause (i.e., infection, malignancy, drugs, surgery), fluid restriction, IV hypertonic saline with furosemide (Na^+ level should be allowed to rise slowly to 0.5 mEq/L/hour as aggressive Na^+ therapy may precipitate central pontine myelinolysis), demeclocycline, vasopressin-receptor antagonists (tolvaptan and conivaptan)[3]
  - Diabetes insipidus: Common following pituitary surgery. Usually transient but can be permanent in extensive transfrontal resections. Head trauma and tumors are other etiologies.
    - Signs and symptoms: Polyuria, polydipsia, hypernatremia. Differential diagnosis includes excessive fluid therapy and diuresis.
    - Therapy includes water replacement, electrolyte monitoring/therapy, and DDAVP administration (Table 40.1).[3]

Biochemistry of Normal Body Metabolism

- Carbohydrates
  - Aerobic utilization
    - Requires O_2
    - Glycolysis → citric acid cycle → oxidative phosphorylation
    - Results in 38 molecules of adenosine triphosphate (ATP)
  - Anaerobic utilization
    - No O_2 in setting of ischemic tissue
    - Only glycolysis → only 2 ATP/glucose molecule

Table 40.1 Summary of hormones and their functions

Gland/tissue	Hormone	Function
Hypothalamus	Thyrotropin-releasing hormone (TRH) Corticotropin-releasing hormone (CRH) Growth-hormone releasing hormone (GHRH)	Stimulates secretion of TSH and prolactin Stimulates release of ACTH Stimulates release of growth hormone
Anterior pituitary	Growth hormone (GH) Thyroid-stimulating hormone (TSH) Adrenocorticotropic hormone (ACTH)	Stimulates protein synthesis, fatty acid mobilization, and tissue growth Stimulates synthesis and secretion of thyroid hormones (e.g. T4 and T3) Stimulates synthesis and secretion of ACTH (e.g. cortisol, androgens, aldosterone)
Posterior pituitary	Antidiuretic hormone (ADH) Oxytocin	Increases water reabsorption by kidneys and causes vasoconstriction Stimulates milk ejection and uterine contractions
Thyroid	Thyroxine (T4) and Triiodothyronine (T3)	Increases rates of chemical reactions in most cells, increases metabolic rate
Adrenal cortex	Glucocorticoids (Cortisol) Mineralocorticoids (Aldosterone)	Multiple metabolic functions, anti-inflammatory effects Increases renal Na^+ reabsorption, K^+ secretion, H^+ secretion
Adrenal medulla	Norepinephrine, epinephrine	Sympathetic stimulation
Pancreas	Insulin Glucagon	Promotes glucose entry into cells Increases the synthesis and release of glucose from liver into body
Parathyroid	Parathyroid hormone	Controls serum Ca^{2+} concentration by increasing Ca^{2+} absorption from gut, kidney and release Ca^{2+} from bone

- End product pyruvate → lactic acid → lactic acidosis
  - Relationship to hormones
    - Insulin – decrease blood glucose
    - Human growth hormone – increase glucose
    - Glucocorticoids – increase glucose
    - Glucagon – increase glucose
    - Epinephrine – increase glucose
  - Stress/surgery – increase blood glucose[2]
- Protein function
  - Provides structure of cells and enzymes
  - Intracellular signaling molecules – cAMP (cyclic adenosine monophosphate), cGMP (cyclic guanosine monophosphate)[2]
- Selected plasma proteins
  - Albumin
    - Provides oncotic pressure to maintain intravascular volume
    - Transports many anesthesia drugs
  - Globulins
    - Provide cellular immunity
    - Fibrinogen
      - Involved with coagulation cascade[2]
- Lipids
  - Triglycerides, lipoprotein, cholesterol
    - Lipoprotein – transport form of lipids in plasma
    - Adipocytes and liver store triglycerides until needed to provide energy
    - Cholesterol – forms cholic acid/conjugates to form bile salt, synthesis adrenal hormones
  - Specific organ metabolism
    - Brain – glucose virtually sole fuel, uses ketones during starvation. No fatty acid metabolism
    - Heart – fatty acids are main source of energy. Can also use ketone bodies and lactate. Virtually no glucose metabolism.
    - Liver – stores fatty acid that are secreted primarily as very low density lipoproteins (VLDL) during fed state; converts fatty acids into ketone bodies during fasted state
    - Muscle – metabolize glucose, fatty acid, ketones[2]

References

1. Hall J. *Guyton and Hall Textbook of Medical Physiology.* Saunders; 2016.
2. Berg J. M., Tymoczko J. L., Stryer L., et al. *Biochemistry*, 7th edn. Palgrave MacMillan; 2011.
3. Barash P. G., Cahalan M. K., Cullen B. F., et al. Clinical Anesthesia. *LWW*, 2013.
4. Butterworth J. F., Mackey D. C., John D., et al. *Morgan & Mikhail's Clinical Anesthesiology.* McGraw-Hill Education; 2013.

Chapter 41

Neuromuscular Physiology and Disorders

Jamie Metesky and Jacqueline Geier

Anatomy and Physiology of Neuromuscular Transmission

Prejunctional events: The neuromuscular junction (NMJ) consists of a presynaptic motor nerve terminal and a postsynaptic skeletal muscle membrane. The space between the presynaptic junction and postsynaptic membrane is called the *synaptic cleft*. Acetylcholine (ACh) is stored in the nerve terminal in synaptic vesicles. ACh receptors (AChR) are located in the postsynaptic motor endplate opposite the nerve terminal. In the adult NMJ, there are approximately 5 million AChRs.[1] The NMJ is the location at which electrical signals are effectively transformed into chemical signals which in turn produce muscular contraction (Figure 41.1)

- **Acetylcholine synthesis and release**
  - The choline and acetate used to form ACh are located in the environment of the nerve terminal.[1]
  - Choline is transported from the extracellular fluid and acetate is obtained from acetyl coenzyme A in the mitochondria.[1]
  - Choline acetyltransferase is responsible for the production of ACh from choline and acetate.[1]
  - ACh is then stored in vesicles within the nerve, both at the nerve terminus and deeper within the nerve as a reserve supply.[1]
  - Movement of and release of vesicles is dependent upon calcium flow into the nerve.[1]
  - Calcium ions enter the nerve via P-channels where they interact with SNARE proteins to create a pore through which the ACh may enter the synaptic cleft in a process known as exocytosis.[1]
  - During continuous stimulation, calcium penetrates the nerve more deeply via L-type calcium channels where it activates the VP1 vesicles (reserve supply) to be moved to the nerve terminal.[1]
  - The rate-limiting step of this entire process is thought to be choline uptake and activity of choline acetyltransferase.[1]
  - All of the components needed to make, store, and release these chemical signals are made in the cell body of the neuron and brought to the nerve terminal by axonal transport.[1]
  - ACh is stored in the cytoplasm until it is transported and stored in synaptic vesicles.[1]

- There are two types of synaptic vesicles:
  - Smaller VP2 vesicles are positioned at the nerve terminal where they are ready for release of ACh.[1]
  - Larger VP1 vesicles are located further from the nerve terminal and are moved to the terminal when the VP2 vesicles have depleted their stores.[1]

- **Modulation of nicotinic and muscarinic prejunctional receptors**
  - ACh release into the synaptic cleft is modulated via both *positive and negative feedback loops.*[2]
  - Presynaptic *nicotinic* receptors modulate ACh in a positive feedback loop with *increasing ACh leading to increased release.*[2]
  - Presynaptic *muscarinic* receptors modulate ACH in a negative feedback loop with ACh *leading to decreased ACH release.*[2]
  - When the nicotinic response is in full effect, the muscarinic response is less capable of producing a negative response.[2]

Postjunctional Events: The AChRs are formed by a five-subunit glycoprotein in the form of a cylindrical channel consisting of two alpha (α) subunits and one each of beta (β), gamma (γ), and delta (δ) subunits.[1,3] The fetal receptor has a similar composition with the epsilon (ϵ) subunit substituted for the γ subunit.[1,3] Alterations in the conventional AChR occur in pathologies including muscle denervation which leads to increased membrane permeability associated with hyperkalemic cardiac arrest.[1,3] The receptor complexes extend through the membrane of the muscle cell, linking the cytoplasm with the extracellular fluid. ACh binds the α subunits on the extracellular side of the receptor, and channel activation requires binding of *both α subunits* in order to effect conformational change and allows passage of ions.[1,3]

- **Acetylcholine binding to acetylcholine receptors**
  - The amount of ACh stored in each vesicle is referred to as a quantum (10^4 molecules).[1]
  - Each nerve impulse releases approximately 200 quanta.[1]
  - This process is enhanced by increasing calcium concentration.[1]
  - As stated above, ACh binds to the *alpha subunits* of the receptors and *both alpha subunits* must be bound by ACh to evoke a conformational change in the receptor.

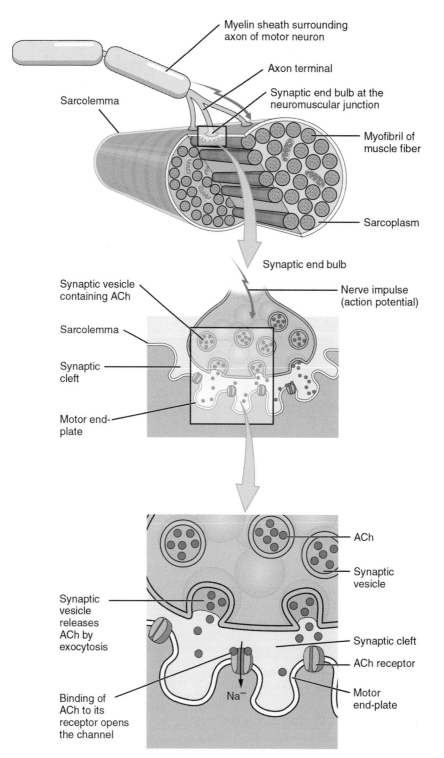

Figure 41.1 OpenStax College. "Anatomy and Physiology." OpenStax CNX, OpenStax College, June 19, 2013, cnx.org/content/col11496/1.6/.

- The conformational change involves a brief opening of the receptor core allowing ion flow through the receptor.[1,3]
- **Ion flow through acetylcholine receptor**
  - Sodium and calcium flow into the receptor; potassium flows out of the receptor, creating an end plate potential.[1]

- When enough receptors are bound, the end plate potential becomes strong enough to depolarize the membrane, which opens voltage-gated sodium channels.[1]
- The action potential then propagates by sodium channels opening, leading to release of calcium from the sarcoplasmic reticulum and binding of contractile proteins leading to muscle contraction.[1]

Perijunctional Voltage-Gated Channels

- P-type calcium channels are located at the nerve terminal.[1]
- Voltage-gated and calcium-gated potassium channels are also present, and regulate the duration of depolarization.[1]
- High concentrations of magnesium, cadmium, and manganese can block entry of calcium through P channels.[1]
- Nerve endings also contain slower, L-type calcium channels.[1]
- Verapamil, diltiazem, and nifedipine block L-type calcium channels but do not affect P-type calcium channels.[3]

Neuromuscular Pathology

Multiple sclerosis is a demyelinating disorder of the optic nerves, cerebrum, and spinal cord, particularly the spinothalamic tract and posterior columns, characterized by a variable course.

- MS has autoimmune pathophysiology that ultimately leads to the disruption of the blood–brain barrier and demyelination.[4,5]
- Anesthetic management should focus on keeping patients normothermic as hyperthermia has been shown to increase the risk of a flare-up. Previous thought was that spinal anesthesia should be avoided, however current literature has shown successful use, particularly for scheduled caesarean deliveries. It seems that dose and duration of local anesthetic may play a more important role than spinal versus epidural. General, spinal, and epidural anesthesia have all been shown to be safe options.[4]

Amyotrophic lateral sclerosis is a demyelinating disorder of both the anterior gray horn matter and the corticospinal tracts, and thus affects both upper and lower motor neurons.

- Clinically, patients present with progressive weakness, fasciculation, and spasticity of the extremities, as well as oropharyngeal dysfunction.[5–7]
- Anesthetic management must balance the risk of enhanced respiratory depression, exaggerated response to muscle relaxation, potential risk of furthering neurologic damage with regional anesthesia, and risk of pulmonary aspiration. Furthermore, depolarizing anesthetics are discouraged due to the risk of hyperkalemic response. Despite these concerns, both general and epidural anesthesia techniques have been described with success.[5–7]

Guillain Barré syndrome is characterized by a sudden onset of lower extremity flaccid paralysis that spreads cephalad affecting the diaphragm, upper extremities, face, and bulbar muscles, with spontaneous resolution usually within weeks.[5,6]

- Autonomic dysfunction is a prominent feature with wide swings in blood pressure, resting tachycardia, cardiac conduction abnormalities, and orthostatic hypotension being described.[5]
- Anesthetic management should focus on maintaining hemodynamic stability which can prove difficult due to autonomic dysfunction.[5]

- Indirect acting vasopressors are not recommended as they may produce exaggerated responses due to up-regulation of receptors.[5]
- Additionally, exaggerated hyperkalemic responses can be caused by depolarizing muscle relaxants and exaggerated hemodynamic responses can be seen with non-depolarizing muscle relaxants that have cardiac side effects.[5]

Duchenne muscular dystrophy (DMD) results from an absence in the dystrophin protein as well as dysfunction of the dystrophin-associated protein complex, leading to instability of the sarcolemma and muscle membrane.[5]

- Clinically, symptoms emerge between ages 2 and 5 years of age and include gait instability, toe walking, difficulty climbing stairs, calf hypertrophy, and Gower's sign using the hands to walk up the legs in order to stand.[5]
- Loss of skeletal muscle function leads to spine instability and scoliosis which can have profound effects on pulmonary function and diaphragm involvement, which further deteriorates pulmonary function.[5]
- The loss of dystrophin, also found in smooth and cardiac muscle, eventually causes fibrosis of the basal segment of the left ventricle, ventricular hypertrophy, fibrosis of the posterior papillary muscle, and mitral regurgitation, as well as significant cardiac arrhythmia.[5]
- Electrocardiogram changes are seen and include tall R waves in V1, deep Q waves in leads 1, V5, and V6, sinus tachycardia, and right-axis deviation.[5]
- Patients with DMD have a frequent need for surgical procedures including scoliosis correction, muscle biopsies, contracture releases, and reduction or fixation of fractures.[5]
- Anesthetic management should include careful pre-operative planning with a multi-disciplinary team to manage the risk of pulmonary and cardiac complications.[5,8]
- Pulmonary function testing, resting EKG, and echocardiogram are all recommended due to the high risk for perioperative respiratory and cardiac sequelae, most notably respiratory failure and cardiac arrhythmias.[5,8]
- Patient's with DMD are also at risk for difficult intubations owing to macroglossia, limited cervical spine mobility, and small mouth opening.[5]
- Additionally, diminished airway reflexes and gut motility predispose to pulmonary aspiration.[5]
- In terms of anesthetic choice, succinylcholine and volatile anesthetics should be avoided due to risk of hyperkalemia and rhabdomyolysis.[5]
- It was previously thought that these children were at risk for malignant hyperthermia (MH), however, this is now thought to be unlikely as the genes are located on different chromosomes.[5,8]
- It has also been noted that hyperkalemia and rhabdomyolysis present without the hyper metabolism seen in MH and thus dantrolene is not an effective treatment.[5]
- Regional anesthesia techniques may be preferable in these patients both to avoid the use of general anesthesia and for post-operative pain management.[5,8]

Becker's muscular dystrophy (BMD) is nearly identical to DMD, except that it presents later in life (adolescence) and is much less common (1 in 30,000).[8]

Myotonic dystrophy can be classified into two types DM1 and DM2, with DM2 presenting later in life and with milder symptoms. Both are due to CTG repeats on the 3' untranslated region of the dystrophia myotonica-protein kinase gene on chromosome 19.[9]

- This results in a characteristic wasting facial muscles as well as weakness of neck extensors and the external rotators of the arm.[9]
- Additionally, proximal muscle weakness of the lower extremities, as well as hands, ankles, and pharyngeal muscles, can be seen.[9]
- Significant cardiac involvement is common with conduction delays, arrhythmias, cardiomyopathy, and valvular abnormalities.[9]
- Anesthetic management should include assessment of cardiac function as well as pulmonary function and risk of aspiration.[9]
- Muscular weakness, number of CTG repeats, and duration of surgery all correlate with the risk of post-operative respiratory complications in a series of pediatric patients with DM1.[9]

Mitochondrial myopathy presents a challenge due to its clinical heterogeneity, but can essentially be classified based on the five main components of mitochondrial metabolism.

- Common symptoms that are 'red flags' of mitochondrial diseases include sensorineural hearing loss, short stature, diabetes mellitus, hypertrophic cardiomyopathy, axonal neuropathy, and external opthalmoplegia.[5]
- Anesthetic considerations for these patients involve a thorough preoperative evaluation of muscle weakness, respiratory and cardiac involvement, and degree of metabolic and endocrine abnormalities.[5]
- All anesthetic choices have a theoretical risk in these patients.
- Extended propofol infusions may predispose to propofol infusion syndrome as both propofol and midazolam have been shown to affect mitochondria in a dose-dependent fashion.[5]
- Volatile anesthetics and succinylcholine confer a risk of malignant hyperthermia and hyperkalemia.[5]
- Non-depolarizing muscle relaxants predispose to extended respiratory depression as do narcotics.[5]
- Despite this, all manner of anesthetic combinations have been described with success in the literature.[5]

Hyperkalemic periodic paralysis (hyperKK) is a sodium channelopathy and presents with myotonia and paralysis. The hyperKK periodic paralyses are a group of autosomal-dominant disorders characterized by episodes of flaccid paralysis often triggered by an alteration in serum potassium concentration.[5,10]

- During the episode of muscle weakness or paralysis, potassium ions are released from the muscle and serum potassium rises, though not always above normal levels.[5,10]
- Administration of potassium, potassium rich foods, and rest after exercise precipitate attacks.[5,10]
- Patients with hyperKK should be admitted preoperatively for electrolyte management and potassium-free fluid administration.[5]
- Potassium, succinylcholine, and anticholinesterases should be avoided as they can all trigger episodes.[5]

Hypokalemic periodic paralysis (hypoKK) has two subtypes. Type 1 is caused by a defect in L-type calcium channels, whereas type-2 is caused by a defect in the same gene that affects the sodium channel in HyperKK.[11]

- The disease presents up to the third decade of life and affects proximal muscles with bulbar and ocular muscle involvement occurring rarely.[11]
- HypoKK is not associated with myotonia, presents with hypokalemia, and is triggered by glucose, unlike HyperKK.[5,11]
- Trigger avoidance is a mainstay of treatment along with acetazolamide for type-1. Acetazolamide can precipitate attacks in type-2 hypoKK.[11]
- Triggers often include high carbohydrate meals, alcohol, viral infections, prolonged rest, menstruation, and pregnancy.[5,11]
- Anesthetic management should exclude succinylcholine, dextrose containing solutions, and focus on maintaining normothermia.[5]
- Patients with hypoKK have an increased risk of post-operative pulmonary complications and thus long-acting muscle relaxants should be avoided.[5]
- Furthermore, there have been numerous accounts of malignant hyperthermia in patients with hypoKK and therefore an association cannot be ruled out.[10]
- A non-triggering anesthetic and extreme vigilance is prudent.[5,10]

Myasthenia gravis (MG) is an autoimmune disease affecting the alpha subunit of the muscle type nicotinic AChR at the neuromuscular endplate.[5]

- Antibodies may be associated with thymoma or thymic hyperplasia in approximately 50% of patients.[5]
- Skeletal muscle weakness ensues and can include bulbar and oropharyngeal weakness. Classically, weakness becomes worse with repetition or throughout the day and the course of the disease is punctuated by periods of relapse and remission.[5]
- Cardiac manifestations have been described and include cardiomyopathy, arrhythmias, myocarditis, heart block, and sympathetic hyperactivity leading to wide swings in heart rate and blood pressure.[5]
- Anesthetic management should focus on preserving neuromuscular function.
- Risk of post-operative mechanical ventilation is increased with the following: disease for more than 6 years, pyridostigmine dose greater than 750 mg total/day, previous

or coexisting lung disease, and forced vital capacity less than 2.9 L.[5]

- Risk of post-operative MG crisis has also been demonstrated with the presence of bulbar symptoms, serum antibody level greater than 100 nmol/L, current MG crisis, and estimated blood loss greater than 1 L.[5]
- It should be noted that patients are exquisitely sensitive to non-depolarizing muscular relaxants and resistant to succinylcholine.[5]
- Train of four monitoring may be difficult and less accurate due to uneven distribution of muscular relaxation, , particularly with monitoring the orbicularis oculi muscle.[5]
- Potent volatile anesthetics have been used alone successfully without the need for paralysis in many patients.[5]
- If choosing a regional anesthetic technique, ester-type local anesthetics may show extended duration of action due to the anticholinesterases patients are using preoperatively.[5]

Lambert-Eaton Myasthenic syndrome (LEMS) is caused by antibodies to voltage-gated calcium channels at the presynaptic terminal of the motor endplate preventing the release of ACh and subsequent weakness.[5]

- Unlike MG, weakness improves with repetition as use of the muscle increases the amount of ACh released.[5]
- LEMS is commonly from a paraneoplastic syndrome with small cell lung cancer found in 50–60 percent of cases.[5]
- Proximal lower limb weakness is the most common symptoms though the upper extremities, respiratory, and bulbar muscles may be affected.[5]
- Additionally, cholinergic symptoms such as dry mouth and decreased lacrimation can be seen.[5]
- Patients are exquisitely sensitive to both depolarizing and non-depolarizing NMBDs.[5]
- Reversal of NMBDs may also be insufficient with anticholinesterases.[5]
- Epidural anesthesia has been successfully described but also requires careful titration and preparedness for post-operative weakness and respiratory monitoring much like MG.[5]

References

1. Martyn J. J. A. Neuromuscular physiology and pharmacology. In: Miller R. D. (ed). *Miller's Anesthesia.* Elsevier: NYC; 2015, 423–43.

2. Südhof T. C. The molecular machinery of neurotransmitter release (Nobel lecture). *Angew Chem Int Ed Engl.* 2014 Nov 17; 53(47): 12696–717.

3. Neuromuscular blocking agents. In: Butterworth J. F., IV, Mackey D. C., Wasnick J. D. (eds). *Morgan & Mikhail's Clinical Anesthesiology*, 5th edition. New York, NY: McGraw-Hill; 2013.

4. Makris A., Piperopoulos A. K. Multiple sclerosis: basic knowledge and new insights in perioperative management. *J Anesth.* 2014; 28: 267.

5. Nozari A. B., Saxena R., Bateman B. T. Neuromuscular disorders and other genetic disorders. In: Miller R. D. (ed). *Miller's Anesthesia.* Elsevier: NYC; 2015, 1266–86.

6. Xiao., Zhao L., Wang F., et al. Total intravenous anesthesia without muscle relaxant in a parturient with amyotrophic lateral sclerosis undergoing cesarean section: A case report. *J. Clin. Anesth.* 2017; 36: 107–9.

7. Shaw. Amyotrophic lateral sclerosis and other motor neuron diseases. In: Goldman L., Schaffer A. I. (eds). *Goldman–Cecil Medicine.* Elsevier: NYC; 2015, 2522–6.

8. Segura L. G., Lorenz J., Weingarten T., et al. Anesthesia and Duchenne or Becker muscular dystrophy: review of 117 anesthetic exposures. *Pediatr. Anaesth.* 2013; 23: 855–64.

9. Sinclair J. L., Reed P. W. Risk factors for perioperative adverse events in children with myotonic dystrophy. *Paediatr. Anaesth.* 2009; 19: 740–7.

10. Marchant C. L., Ellis F. R., Halsall P. J., et al. Mutation analysis of two patients with hypokalemic periodic paralysis and suspected malignant hyperthermia. *Muscle Nerve.* 2004; 30: 114–17.

11. Raja Rayan D. L., Hanna M. G. Skeletal muscle channelopathies: nondystrophic myotonias and periodic paralysis. *Curr. Opin. Neurol.* 2010; 23: 466–76.

Chapter 42

Special Problems or Issues in Anesthesiology

Martha Schuessler and Sanjana Vig

Physician Impairment or Disability

Substance Abuse

Definition(s)[1]:

Abuse	Addiction	Dependence	
"Use of psychoactive substance in a manner that is *detrimental* to the user or society, but does not meet the criteria for dependence".[1]	Disease state: *"Compulsive* use of an addictive drug," with *"loss of control* and *irrepressible craving* of the drug".[1]	Physical: *Withdrawal* occurs with abstinence from the substance.	Psychological: There is a sense of *"need" for the substance* either for positive effects or prevention of withdrawal.

Facts

- Risk of addiction with physicians is the *same* as in the general population
- Specific risk factors in physicians:
  - Family – Genetics, positive family history of substance abuse, dysfunctional familial interactions
  - Work
    - Residency training (including resultant alienation from friends and family)
    - Personal identity suppression by professional identity, dehumanization of physicians
    - Excessive fatigue, use of stimulants, insomnia
    - Self-medication for physical/psychological pain
    - Access to medication
- Characteristics of addicts
  - >2/3 male, >3/4 Caucasian
  - Bimodal age distribution (with 50 percent less than 35 years old), 33–50 percent with polysubstance abuse, 33 percent with family history of addiction.

Anesthesia and Addiction

- Anesthesiologists make up 4 percent of physicians, however, represent 12–15 percent in rehabilitation facilities.[1]
  - Incidence approximately 0.4 percent residents, 0.1 percent faculty[1]
- Methods of obtaining illicit substances
  - False recording on anesthesia record
  - Substituting syringes
  - Keeping waste

- Breaking ampules
- Poor accountability
- Figure 42.1 shows commonly abused medications among anesthesiologists and the time it takes to detect abuse.[1]
- Risks of substance abuse
  - Physical
    - Loss of life or health. High mortality rate for anesthesiologists (2.21× more likely to commit suicide by drug overdose, and 2.79× more likely to experience drug-related death)[2]
    - Death can be the presenting symptom of relapse.
  - Patients
    - Increased malpractice claims, decline in quality of patient care
  - Work
    - Loss of licensure, professional standing, career
  - Life
    - Loss of family, self-esteem
    - Loss of ability to gain health or disability insurance
- According to the ASA, of residents allowed to return to training after rehabilitation, 56 percent completed their residency, 44 percent achieved American Board of Anesthesiology certification, and 29 percent relapsed at least once (13 percent of those having death as the first sign of relapse).[2]
  - There is an overall relapse rate of 43 percent over a 30-year period.

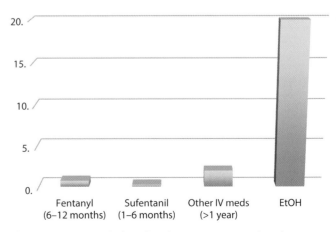

Figure 42.1 Commonly abused medications among anesthesiologists and time to detection (years)

American Disabilities Act (ADA)

- In regard to drug abuse: "The Americans with Disabilities Act (ADA) offers some protection to a previously addicted anesthesiologist, *provided he or she is enrolled in a treatment or monitoring program*. However, if the person is not enrolled in a program, no protections are provided. Also, the ADA does not protect against the legal consequences of drug diversion".[2]

Fatigue

Definition(s)[3]:

Fatigue	Chronic partial sleep deprivation	Sleep inertia
Extreme tiredness, typically resulting from *mental or physical exertion* or illness	Sleep duration of *less than five or six hours* for several consecutive nights	Awakening at certain parts of the circadian cycle creating similar effects to a period of 26 hours awake

ASA Statement on Fatigue[3]

- Sources of fatigue: Sleep deprivation, patient severity, case volume and turnover, facility conditions, personal stressors, age, work patterns, breaks, meals, scheduling changes, wait times, and handover procedures
- Sleep deprivation causes significant, measurable cognitive impairment, as well as a decline in self-assessment ability, quality of decision-making, clinical performance, vigilance, memory, motor skills, and attention.

Facts

- Libby Zion Case: 1984 Libby Zion was killed after being prescribed intramuscular meperidine while on monamine oxidase inhibitor. In court, this was attributed to negligence due to fatigue and undersupervision of residents.
- Highest risk physicians
  - Frequent 24-hour calls, those who experience chronic partial sleep deprivation and sleep inertia

Aging, Visual, and Auditory Impairment

Facts[4]

- As the life expectancy of the population at large increases, the number of physicians in practice over the age of 65 has increased by 2.3 percent between 1985 and 2005.
- Aging causes physiological changes which may or may not affect a clinician's ability to deliver the standard of care and is a factor that may impact clinical competence.
- In the practice of anesthesia dexterity, visual–spatial acuity, memory, problem-solving, data analysis, life-long learning are among the most important areas which may be compromised.
- The aging process is extremely variable. Physicians should be regularly and routinely assessed. Often this does not happen until an incident occurs.

Ethics, Practice Management, and Medico-legal Issues

Professionalism and Licensure

Professionalism[5,6]

- The ASA adheres to the ABIM Foundation's 2002 statement on professionalism, "Medical professionalism in the new millennium: A physician charter."
- Three main principles:
  - Primacy of patient welfare
    - Dedication to service of patients regardless of societal or economic pressures
  - Patient autonomy
    - Empowering patients to make informed decisions regarding their own care
  - Social justice
    - Fair distribution of health-care resources regardless of socioeconomic, racial, gender, religious, ethnic factors
    - Includes commitment to professional competence, honesty with patients, patient confidentiality, appropriate relationships with patients, improving quality of and access to care, just distribution of finite resources, scientific knowledge, professional responsibilities, maintaining trust by managing conflicts of interest

Licensure[7]

- Varies state by state, required for ABA certification
- Application for license requires completion of USMLE boards, anesthesia residency, and passing of anesthesiology written and oral exams.
- Any and all disciplinary action filed against a practitioner must be disclosed when applying for new, or maintaining, licensure.

Advanced Directives/DNR/DNI

Advanced Directives

Definition(s)
- Healthcare Proxy (HCP) – A person or persons to make decisions for the patient if patient is unable (cannot be a treating physician).

Facts

- Serve as a way to prevent costly and unwanted interventions to patient
- Decision tree for HCP (Figure 42.2)
- Only go into effect when patient loses capacity for decision-making
- 2009: *America's Affordable Health Choices Act* authorized reimbursement for these discussions
  - Not included in *Affordable Care Act (ACA)*, due to fear of creation of "death panels"

- *Physician Orders for Life Saving Treatment (POLSTs)* can serve as a way to provide framework especially in patients without advanced directives, but do not supersede the advanced directive.

DNR/DNI

Definition(s)

Do Not Resuscitate (DNR)	Do Not Intubate (DNI)
May NOT resuscitate with medications and chest compressions May intubate	May resuscitate with medications and chest compressions May NOT intubate

Facts

- DNR/DNI is a type of advanced directive
- In an operating room setting, advanced directives may be suspended (Table 42.1)

Patient Privacy

Facts

- Health Insurance Portability and Accountability Act (HIPAA): 1996[9]:
  - Set standards for protection of privacy of health information
  - Addresses use of protected health information (PHI)
    - Requires patient's permission for use, except in instances listed in Table 42.2

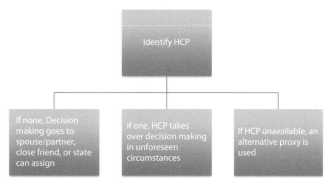

Figure 42.2 Decision tree for HCP

- Applies to providers, healthcare clearinghouses, health plans
- Includes all past/present/future physical or mental health problems and care received, including common identifiers

Informed Consent

- Definition: As highlighted in Figure 42.3, there are multiple elements required to complete consents appropriately and accurately.

All discussions with patients or families must be documented within the patient chart. All documentation regarding consent must be placed in the patient chart. Patient's wishes must be clearly delineated and communicated with all operating room team members.

Patient Safety

- Medical errors: Assessment and prevention[11,14]
  - Fall into three categories:
    - Slips – failure to execute
      - Lapses – memory failure
      - Mistakes – rule-based or knowledge-based
  - Include wrong patient, surgery, site, failure to diagnose, wrong drug/dose

Table 42.2 Exceptions to PHI permission requirement

Instances where patient's permission is NOT required when disclosing PHI
• Legal proceedings • Prevention or control of disease/injury/disability, child/elder abuse/neglect, persons at risk for spreading or contracting a disease • Workplace surveillance OSHA/workman's compensation • Research/IRB approval • Cadaveric organ donation • Historical purposes >50 years after death

Threshold elements	Information elements	Consent elements
• Competency and capacity • Voluntariness	• Discussion with patient • Disclosure: treatment and alternatives, material	• Decision by patient • Autonomous authorization

Figure 42.3 Elements of informed consent[10]

Table 42.1 Alternatives to advanced directives in the operating room[8]

Suspension options		
Limited attempt at resuscitation defined with regard to *specific procedures*	**Limited attempt at resuscitation defined with regard to *patient's goals and values***	**Full attempt at resuscitation**
Patient or surrogate may elect to continue to refuse certain resuscitation procedures. Anesthesiologist must indicate which are necessary for successful anesthetic and which are not essential (i.e., must suspend DNI in order to provide anesthetic; however, chest compressions as part of a resuscitation effort are not necessarily essential).	Patient or surrogate allows anesthesiologist and surgical team to use clinical judgment when determining which resuscitation procedures are appropriate based on patient goals of care (i.e., patient is ok with intubation if needed, so long as can be extubated in the immediate postoperative period).	Patient or surrogate may fully suspend DNR/advanced directives in perioperative period.

- Malpractice and negligence[11]
  - Malpractice is defined as professional misconduct, but specifically is referring to negligence
  - Negligence
    - Four components required to prove:
      - Duty
        - Anesthesiologist owed a particular obligation to patient.
      - Breach of duty
        - Anesthesiologist failed to fulfill this specific obligation to the patient.
      - Causation
        - There is a reasonably direct correlation between the actions of the anesthesiologist and the reason for the suit
      - Damages
        - Damages occurred as a result of the specific actions of the anesthesiologist.
- Sentinel events[12]
  - Defined by the Joint Commission as "an unexpected occurrence involving death or serious physical or psychological injury, or the risk thereof."
  - Require immediate investigation and response
  - Not synonymous with the term "error"
  - Hospital review of sentinel events is a component of the Joint Commission review.
- Disclosure of errors to patients[11]
  - Full disclosure is controversial among hospitals, attorneys, and physicians because of "potential medico-legal consequences." This is because often times, the underlying medical condition of the patient is contributory to the complications.
  - However, often a full disclosure and formal apology will decrease the likelihood of litigation.
  - Should seek advice from risk management and/or malpractice carrier prior to disclosure.
  - Disclosure in absence of a bad outcome is equally controversial. Many experts argue against disclosure in these instances.
  - Careful preparation with risk management and all involved parties should occur prior to disclosure. Disclosure should occur in private environment with all necessary parties (including family, social workers, language interpreters, clergy, etc.). Disclosure should

be limited to the medical error itself, and blame should not be assigned to others. Focus should be on answering questions, the relationship with the patient, and coordinating further care.

Core Competencies

There are multiple core competencies required for residents as they progress through their training programs. They are defined below along with examples[13]:

- Patient care
  - Pre-anesthesia care: patient evaluation/assessment/preparation, anesthetic plan, peri-procedural pain management
  - Management of perioperative complications
  - Crisis management, triage, and management of the critically ill in non-operative setting
  - Acute/chronic/cancer pain management
  - Technical skills including airway management, use and interpretation of monitoring and equipment, and regional anesthesia.
- Medical knowledge
  - Biomedical sciences and clinical sciences
  - Epidemiology, social–behavioral science
- Practice-based learning and improvement
  - Incorporation of QI and patient safety initiatives into personal practice
  - Self-analysis and identification of areas of improvement
  - Self-directed learning
  - Education of patients/families/students/residents/other health-care providers
- Interpersonal and communication skills
  - Communication with patients and families
  - Communication with other professionals
  - Team leadership
- Professionalism
  - Responsibility to patients/families/society to work with honesty, integrity, and ethical behavior
  - Commitment to institution/department/colleagues, receiving and giving feedback
  - Responsibility to maintain personal emotional/physical/mental health
- Systems-based practice
  - Coordination of patient care, patient safety, QI

References

1. American Society of Anesthesiologists. ASA Substance Abuse Education Guidelines http://uthscsa.edu/gme/documents/ModelCurriculumonDrugAbuseandAdditionforResidentsinAnesthesiology.pdf

2. American Society of Anesthesiologists. ASA Ethics Syllabus. 2015. www.asahq.org/~/media/sites/asahq/files/public/resources/asa%20committees/syllabus-on-ethics-2016.pdf?la=en (Accessed January 30, 2017).

3. American Society of Anesthesiologists. ASA Statement on Fatigue. 2015. www.asahq.org/~/media/sites/asahq/files/public/resources/standards-guidelines/statement-on-fatigue.pdf (Accessed January 30, 2017).

4. American Society of Anesthesiologists. The Aging Anesthesiologist. 2013. www.asahq.org/~/media/sites/asahq/files/public/resources/practice%20management/ttppm/the%20aging%20anesthesiologist%20november%202013%20rev.pdf (Accessed March 13, 2017).

5. Waisel, D. American Society of Anesthesiologists: Medical Professionalism. www.asahq.org/resources/ethics-and-professionalism/medical-professionalism (Accessed March 14, 2017).

6. ABIM Foundation. American Board of Internal Medicine. ACP-ASIM Foundation. American College of Physicians-American Society of Internal Medicine. European Federation of Internal Medicine. Medical professionalism in the new millennium: A physician charter. *Ann Intern Med.* 2002; 136:243–6.

7. American Board of Anesthesiologists. Primary Certification Policy Book. 2016. www.theaba.org/PDFs/BOI/2017-Primary-Certification-Policy-Book (Accessed March 14, 2017).

8. American Society of Anesthesiologists. ASA Statement on Suspension of DNR. 2013. www.asahq.org/~/media/sites/asahq/files/public/resources/standards-guidelines/ethical-guidelines-for-the-anesthesia-care-of-patients.pdf#search=%22advanced directives%22 (Accessed March 1, 2017).

9. U.S. Department of Health and Human Services. Health Insurance Portability and Accountability Act of 1996. https://aspe.hhs.gov/report/health-insurance-portability-and-accountability-act-1996 (Accessed February 10, 2017).

10. Waisel, D. et al. Informed consent. *Anesthesiology* 1997; 87: 968–78.

11. American Society of Anesthesiologists. Manual on Professional Liability. 2010. www.asahq.org/~/media/sites/asahq/files/public/resources/asa%20committees/manualonprofessionalliability.pdf?la=en (Accessed March 13, 2017).

12. The Joint Commission. Sentinel Events (SE). 2016. www.jointcommission.org/assets/1/6/CAMH_2012_Update2_24_SE.pdf (Accessed March 22, 2017).

13. American Board of Anesthesiology. ABA Certificate of Clinical Competence Report. 2017. www.theaba.org/PDFs/Clinical-Competence/CCC-Anesthesiology (Accessed February 22, 2017).

14. O'Leary, C. Informed consent: Principles and practice. *ASA Monitor* 2010; 74: 20–45.

Index